MW01445823

DEADLY RIVER

A volume in the series
The Culture and Politics of Health Care Work
Edited by Suzanne Gordon and Sioban Nelson

A list of titles in this series is available at
www.cornellpress.cornell.edu.

DEADLY RIVER

Cholera and Cover-Up in Post-Earthquake Haiti

Ralph R. Frerichs

ILR PRESS, AN IMPRINT OF CORNELL UNIVERSITY PRESS
ITHACA AND LONDON

First published 2016 by Cornell University Press
First printing, Cornell Paperbacks, 2017

Library of Congress Cataloging-in-Publication Data

Frerichs, Ralph R., author.
Deadly river : cholera and cover-up in post-earthquake Haiti / Ralph R. Frerichs.
pages cm
Includes bibliographical references and index.
ISBN 978-1-5017-0230-3 (cloth : alk. paper)
ISBN 978-1-5017-1358-3 (pbk. : alk. paper)
1. Cholera—Haiti—Epidemiology. 2. United Nations Stabilization Mission in Haiti. 3. Earthquake relief—Haiti—International cooperation. 4. Emergency medical services—Haiti—International cooperation. 5. Humanitarian assistance—Haiti—International cooperation. 6. Haiti Earthquake, Haiti, 2010. I. Title.
RA644.C3F74 2016
614.5′14097294—dc23 2015036033

Cornell University Press strives to use environmentally responsible suppliers and materials to the fullest extent possible in the publishing of its books. Such materials include vegetable-based, low-VOC inks and acid-free papers that are recycled, totally chlorine-free, or partly composed of nonwood fibers. For further information, visit our website at www.cornellpress.cornell.edu.

Above all, to Rita, Renaud, and Martine, who embody love, friendship, and unwavering support;

To my and Renaud's immediate families: Peter, Christine, Brigid, Raphaël, Julie, and Loïc;

To contributors large and small: Robert Barrais, Rita Colwell, Scott Cooper, Suzanne Gordon, Paul Keim, Dong Wook Kim, Daniele Lantange, Timothy McGirk, Raymond Neutra, Stanislas Rebaudet, and anonymous reviewers;

To frontline journalists who stayed with the story: Roberson Alphonse, Jonathan M. Katz, and Sebastian Walker;

To inspirational John Snow and close friend and fellow sleuth Douglas Mackintosh (both deceased); and especially

To the people of Haiti, who deserve the truth.

Contents

Preface

As a retired epidemiologist and professor emeritus of epidemiology at the University of California, Los Angeles (UCLA), I had been reading about Haiti's cholera outbreak for several weeks, ever since it began in October 2010. Having never associated cholera with Haiti, nor for that matter with the Caribbean region, I was quickly drawn in by the rapidly spreading outbreak. During my long academic career, I had taught and done epidemiologic research in many less developed countries, mainly in the Americas, Africa, and Asia. Although I had never worked in Haiti and had no connections to the country, I did have a longstanding interest in cholera.

One of my legacies is a popular website on Dr. John Snow, the nineteenth-century British physician best known—because of his early studies of cholera—as the "father of epidemiology" (see Frerichs, "John Snow—A Historical Giant in Epidemiology"). Snow was a successful anesthesiologist who had administered chloroform to Queen Victoria during the births of two of her children.

Snow first faced cholera during his late teenage years while serving as an apprentice with a local physician in rural England. When cholera appeared at a nearby coal mine, he was sent to provide medical assistance to the miners and their families. His experience with the outbreak—seeing the deaths that followed profuse discharges from stomach and bowels—had a lifelong effect on the young man.

In the mid-1800s, John Snow was well regarded for his observations of cholera outbreaks, battling the prevailing notion that the disease arose from miasmas or "bad air" that drifted from decomposed matter in swamps and other locations. Snow believed cholera was propagated from one person to another by faceless germs, but he never identified the disease-causing agent. He also believed the cholera agent existed in water—both in contaminated wells and in rivers polluted by local sewage.

The nature of the cholera disease agent had been mightily debated during Snow's lifetime and in the years that followed. There was no consensus on why cholera spread the way it did. Snow was undeterred, took a fresh look at the etiological disagreements, and decided to test the logic of the different hypotheses, using field observations, maps, and insights derived from the emerging field of epidemiology.

Although for Snow epidemiology was an avocation, he helped define the field. I wondered how he would have viewed the cholera outbreak in Haiti. And as the facts associated with the outbreak trickled out very slowly, I kept returning to the same question: Was there a modern-day John Snow who could unravel the causative complexities of cholera in Haiti and help control the disease?

As I pondered this question, various reports about the Haitian epidemic mentioned someone called Renaud Piarroux, a French physician and epidemiologist based in Marseille whom the Haitian government had asked to investigate the epidemic. At first his name came up only in passing; other, louder voices—which we will hear later in this story—were getting the lion's share of attention as they theorized about why and how cholera had made its first appearance on the Caribbean island.

In early December 2010, a report of Piarroux's field investigation surfaced, shared anonymously by several news organizations. It was written in French, a language I neither read nor speak. With the help of an online program, I laboriously translated the report into English and posted it on my website early one morning.

When I later walked into the kitchen, I told my wife, Rita, about an interesting man who had developed a theory about the origin of the cholera epidemic in Haiti that was generating considerable controversy. With good reason, he seemed to be questioning the views of notable scientists as well as some of the most powerful international organizations in the world. Although I was impressed by the field investigation report of Piarroux, I was also confused—the translation program left much to be desired. Rita suggested I write Piarroux, and I did so in early January 2011.

My electronic message from Southern California reached Piarroux at his home in France, and he responded a few days later, in what would be the first of many messages between us. Over time, we formed a special bond based on similar views of life, values, and science—and particularly over our convictions about the origins of the cholera epidemic in Haiti. We corresponded for about eight months and finally met in August and then several times later. As I learned more about Piarroux's experiences in Haiti, I became persuaded that he was right about the origins of the cholera epidemic, about what should and could be done to manage the current outbreak and prevent future ones. As I listened to his story unfolding in real time and heard more about the role of the United Nations and reputable scientists who were espousing suspect theories about the outbreak's origins, I became convinced that the inside and ongoing story of what Piarroux had encountered in Haiti needed to be told to a wider audience than could be reached through the journal articles that he and then the two of us, with other colleagues, authored. We thus decided to write a book about his experiences.

Once the book decision was made, we wrestled for some time with the question of how best to tell the story. Over dinner one night several years ago in a rural hamlet in France, our families agreed: Piarroux would be the main character and I would be the author and storyteller, appearing sparingly in the book. It seemed to be a good solution to the discomfort Piarroux felt writing about himself. We used frequent e-mail and voice and video calls to address each notion and passage until we forged complete agreement. With such close bonding, we hope the observations and conclusions we made as the cholera tragedy unfolded will more effectively come to life, weaving a vivid tapestry of investigation, science, and politics in the proud but troubled nation of Haiti.

To enhance the reading experience, a gratis website created independent of the publisher is available with supplementary maps, figures, and documents referred to in the book: www.deadlyriver.com.

DEADLY RIVER

Introduction

The Haitian cholera epidemic could not have emerged at a worse moment. In January of 2010 an earthquake of catastrophic magnitude 7.0 hit Haiti. With its epicenter near the port town of Léogâne about twenty-nine kilometers (eighteen miles) west of the capital city of Port-au-Prince, it sent many aftershocks through the southern region of the country. An estimated three million people were affected, according to the International Red Cross and Red Crescent Societies, and the death toll was put at between 80,000 and 230,000, depending on who was doing the counting. The quake left countless numbers without homes, sustenance, or hope. In the following days, anger and impatience intensified as desperate Haitians found the international aid to be too little and too slow to meet local needs.[1] Over time, the sheer number and scope of foreigners working for nongovernmental organizations (NGOs) that swooped in to help the country rebuild became a powerful parallel state, which many felt was not accountable to Haitians.[2]

Nine months after the earthquake, the world's greatest cholera epidemic tore through the country, and in the ensuing years it infected hundreds of thousands and killed upwards of nine thousand. As if the earthquake and cholera outbreak did not create enough devastation and political turmoil, in early November a hurricane passed over the southern region and touched the western shores, causing flooding and misery in communities barely coping with all that had happened.

All of this would fuel even greater anger and create a political tinderbox. The cholera outbreak—now epidemic in size—coincided with Haitian elections for a successor to President René Préval as well as parliamentary deputies and senators.

For many powerful players, finding answers to the latest crisis in Haiti was not only a humanitarian undertaking but also a political imperative.

When the epidemic erupted, the Haitian government called on the French epidemiologist Renaud Piarroux to track the origins of the epidemic. Piarroux was the department chief of the laboratory of parasitology and medical mycology at La Timone academic hospital in Marseille, France, as well as a professor of parasitology and mycology at the medical school of Université d'Aix-Marseille. Through his service on humanitarian missions in Afghanistan, Comoros, Honduras, Ivory Coast, and the Democratic Republic of the Congo, and his studies in microbiology and tropical medicine, he had developed an interest in and a deep understanding of how cholera spreads through regions and communities—and of how epidemics can be controlled and the disease even eliminated. In 1999, the Médecins du Monde team he was leading actually eliminated cholera from Grande Comore, the largest island in the Comoros nation off Africa's east coast. This won Piarroux, on behalf of his team, a nomination in 2000 for the Grand Prix de la Coopération Internationale, an award given by Lionel Jospin, the prime minister of France at the time.

So when the government of France responded to the Haitian government's request for epidemiological assistance as cholera engulfed the country, it asked Piarroux to travel to Port-au-Prince, where under the auspices of the French embassy he would address the epidemic, identify its source, describe its impacts, and offer suggestions for control.

During Piarroux's time in Haiti, two scientific theories vied for dominance when it came to explaining the origins of cholera outbreaks and epidemics. One was the environmental theory promulgated by researchers who studied coastal regions in South Asia and viewed cholera as a waterborne disease.[3] Piarroux was familiar with this theory before he came to Haiti. Many years earlier, researchers had found *Vibrio cholerae* attached to live copepods in the bay waters of Bangladesh. Because the causative microbe lives naturally in brackish waters and estuary environments, the environmental group postulated that cholera was not an eradicable disease—that is, not one that could be eliminated from the world, as smallpox had been declared eradicated by the World Health Assembly in 1980.[4]

The environmental theory maintains that seasonal patterns of cholera arise from changes in factors such as water temperature and salt level, transforming waterborne *Vibrio cholerae* into disease-causing microbes. When contacted by humans, the altered cholera bacteria cause human outbreaks that abate with time. This gives the organism a sort of Dr. Jekyll and Mr. Hyde quality, with two existences: an inoffensive bacteria living on copepods in brackish water, and then after periodic changes, a virulent germ that causes disease and death in humans. The theory also fits well with existing global warming concerns: rising coastal water temperatures stimulate microbial change and unleash deadly cholera epidemics, affecting human populations.

Piarroux considered this an important and interesting theory, but the more he went to the field, especially in African settings, the more he found that it simply did not fit the cholera patterns he observed. Instead, he found that in many epidemics the cholera organism was spread more by human contact with cholera-infected feces that then contaminated food or drinking water than by cholera-ridden estuaries. Human travelers, whether on land or sea, or fecal-contaminated food and water brought the toxic organism into contact with new susceptible hosts, thereby creating an outbreak or epidemic.

As Piarroux investigated cholera in Haiti, he discovered that the sources of the epidemic were not environmental but human—in this case Nepalese troops who were stationed in Haiti as part of MINUSTAH, the Mission des Nations Unies pour la Stabilization en Haiti (the United Nations Stabilization Mission in Haiti), which had been in Haiti since 2004 under a mandate from the UN Security Council.

As we shall see in this book, the consequences of the scientific debate over the importance of these two hypotheses—environmental versus human activity—were and remain significant. The environmental theory is based on the belief that the island and its coastal estuaries are a permanent breeding ground for the cholera disease. Earthquakes and hurricanes, or even just the rainy season, provoke the cholera monster to rise and attack. According to this theory, the Haitian people are helpless before the onslaught of cholera, ever present in the Haitian aquatic environment, ready to be churned up by earthquakes and turbulent weather that threaten the land. Indeed, under this theory, even the underdeveloped Haitian economy, health care system, and its impoverished people can be held as more responsible for cholera's persistence than anything else.

Piarroux's human activity theory, by contrast, forms the basis of a concerted strategy for eliminating the disease altogether, proven in other countries. He realized that vast sanitation and water projects—advocated by many to control cholera—would take decades to complete. Instead, Piarroux has tried to promote and implement disease-control strategies that are affordable in developing nations. He worries that sanitation and water for all—highly effective in the economically advantaged world—might be hard to come by in less developed regions, where outside financial assistance is a sometimes thing. If cholera were to become endemic in Haiti, even popular vaccination programs might be difficult to finance for the country's ten million people if large-scale and continued revaccination were deemed necessary. To Piarroux, a better strategy was to attempt to eliminate the disease from the population. This could be done if there was a clear understanding of how cholera first arrived and settled in the country, assessing whether or not the causative microbe found a sustainable home in the surface waters of Haiti.

The timing and spatial distribution of past outbreaks would tell much about the capacity for spread, as would seasonal patterns of the disease, related to wet and dry seasons. While economical water and sanitation systems should certainly be put in place, planning should follow better understanding of how cholera outbreaks emerge and spread. Typically during a dry period when rains stop, there is a lull in cholera cases. Piarroux's strategy was to take advantage of the lull with cost-effective interventions to eliminate the local pathogen. That's what he tried to do in Haiti in 2014 after discovering that disease-causing *Vibrio cholerae* did not settle at a significant level in the aquatic environment.

Piarroux's views on the origin and elimination of cholera met consistent but often-subtle opposition from the United Nations, aided by the proponents of the environmental theory. Tragically, this set back the fight to eliminate the disease. When the rainy season returned to Haiti in May 2014, cholera found new vigor. The disease had been nearly eliminated, maintained for months at a low equilibrium with only a few persistent foci remaining in Haiti's northern regions. Efforts to permanently halt cholera spread proved insufficient, however, leaving untended foci of the disease. By late 2014, the epidemic had once again rejuvenated, mainly attacking in areas where little or nothing had been done to reduce local vulnerability. Cholera once more made its way into Port-au-Prince.

In a letter on the Haitian cholera epidemic written to the United Nations General Secretary in September 2014, four special UN rapporteurs described the situation quite bluntly, offering a glimmer of hope while citing chilling impact and challenges:

> Despite the reduction of overall incidence by 50%, and the first months of 2014 registering the lowest number of cases and cholera related deaths since the beginning of the epidemic, the figures remain of deep concern: from October 2010 to July 2014, around 703,000 suspected cholera cases and estimated 8,500 deaths were reported by the Haitian Ministry of Health.
>
> Despite ongoing efforts, lack of access to safe water, adequate sanitation and health systems in Haiti are causing cholera to persist. Over the past four years, cholera has infected about one in twenty Haitian men, women and children. It has disproportionately impacted the poor and the vulnerable. Victims include farmers, teachers, and caretakers whose illness or deaths have left families without means to meet their basic needs.[5]

By 2015 at this writing, Piarroux and his team have returned to Haiti and investigated the causes of the late-2014 cholera rebound. The wily epidemic had changed once more. Although control measures in general were effective in rural areas and in most provincial towns, the situation had deteriorated in Port-au-Prince. In the southern district of the city, the water system had become so degraded that fecal contamination followed rainfall, bringing the cholera microbes to those served by the water network. Although Piarroux immediately alerted the authorities and they took the matter seriously, fixing the problem was complicated, and the dr, particularly short in 2015—provided no help to the elimination campaign.

This book covers approximately the first four years of the cholera epidemic in Haiti, weaving in the social, political, and cultural milieu of this complex but vibrant country. In some respects it is detective story, relating how Piarroux's work in the field unfolded, how his conclusions about the origins of the epidemic in Haiti developed, and what happened when the UN opposed them. Unlike traditional detective stories, however, we know from the beginning of this one not only what was done but who done it. Many reports and articles have been written about the controversy that erupted regarding the origin of the Haitian cholera epidemic. News reports have highlighted that Piarroux identified UN peacekeepers from Nepal as having brought the disease to Haiti, and scientific analyses have confirmed that the strain of *Vibrio cholerae* was indeed the one found in a preceding cholera outbreak in Nepal. Also widely known is that the UN has consistently denied that its peacekeepers played any role in the epidemic's origins and has found support from prominent scientists who promote an entirely different view of how and why cholera suddenly appeared.

What this book offers is an in-depth portrait of how scientific investigation is conducted when it is done right. It explores a quest for scientific truth and dissects a scientific disagreement involving world-renowned cholera experts who find themselves embroiled in turmoil in a poverty-stricken country. It describes the impact of political maneuvering by powerful organizations such as the United Nations and its peacekeeping troops in Haiti, as well as by the World Health Organization (WHO) and the US Centers for Disease Control and Prevention (CDC). In so doing, it raises issues about how the world's wealthy nations and international institutions respond when their interests clash with the needs of the world's most vulnerable people. In an era when there is more focus than ever before on global and population health, the story poses critical questions and offers insights not only about how to eliminate cholera in Haiti but about how nations and international organizations such as the UN, WHO, and CDC deal with deadly emerging infectious diseases.

At the time the writing of this book was concluded, some of the same issues it illuminates surfaced in the epidemic of Ebola in West Africa. International health officials were unprepared for the dramatic onset and scope of Ebola, rejected input and suggestions from those working in the field who had direct contact with the disease, and were unable for months on end to contain the fear and disorganization that contributed to the spread of the deadly virus.[6]

The nagging question of how cholera came to Haiti and what powerful actors were willing to do with that knowledge is therefore an inquiry with implications well beyond one island nation in the Caribbean Sea.

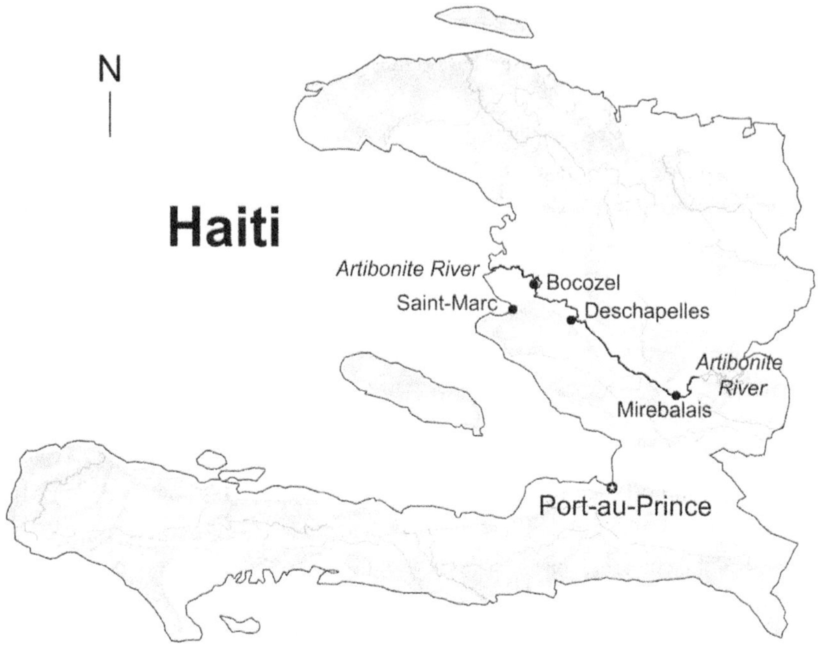

FIGURE 1.1. Artibonite River, Haiti's life source that nourishes the central agricultural valley

1

UPHEAVAL

It all seemed to start in the delta of Rivière de l'Artibonite, the Artibonite River, Haiti's main watercourse. That morning in Bocozel village, two young boys—we'll call them Paul and Jean, both primary-school age—followed their usual path to school, crossing the canal bridge over the water that flowed to the nearby rice fields. It was hurricane season, but the weather had been mild for a few weeks. Early mornings were cool, but now the sun warmed the air.

The long, grand Artibonite River originates in the mountains of neighboring Dominican Republic and flows west 240 kilometers (150 miles) through central Haiti and on to the ocean waters of the Gulf of La Gonâve. Along its course, mountains rise on both sides until farmland spreads out fan-shaped closer to the coastal plain. Many who live by the river are subsistence farmers growing rice in the fertile valley.

That particular day, Paul and Jean drank from the canal—just as most area youngsters did—to quench their thirst before beginning the school day. The flowing water looked the same as always, but something was very different that morning. Far too small for the eye to see, deadly microbes floated in the murky water.

The boys arrived at school and settled in to their daily routine of lessons. As the morning wore on, they began to feel queasy and asked their teacher for permission to use the toilet. Both had watery diarrhea but felt no pain—at least at first. By early afternoon, though, their diarrhea intensified. They felt nauseous and began to vomit. They became severely dehydrated, and their heads throbbed with intense pain.

More time passed. The two became very thirsty and progressively weaker. They could feel their hearts beating faster and faster. The afternoon grew warmer, but their feet and hands were very cold. They became lightheaded, dizzy, and increasingly sleepy.

Soon, other children in the school became sick with similar symptoms. The alarmed teacher, sensing something was very wrong, took them all to a small clinic a short distance away. The symptoms grew worse, and right before the eyes of the caregiver young children underwent frightening transformations. Paul and Jean were most severely affected—by then, they were almost unrecognizable. Their breathing was labored. In a few short hours, the bloom of their youth gave way to sunken eyes, grayish wrinkled skin, and a deathly pallor resembling that of the very old. They were thirsty but could not drink. They became unresponsive and lapsed into unconsciousness.

Within an hour of arriving at the clinic, the two boys were dead. A third schoolchild from a neighboring hamlet died an hour later. A pained message was sent to the health director of Artibonite *département* (one of Haiti's ten administrative units): three children dead from acute watery diarrhea. It was only the beginning of a long list of deaths.

The date was Tuesday, October 19, 2010, and cholera had broken out in Haiti.

Although new in Haiti in 2010, cholera is not a new disease. In the ancient world, it was found mainly on the Indian subcontinent. Toward the middle of the nineteenth century, it began to move around the globe in a series of waves or pandemics.[1] The most recent pandemic—the seventh—began in Indonesia in 1961 and gradually spread throughout Asia and on to Africa.

Researchers had shown the presence of cholera in the Caribbean region three times but only in the 1800s and never before in Haiti itself—at least not in recorded history.[2] So when the disease was first confirmed in Haiti in 2010, scientists could link the outbreak to the seventh pandemic but knew little more.

Why had Haiti been spared before 2010? Historical investigators had long considered infected travelers the primary mode of cholera introduction,[3] but Haiti had not had any such visitors. Haitians had overthrown their French colonizers in what was then called Saint-Domingue in a slave revolt (the Haitian Revolution of 1791–1803), which led to the founding of the Republic of Haiti. With slavery eradicated, the island nation no longer had boatloads of disease-carrying Africans arriving on its shores. And while over time Haiti found itself occupied by foreign troops (including U.S. Marines from 1915 to 1934), it was spared the scourge of invading cholera-ridden troops, a frequent event during the first six pandemics. Finally, Haiti had never been a destination for overseas agricultural or factory workers. No one traveled to the poorest country in the Western Hemisphere seeking work.

What changed that October?

As events unfolded in Bocozel, a small town of about fourteen thousand people some fifteen kilometers southeast also faced a dire situation. Deschapelles, in the agricultural valley where the Artibonite River branches into the Artibonite plain, is near a dam that distributes water from the river to the canals that irrigate downstream lands. It's also home to Hôpital Albert Schweitzer (Albert Schweitzer Hospital), which was suddenly inundated with an influx of people with similar symptoms. Almost all the patients came from the areas bordering the Artibonite River. Many reported they had drunk from the river. The hospital staff of fourteen doctors and fifty nurses, although fairly well equipped, was about to be overwhelmed that Tuesday afternoon and the next day.

Dr. Ian Rawson, the hospital's managing director and a medical anthropologist and public health specialist, blogged regularly about the comings and goings at the hospital. That evening and the following day he faced the disease firsthand when he saw dozens of newly arrived diarrhea patients. Late Wednesday evening, October 20, 2010, on the hospital blog Rawson wrote, "The causative organism has not been identified and the initial suspicions have focused on typhoid"—a gastrointestinal disease caused by a bacterium.

Specimens collected from diarrhea cases were sent to the Laboratoire National de Santé Publique (LNSP, National Public Health Laboratory) in Port-au-Prince, Haiti's capital city. Awaiting the lab's diagnosis, Rawson's medical staff focused on hygiene and rehydration. Most patients needed intravenous fluids to replenish what they had lost from the diarrhea and to prevent death from severe dehydration. Some needed daily infusions of ten liters or more. Hospital staff worried supplies might not last very long.

The Albert Schweitzer doctors didn't even have a dim thought of cholera.

What had spared Haiti before from deadly cholera? Past policies? Good luck? Surely public officials and scientists would soon begin the appropriate investigation to unravel how cholera had come to the country. Scientists who study diseases such as cholera seek out origins so they can inform public officials needing to implement new policies and correct past mistakes so future generations can be spared.

Haiti had experienced many calamities. A devastating earthquake struck its most populated area the afternoon of Tuesday, January 12, 2010. In the aftermath of the earthquake, many predicted the occurrence of epidemics, including cholera. But for nine months, there were no epidemics.

Among the quake's casualties were three of the top commanders of MINUSTAH. They died when the headquarters in Port-au-Prince collapsed. MINUSTAH's presence in the country for the past six years—with about nine thousand military personnel and nearly four thousand police—was a source of comfort for some but anger and frustration for many others, and it spurred periodic protests and unrest. From time to time, those feelings spilled into the streets, as they did in September 2010 when protesters rallied against MINUSTAH after a teenage boy was found hanging from a tree at a MINUSTAH base.

In October, as fear of cholera increased and the mysteries of origin and transmission remained unsolved, people raised questions and spread rumors that in turn stimulated social tensions and violence. Fear, panic, and anger set in. Who was to blame for cholera's arrival? Haitians wanted to know. Who was causing the disease to spread? Who was telling the truth? Lying? Who was saving lives? Causing deaths? Answers were not forthcoming.

Later, when more rumors began to spread that linked UN peacekeepers to the outbreak, cities and villages in some regions of Haiti erupted in protests. On Monday, November 15, as the epidemic continued to rage through the country, street protests broke out in Cap-Haïtien, the country's second-largest city. When a Haitian protester was shot dead, MINUSTAH officials insisted that peacekeepers had shot in self-defense.[4] Since the violence was occurring in the midst of a campaign for the nation's presidency and parliament, a MINUSTAH spokesperson insisted it had been provoked by political forces "that do not want elections to happen" and that UN forces providing logistical support for the upcoming vote were being targeted as a "way of hampering the electoral process."[5] He made no mention of the UN cholera rumor, nor did he acknowledge the bitter frustration of people exposed to a terrible disease who had to live without the benefit of toilets and safe water.

Throughout that fateful Wednesday, October 20, Dr. Rawson maintained contact with a colleague, Dr. Scott Dowell, a hospital board member and prominent physician at the United States Centers for Disease Control and Prevention in Atlanta, Georgia. CDC had people in Haiti who would soon be investigating the sudden outbreak and offering medical assistance to those in need.

"We are waiting to see what the morning brings," Rawson blogged late that evening, likely weary from work and probably without the warm smile he had in almost every photograph. But before morning, word came that Bocozel and Deschapelles were not the only areas affected by the violent outbreak of enteric disease. By Wednesday evening, the emerging epidemic was overwhelming people at an unprecedented level, striking all communities along the banks and delta of the Artibonite River. The fifty-two hospitals and clinics serving the lower river communities were overwhelmed with cases—thousands appeared at health facilities, and hundreds were dying. Local medical staff had never seen such a wave of patients. Throughout the region, people were suddenly experiencing explosive diarrhea, quickly becoming dehydrated, and suffering intense headaches, dizziness, and lethargy.

Diarrheal diseases in tropical countries typically affect the very young, but patients in Haiti spanned all ages. What they had in common was living near the Artibonite River. Most bathed in river water and drank from the river, either directly or through household water containers. They ate food splashed with river water or handled by family members who had touched the river but then left their hands unwashed.

The worst of the epidemic's early days occurred at Hôpital St. Nicolas (Saint Nicolas Hospital), a major referral hospital in the coastal town of Saint-Marc. As at clinics in the surrounding regions, the rush of patients began on Tuesday afternoon. A typical day brought a few patients needing urgent care, but soon Saint Nicolas was seeing hundreds. Throngs of sick people and family members choked the hospital's main entrance trying to get inside for medical attention. Explosive vomitus and diarrhea flowed from the infirm in the crowded courtyard outside; many died waiting. Those who managed to get in found conditions even worse. The stricken were everywhere, filling hospital wards, corridors, and even the spaces between buildings.

Cholera seemed to strike people at random. Some had seizures and died within hours. Others suffered acute dehydration and became dried-up caricatures of their former selves. Respiratory difficulties increased as death approached, the lack of oxygen turning the skin of black Haitians a grayish color. Neurological symptoms among some gave the impression of demonic possession. Panic, fear, and the face of death were all haunting realities. Because of the explosive nature of the epidemic and the fear of cholera symptoms and deaths, many Haitians reacted as did Europeans during nineteenth-century epidemics, when fear of *la peur bleue*—the blue skin of cholera—terrorized many and riots were all too frequent.[6]

By Thursday, the emerging epidemic had reached an unprecedented scale, involving many communities along the riverbanks and delta of the Artibonite valley. The main Haitian river had always been a life source, but now it had become a source of death.

Haitian newspapers immediately understood the seriousness of the situation. The diagnosis was not official, but the press still wrote of cholera,[7] reporting the official death toll at 49 but unofficially telling of 1,500 cases and 135 deaths—so far. The figures came from the president of the Haitian Medical Association, who may have heard it was cholera from Haitian epidemiologists and scientists at LNSP.

Dr. Gabriel Thimothé, director general of the Ministry of Public Health and Population (MSPP), focused reporters on the dire situation in coastal Saint-Marc. He said experts were seeking the point of the river's contamination. Dr. Alex Larsen, minister of health, pinpointed the affected area as Artibonite département and upriver Centre département. "The causative organism was likely an imported microbe that flowed in the Artibonite River," he explained. When a reporter asked whether the imported microbe could be cholera, Larsen said it was doubtful but advocated caution.

The reporter's question was answered officially when a cholera diagnosis was confirmed. On October 19 and 20, stool specimens from patients in health facilities in Artibonite and Centre départements had been brought to LNSP, where rapid tests—typically not as good as regular laboratory tests but useful for immediate diagnosis—were conducted on eight specimens found positive for *V. cholerae* O1.[8] LNSP further analyzed three of the specimens and, on October 22, provided a more complete identification of the organism as toxigenic *V. cholerae serogroup O1, serotype Ogawa, biotype El Tor.*

In Washington, D.C., the Pan American Health Organization (PAHO) was immediately told of the outbreak, was closely monitoring the situation, and issued a press release on Thursday, October 21 informing the world that cholera had come to Haiti.[9] It confirmed the cholera diagnosis by Haiti's national laboratory and presented the epidemiological situation. The report focused on Artibonite département but mentioned other areas, including Mirebalais in Centre département.

After drawing attention to the need for immediate medical care (without rehydration, fatalities reach close to 50 percent), PAHO's statement briefly addressed the epidemic's cause, focusing on a possible link between the spread of cholera and an *environmental* cause: the terrible January earthquake, noting that in its aftermath "more than 1.5 million Haitians were settled in temporary sites throughout Port-au-Prince and beyond."

But why would an earthquake nine months earlier cause cholera in Haiti? PAHO offered only a vague response: cholera transmission is "closely linked to inadequate environmental management." Risky areas include urban slums and camps for internally displaced persons, the release stated. The lack of "clean water and sanitation" is a major risk factor.

PAHO did not speculate further about how cholera might have arrived in the country.

The people of Haiti were increasingly eager to identify the source of their new misery. And when public officials showed no interest in the quest for that particular truth, Haitians felt disrespected and devalued. They wondered whether their suffering meant anything to anyone. Not surprisingly, anger, suspicion, and social unrest followed. As many European populations did during the nineteenth-century cholera epidemics, people in Saint-Marc became violent. Doctors and nurses of Médecins Sans Frontières (MSF, Doctors without Borders), were there to provide medical care for cholera patients at overcrowded L'Hôpital St. Nicolas and wanted to expand their vital services with a new four hundred-bed center.[10] But unexpected riots forced them to abandon the project.

Local residents revolted when they learned the new treatment center would be built near two schools, fearing cholera would spread to their children. Angry and frustrated, they threw stones and burned several tents, but fortunately there were no serious injuries. Nevertheless, the local government called MINUSTAH for help, and Argentine UN peacekeepers were sent to intervene. The violence kept the new cholera treatment center from opening, so care continued at the greatly overcrowded facility.

On Wednesday, October 27, at Hôpital Albert Schweitzer, Dr. Rawson blogged that CDC investigators—active in the epidemic's early weeks—were planning to spend a week or more researching the disease, "visiting the homes and courtyards of patients, and taking samples from water sources, wells, rivers and canals." He wrote that hospital staff had visited many patients' households and "found concentrations of cases in courtyards where the water table is quite high (it is possible to dip water out of the well with a cup), and the wells are very near to latrines and canals." Recognizing the transmission potential, Rawson continued, "The wells are treated with chlorine powder, but it is apparent that exposure to the pathogen will continue in the absence of a dependable potable water source."

His forecast was bleak.

At the end of the first week of the epidemic, some 4,722 cholera cases were reported. MSPP further reported that hospitalizations for cholera dramatically increased for two days, then declined to a lower, steady level.[11] More than three-quarters of the cases came from Artibonite département, another fifth from Centre département, and the remaining few from Nord (north of Artibonite) and Nord Est (northeast of Artibonite) départements. These numbers, though, did not even include nonhospitalized patients with watery diarrhea.

The official death toll stood at 303. There would be many more.

The Haitian people were demanding answers about where the disease came from and how long it would continue to attack them and their families. Some sensed that whether one lived or died from cholera was a fluke of time. Anger gripped many, while many others were overcome with feelings of powerlessness and despair. Most had no choice but to continue to lead their daily lives as best they could.

2

VIBRIO CHOLERAE

Vibrio cholerae, the bacterium that causes cholera, has many relatives, some more welcome than others. Like most bacteria, the cholera microbe is minuscule in size, no more than one to three thousandths of a millimeter in length. Moreover, it does not cause much damage to people unless swallowed in a gulp that contains a large number of microbes.

While using the same general name, *Vibrio cholerae* is classified into more than two hundred serological groups based on the O antigen present in the outer membrane of the microscopic comma-shaped rod with a whip-like tail, or flagellum, on one end. Only two of these many groups, however, are associated with epidemic cholera, namely O1 and O139. Yet the many non-O1 and non-O139 groups living harmlessly in coastal waters and estuaries still find their reputations tainted by the dreaded *Vibrio cholerae* name. Some scientists, however, believe the tainted reputation is warranted, postulating that segments of genetic material in environmental vibrios living in estuaries are periodically rearranged and combined—through genomic recombination—making a harmless *V. cholerae* into a disease-causing bacterium able to cause a cholera outbreak.[1]

The cholera organism loves water. In many regions of the world, cholera bacteria thrive independent of humans in coastal waters or estuaries and often reside in shellfish and the group of small crustaceans called copepods.[2] Swimming is easy for the cholera microbe; it uses its tail to move effortlessly in aquatic environments.

Even within the two troublesome groups, O1 and O139, only some cause the severe diarrhea, vomiting, dehydration, and death that typify the disease called "cholera." The pathogenic group of cholera-causing microbes produces a toxin that alters the gastrointestinal walls, leading to a rapid loss of body fluids. Residing in these fluids are thousands to hundreds of thousands of *Vibrio cholerae.* Having the toxin is what gives human-infecting *Vibrio cholerae* the survival advantage, allowing the organism via feces and vomitus to move from one host to another. Without the toxin, the microbe can still live in aqueous environments, but it is not able to cause epidemic disease.

When Haitian and CDC laboratory scientists analyzed the cholera organism found in Haiti, they reported it to be the toxigenic form of the O1 serogroup, further classified as serotype Ogawa and biotype El Tor.[3] Though the long name identifies one form of *Vibrio cholerae,* it does not tell where the organism came from, other than from South or Central America, Asia, or Africa, where similarly named microbes have been reported in the past. With the use of newer molecular techniques, the Haitian organism was subsequently uniquely identified with a more descriptive complex name. That made it easier to find the origin.

While deadly in some, most infections with toxigenic *Vibrio cholerae* are asymptomatic, meaning without symptoms. A small percentage of infected persons develop mild or moderate diarrhea, and an even smaller percentage exhibit the dramatic signs of severe cholera. Such severe cases first become dehydrated, then develop leg cramps and shock, and if untreated, die in a few hours.

A similar symptomatic pattern was observed in Haiti. In a large serological survey done six months after the epidemic onset in Grande Saline (one of six *communes* in the Artibonite plain), investigators found that 74 percent of cholera-infected persons reported no diarrhea, 7 percent reported mild disease (diarrhea without a health facility visit), 10 percent had moderate disease (diarrhea and a visit to a health facility but not meeting criteria for severe disease), and 9 percent had severe cholera, needing intravenous fluids and overnight hospitalization.[4] The survey findings suggest that while thousands of cholera cases were reported by health facilities in the Artibonite plain, many more infected persons were not counted because they did not experience diarrhea or because they did not seek care in health facilities.

When epidemic cholera occurs in different regions of the world, the disease pattern is termed a "pandemic." The Indian subcontinent has been the site of cholera since ancient times. In 1817, cholera began spreading around the world in seven different pandemics. The third of these occurred in the mid-1800s in a broader area including London, where Dr. John Snow gained fame for his cholera research. The seventh, most recent, pandemic began in 1961 in Indonesia, featuring the El Tor biotype of *Vibrio cholerae*. The pandemic spread through Asia to Africa, Europe, and Latin America.[5] By 1991, cholera had come to Peru, then moved on to other countries in Central and South America—although skipping Haiti—before ending a decade or so later.

In the seventh pandemic, the El Tor form of *Vibrio cholerae* arises from a common lineage or ancestral group. The ancestors of this pathogen are different from the *Vibrio cholerae* forbearers of the non-disease-causing strains that are present in environmental waters throughout the world. Recent analyses suggest that travel and poor sanitation, both associated with human activity, are the likely sources of the disease-causing El Tor clones, threatening worldwide populations.[6]

The cholera organism moves from infected host to susceptible person mainly in two ways: through contaminated water and food and by close contact with infected persons. The exact number of microbes needed to cause cholera was determined in studies of prisoners during the 1970s in the United States.[7] After ingesting ten thousand cholera organisms mixed with a solution for neutralizing stomach acid, some of the "volunteer" prisoners had mild cholera-ridden diarrhea. When the scientists increased the numbers to between one hundred thousand and one million organisms, the diarrhea became more severe, requiring intravenous injections to maintain fluid balance. These two earlier studies, while useful, will not be repeated or refined because of contemporary ethical concerns. Hence, the infective dose numbers here presented for cholera remain the best available.

To unravel how infectious diseases are spread from one person to another, field epidemiologists use knowledge of incubation periods, or the time from onset of infection (i.e., swallowing the ten thousand or more organisms) until the beginning of symptomatic disease. Once a symptomatic case appears, the disease detective works backwards using the incubation period to find the location of the case at the time of exposure. For cholera, WHO has stated that the incubation period is two hours to five days.[8] In their 1974 prisoner study, the investigators presented a slightly different evidence-based view of the cholera incubation period. From the exact time of exposure, the first cases of diarrhea did not appear until 10 hours later and the last cases until nearly 150 hours later, or just over six days. When the observations of other cholera experts are taken into account, the minimum incubation of 10 hours seems greater by several hours than it should be, perhaps because the strain of cholera the investigators used was not overly pathogenic and the inoculums were only moderate in size. The investigators of the two 1970s prisoner studies suggested as much when they noted that that those who consumed larger doses of cholera organisms had shorter incubation periods, as did those cases with more severe cholera. These seminal studies suggest that a more complete definition of the cholera incubation period is from a few hours to six days, usually one to two days.

The toxigenic microbes can live for long periods in water and sometimes multiply in moist foods or clothing. Lately scientists have questioned, but have yet to resolve, whether toxigenic *Vibrio cholerae* occasionally found in water environments in endemic areas are living and multiplying there or are there temporarily as a result of contamination of the environment by nearby cholera cases.[9] To infect a susceptible person, the necessary dose of comma-shaped organisms must first enter the mouth and then pass through the stomach, where locally produced acidic fluids cause them harm. If the number of cholera microbes in the ingested food or water is great enough (perhaps ten thousand or more), many will be able to move on to the small intestine. There they multiply and create the powerful toxin that affects the intestinal lining, allowing electrolytes—various ions such as sodium, potassium, or chloride—and water to leave the host and come streaming out as "rice-water" diarrhea, containing flecks of mucus and some epithelial cells about the color and size of pieces of rice. Included in this are about ten million to one billion vibrio per milliliter of stool, or fifty million to five billion microbes per teaspoon of liquid diarrhea.[10] If sufficient diarrheic fluid contaminates other food or water, a new inoculum containing thousands of microbes moves on and infects another person.

The crafty cholera organism has another feature that eases transmission. Rather than causing diarrhea in each infected host, about three-quarters of human hosts show no disease signs or symptoms. Transmission is certainly more difficult in this asymptomatic group since the concentration of organisms in their stools is much lower than in those with free-flowing diarrhea. Yet if the asymptomatic person lacks personal hygiene or, say, defecates in a communal stream, on occasion the stealthy cholera microbe can still be transmitted.

Once cholera arrives, diarrhea of the affected person provides the most common form of spread, transmitting the organism to the oral cavity and stomach of other susceptible individuals. Farmers in the fertile Artibonite valley, for instance, practice what scientists call "open defecation": they typically defecate in the fields and rice paddies, which allows fecal waste to meld with the water. Four years earlier, a nationwide survey noted that open defecation was practiced by about half of Haiti's rural population,[11] not unlike 43 percent in rural Nepal[12]—the equally poor country that provided troops to the MINUSTAH camp near Mirebalais. In their initial study of midvalley cholera patients, CDC investigators reported that more than three-quarters had practiced open defecation, and two-thirds drank untreated water from rivers or canals.[13]

Such defecation practices and water exposure likely increased the occurrence of local cholera, facilitating transmission from infected to susceptible.

Once infected and showing disease, surviving cholera patients become partially immune to future infection, at least for a few years. In 1981, cholera was induced in four volunteers, then after thirty-three to thirty-six months, they were again challenged with *Vibrio cholerae*. None of the four developed diarrhea, whereas four of five susceptible volunteers who also were challenged with the microbe developed clinical cholera.[14]

Years later, a much larger study was conducted in a cholera-endemic population in Bangladesh.[15] The investigators compared two groups gathered between 1991 and 2000—patients with clinical cholera and same-aged persons who did not have cholera. Both groups were observed during the following three years for onset of new cholera. Apropos to the El Tor cholera strain in Haiti, patients who had developed cholera three years earlier from the El Tor biotype had a 65 percent lower risk of again developing El Tor cholera than those in the control group. Natural cholera infection stimulated protection, but not overwhelming protection, in the coming three years.

The issue of natural cholera infection remains the subject of ongoing research. As a 2012 review article noted, "The precise immunological effectors that mediate protection against *Vibrio cholerae* are not fully understood."[16]

The severe damage cholera does to human hosts is measured by case-fatality, or the proportion of patients diagnosed with cholera who subsequently die of the disease. While death is easy to determine, there is typically some confusion over the precise definition of a cholera case.

The situation in Cité Soleil, a poor area near Port-au-Prince, provided an example of such confusion, giving the impression—using case-fatality—that cholera was more severe than it really was. During the epidemic's first weeks, the case-fatality in Cité Soleil seemed quite high, suggesting that cholera was very deadly among cases. From all appearances, local medical staff had correctly counted the number of cholera deaths and correctly identified new cases. But their initial reports had tallied only the number of hospitalized cholera cases given intravenous fluids for at least one night—the more severe group—and omitted the milder cases treated in the hospital with either intravenous fluids or oral rehydration solutions and then sent home. Therein was the discrepancy.

Later, in mid-November, the reporting staff changed the government submissions to the DELR (Direction d'Epidémiologie, Laboratoire et Recherche, or Department of Epidemiology, Laboratory and Research) to include both the more severe hospitalized cholera patients and the milder, nonhospitalized cases. When the latter were included, the case-fatality appeared to decline, giving the impression that medical care was increasingly successful. Reality, though, was something different. The severity of the disease (as measured by the case-fatality) appears not to have changed much over time in the cared-for population, only the reporting method.

3

RUMORS

The day after the Pan-American Health Organization issued its October 21 press release confirming cholera in Haiti, MINUSTAH posted a notice on its website with an origin time for the outbreak: "The first case of cholera was recorded on September 24, occurring in the Lower Artibonite region, a populated place where people live in precarious conditions without drinking water or latrines."[1] The source for this information was identified as the MSPP—but the September 24 origin date in the Artibonite region near the coast had never been mentioned in any press release, nor had it been acknowledged or cited by anyone in the news media.

Meanwhile, Dr. Ian Rawson in Deschapelles was writing yet again on the Albert Schweitzer Hospital blog. The hospital was facing an influx of cholera cases, and staff members were frantically making changes to improve patient management and care. Fortunately, most patients were cared for in two to three days and could be discharged with a supply of oral rehydration powder to use if their diarrhea reappeared. Several international relief agencies had come by with resupplies of gloves, oral rehydration packets, antibiotics, and buckets, which were shared with the health facility in nearby Verrettes.

On Thursday evening, a few hours after the PAHO press release was issued, a team of CDC investigators appeared at Albert Schweitzer Hospital. The diarrhea outbreak throughout the Artibonite region had been confirmed as cholera, they told the medical staff. The CDC team was particularly interested in maps that could help pinpoint the disease and its course. At first glance, it appeared most patients had contracted the disease near the river and canals, a few kilometers from the hospital, rather than in the immediate area.

Friday and Saturday were busy days for the CDC team as it identified cases of severe diarrheal disease and verified *Vibrio cholerae* as the causative organism. Team members also set out to interview cases, looking for where they had been infected. Knowing time and place is key to an epidemiological investigation. Since the incubation period—or time from infection to the onset of symptoms—for *Vibrio cholerae* is usually one to two days but may range from a few hours to six days,[2] CDC team members planned to ask where the cases had been living (and likely where they'd been working or traveling) in the previous week, focusing on when they were probably infected. They would also ask about water and food consumption practices.

The epidemiologists used a standardized questionnaire to interview a convenience sample of twenty-seven patients in five hospitals, four in Artibonite département and one to the south in Ouest département, another administrative area surrounding Port-au-Prince. Patients in a "convenience sample" are not selected randomly, and so any findings may not be representative of all cholera cases in the population. But this was a crisis, and the CDC epidemiologists may have been more concerned with feasibility and speed than with complete accuracy.

The epidemiologists found that most patients resided or worked in rice fields in communities located alongside a twenty-mile stretch of the Artibonite River. Rice has been cultivated in Haiti for more than two hundred years. It is a staple food in the country, and locals proudly refer to the Artibonite valley as "Haiti's largest granary."

The Artibonite River in Haiti is 150 miles long, but the patients interviewed were from a relatively narrow area mainly in downriver Artibonite département. Still, the findings were revealing. The investigators stated, "18 (67%) of the 27 hospitalized patients reported consuming untreated water from the river or canals before illness onset, 18 (67%) did not routinely use chlorine for treating water, and 21 (78%) practiced open defecation" somewhere other than a toilet.[3]

As CDC's activities became known, they raised a red flag in my mind. While officially retired from the institution, I was still teaching the occasional UCLA epidemiology course and was always looking out for interesting outbreaks, sample surveys, or field investigations. I wondered why CDC had opted for a convenience sample rather than randomly selecting patients. Charitably, I figured the team must have been doing its best under difficult circumstances. Still, though, I was more troubled by its failure to seek—*early on*—the starting point of the cholera epidemic. That would soon raise another red flag.

The CDC investigators did seem to understand the potential importance of the Artibonite River as a transmission vehicle. The initial PAHO report indicated that some of the first wave of severe diarrhea samples and deaths came from the town of Mirebalais in Centre département, upriver from Artibonite département.[4] Perhaps they also knew that stool specimens had been collected in Centre département, with rapid tests for cholera showing some as positive. But why did they interview residents of Artibonite département but no one who lived in Centre département? Moreover, why did they choose to interview patients from Ouest département, an area south of Artibonite département and some distance from the river?

Academic epidemiologists routinely teach that in outbreak investigations there is "great urgency to find the source."[5] I am no different. That's how you find out what went wrong, how to stop transmission and prevent future outbreaks. The source of an epidemic can be as varied as eating contaminated whale and dolphin meat, which can lead to mercury poisoning, or consuming chickens from a filthy farm, which can result in a widespread *salmonellosis* disease. It's something investigators need to know.

Dr. Gabriel Thimothé, the MSPP director general, reiterated this point when early on he told a reporter that "experts are seeking to determine the point of contamination of the river."[6] To that end, local maps were given to the CDC team to chart the Artibonite River, identify where suspected cases probably first arose, and help determine how the outbreak got under way.

PAHO included a map with its fourth and sixth situation reports, both later cited by CDC in its own initial report on cholera in Haiti.[7] The two maps clearly showed the Artibonite River, the upriver Centre département, and the downriver Artibonite département.[8] An inquisitive epidemiologist, knowing cholera's water-loving nature, should have been drawn to Centre département and looked there for additional cases.

I also wondered why CDC had not used a spot map to show the location of the various positive stool samples and cholera patients. It would have allowed the team to glean so much more information. Spot maps are an important tool for disease detectives. It wouldn't be at all unusual to see a team of epidemiologists huddled around a spot map on the wall, using colored ball-top pins to identify cases. More likely, computer-savvy CDC epidemiologists would create and share a spot map on their computers. So why had the CDC team failed to offer such a map for the eight stool samples that tested positive with a rapid test and the twenty-seven patients interviewed in the convenience sample? Why describe their macrolocation in the mid-November report only as being somewhere in the Artibonite and Ouest départements?

There also seemed to be a problem with the design of the CDC study: investigators had gathered responses only from patients as a case series. Disease detectives recognize that information on cases alone does not tell the whole story. For instance, learning that two-thirds of the hospitalized cholera patients drank water from the river or canals before illness onset was of limited use. Is that percentage among cases high or low? What about the percentage of all people in the area who drink from the river? To answer, epidemiologists would need to know the water consumption patterns of noncholera patients, termed "controls," and then compare the two values.

Why didn't the CDC team conduct a case-control study? Individuals without cholera, the control group, should have been selected from the same locations as the respective cases. Such a study, common to acute outbreak investigations, would have been very useful with the initial wave of cases. The hastiness of relying on a convenience sample had already caught my eye. Was haste behind CDC's choice of a case-only study too?

Morbidity and Mortality Weekly Report (*MMWR*), which published the initial CDC team's findings, included this editorial note: "A case-control study is under way that will provide additional information about risk factors for illness in Artibonite."[9] This pleased me, although the study findings were not published until a year later, not offering much assistance to those wanting to utilize the results. The investigation was done in October–November 2010 in Petite Rivière, a town near the Artibonite River, close to Albert Schweitzer Hospital.[10]

On Sunday, October 24, blogger Rawson noted the arrival of a second CDC team at his hospital, this time a group of epidemiologists planning for surveillance of the disease. Before the surveillance system could be implemented, though, they had to learn more about mapping the cases and describing the course of the epidemic.

There was a curious shift regarding the question of cholera's origin on the hospital blog on Monday, October 25. "The origins of this outbreak are a mystery, but are not a primary question at this time. What is of most concern will be the modes of transmission," wrote Rawson—a view that would be repeated by many other scientists, practitioners, and journalists as the epidemic progressed.

Not so subtly, Rawson had pushed aside the issue of finding the origin or source of a major epidemic in Haiti caused by a deadly microbe never before seen in the country. Limiting transmission became his primary concern. Of course, his hospital was on the front lines, trying to keep patients alive.

Rawson's blog post on transmission continued. "In our area, the initial cases were from men who were working in the rice fields in the lower Artibonite River, who traveled to Hôpital Albert Schweitzer to receive care for the disease," he wrote. "More recently, cases have involved young children. These families, who live closer to the hospital and also near to the river and its canals, report that they had been drinking from wells in their courtyard or at their neighbors." Rawson's informal hypothesis, based on what patients had said, was that cholera came from the water of the Artibonite. No one seemed to be addressing how the cholera organism got into the river in the first place.

In the early days of November, another natural catastrophe hit Haiti. Hurricane Tomas made landfall and battered the western part of the country without mercy. On top of the devastating January earthquake and then the cholera epidemic, it was a brutal reminder of how difficult a year 2010 continued to be. In Port-au-Prince, the intense storm even shut down runways at the main airport and delayed flights until Sunday, November 7. That was the day Renaud Piarroux—a professor of parasitology at Aix Marseille University in Marseille, France, and the chief of parasitology and mycology at a hospital there—arrived to consult on cholera.

Piarroux is a muscular man standing about six feet tall, who travels light. He arrived in Haiti with nothing more than a backpack, a jacket and dress shirt for formal meetings, and his usual attire—a long-sleeved blue denim shirt, black jeans, and *une paire de baskets noires* (a pair of black sport shoes). This was a habit developed during his many global trips. He had embarked on his first such mission in 1994, when he was a thirty-three-year-old pediatrician working on a PhD in microbiology. Piarroux had decided to volunteer with the humanitarian organization Médecins du Monde (Doctors of the World) in Goma, a Central African city in the Democratic Republic of the Congo (DR Congo, formerly Zaire).

In the weeks prior to his arrival in Goma, hundreds of thousands of refugees from Rwanda converged on the city as they tried to escape an intense civil war in their home country. Almost as soon as the refugee camps were established, cholera erupted. It was proving impossible to deal with all the people, let alone address epidemic cholera and other diseases that caused tens of thousands of deaths in a six-week span. The need for help was desperate.

Piarroux's mission was to provide medical care for 2,500 orphans in one of the larger camps. By the time he arrived, the cholera epidemic was already at its peak, striking down countless young children in hours to days. As this enormous loss of young life unfolded before his eyes, Piarroux found himself haunted by the vision of his own three children back in Marseille—then aged eight months, four years, and five years.

Returning to Marseille, he vowed never to forget the tragedy he'd seen in Goma and decided to devote part of his life to understanding and combating epidemics in developing countries. In the ensuing years, while working full time in his clinical activities and his academic career in parasitology, he continued to go on humanitarian missions that would take him—for weeks at a time—to far-flung places such as Afghanistan, Comoros, Honduras, Ivory Coast, and even back to DR Congo. Over time, those field experiences taught Piarroux a great deal about cholera, including how the disease moved through populations. As he observed cholera epidemics during these missions, he found that wars, hurricanes, volcanic eruptions, and many other calamities were associated with the epidemics in certain instances but not in others.

As noted earlier, Piarroux had become skeptical over time about the environmental theory of cholera's origins. He had also become troubled by the role NGOs play in the spread and elimination of cholera. As his voluntary fieldwork continued, it became apparent to Piarroux that many NGOs, relying on both volunteers and outsides funding agencies, had short memories when it came to the successful elements and errors of past disease control efforts.

In 2002, cholera reappeared in DR Congo and spread rapidly to Kongolo District, where Piarroux was leading a Médecins du Monde medical team with the objective of improving access to care. The case-fatality from cholera was very high in the local hospital, about 10 percent. As an organization, however, Médecins du Monde seemed reluctant to embrace the fight against the disease fully and was hesitant to support the local health authorities in their community intervention efforts. Why? The organization's mandate in DR Congo did not include cholera outbreaks. Also, a broader focus on cholera would require additional money, and Médecins du Monde's donors were already being solicited for many other emergency responses all over the world. Raising the additional funds would require considerable time and effort. So the head of Médecins du Monde instead contacted Médecins Sans Frontières to ask for help. MSF, though, was busy dealing with cholera elsewhere in DR Congo, and it would be weeks before a team could come to Kongolo District. Even then, MSF could offer only a few days of care. Reluctantly, Médecins du Monde decided not to address cholera—which incensed Piarroux, who soon thereafter resigned as head of mission.

The following year, he again tried to get Médecins du Monde involved with broader control efforts aimed at cholera epidemics in DR Congo, but no agreement could be reached because of the differing views on what to do. It was becoming apparent to Piarroux that in developing countries, fighting epidemics was too long and complex a mandate for NGOs. It required active collaboration with local public health officials. It meant developing and supporting epidemiologic surveillance systems. There would have to be water and sanitation interventions, and health education programs would have to be developed and implemented.

Most medical NGOs seemed to be at their best when providing care at the peak of epidemics, helping overwhelmed local doctors meet patient needs in their communities. They typically provided medical care and then moved on. Long-term cholera control strategies were not in their bailiwick but rather were the responsibility of the affected countries, regardless of limited capacity, ability, or political will. The problem wasn't just with Médecins du Monde, thought Piarroux, but also with many other humanitarian organizations—all unwilling or unable to address the major shortcomings of government health agencies that were all too common in developing countries. Recognizing these problems, Piarroux decided in 2003 to change his own approach to cholera. He would no longer volunteer for general medical missions. Instead, he decided to build on his academic experience and use research to create affordable strategies that dealt specifically with cholera. His true fight against the disease was about to begin.

In facing this challenge Piarroux is committed to the scientific approach, which is his guide: identify a problem, construct an argument, figure out the tools to fix the problem, obtain results, and sum it all up for presentation. Applying that approach to something significant, like a deadly epidemic, holds particular interest for him. Travel and meeting new people with whom to work makes it even more exciting. He believes the adventure and satisfaction offset, a thousand times over, the discomfort and danger of the situations in which he often finds himself.

His mission in Haiti, as described by the French embassy, was to provide medical and scientific support as well as coordination assistance to the Haitian Ministry of Health. He planned to be in Haiti for ten days.

Joining Piarroux in Haiti was a university colleague from Marseille, Dr. Benoit Faucher, who had volunteered for a UNICEF project that would place an epidemiologist and sanitary engineer in each of Haiti's ten départements. Faucher is a physician specializing in infectious diseases but also skilled in geographic information systems and computer mapping. Piarroux also asked his wife, Martine, a physician and medical geographer, to join the team. She remained in Marseille, working over the Internet.

His small team set, Piarroux was ready to implement a cholera map tracking system, essential for understanding the time course of the evolving epidemic. His first days in Haiti, though, would be spent in meetings. He needed to understand the existing flow of cholera data, clarify what various agencies were doing, and get a sense for how well the work was coordinated. He knew it was important to build relationships and establish trust. Only then would he venture into the Haitian countryside to witness firsthand the dimensions of the epidemic and its impact.

The French embassy in Port-au-Prince, a stately, multifloor building in the heart of Haiti's capital city, stands only a few blocks from the National Palace—the traditional residence of the country's president that sustained heavy damage in the January earthquake. The embassy, too, was damaged. Piarroux met staff there on Monday morning, November 8, and briefed them on his plans. He then phoned officials at the World Health Organization, UNICEF, and Médecins Sans Frontières. Later he spoke with officials at Direction Nationale de l'Eau Potable et de l'Assainissement (DINEPA), the public institution responsible for overseeing the distribution of drinking water, to learn about Haiti's water use patterns.

Piarroux's most important meeting that first day took place in the evening, when he met with Haiti's "presidential cell"—a group that advised President René Préval on matters regarding the earthquake and cholera epidemic. Professor Jean Hugues Henrys, dean of the Faculty of Medicine, Sciences, and Health at the Université Notre-Dame d'Haïti in Port-au-Prince, chaired the meeting. The group also included Dr. Claude Surrena, president of the Haitian Medical Association, and Dr. Daniel Henry, chief of staff for Haiti's minister of health.

From Piarroux's perspective, a step-by-step approach is essential when beginning to investigate an epidemic. It is an issue of both method and self-assurance. Investigatory tasks can be daunting. Sometimes the challenges may seem insurmountable. By carefully taking a first step and then another Piarroux is able to deal with the inevitable frustrations.

First and foremost, he wants to gain a clear understanding of how an epidemic got started and how it continues to evolve. He confesses his lack of any special gifts when it comes to computer applications and complicated epidemic models. His favorite software is a pair of shoes with good strong soles. Some epidemiologists stare all day at a screen, but Piarroux prefers to get his shoes dirty. He planned to work with local Haitian epidemiologists and local health authorities, review medical records, talk to medical staffs, and use the information to understand disease transmission patterns. He values the give-and-take of discussion, especially in local communities where public health colleagues can address specific disease risk factors.

But it wouldn't be all shoe-leather epidemiology, Piarroux told the presidential advisory group. His technologically savvy colleagues on the team would create sophisticated statistical models. He described a surveillance system for cholera that relied on local data collection and computer-generated maps to clarify the force and spread of the epidemic, from which control strategies could be formulated. Congolese officials were using the system to curb a cholera epidemic that had been ravaging broad areas for more than two decades. Piarroux believed it could also work in Haiti.

The presidential advisers liked what they heard, assuring Piarroux they would open whatever doors were necessary.

Haiti's health ministry is located near the Champ de Mars, Port-au-Prince's main square. In the months after the January earthquake, the square housed survivors in a crude camp with row upon row of tents. Many bore the words "P. R. China" and the Chinese flag—they had been donated by the People's Republic of China as part of the world's response to Haiti's humanitarian crisis. Small plastic enclosures, interspersed among the tents, served as toilets. People took showers in the open air, with no privacy from the intruding eyes of passersby on the roadway. Camps like this were places of great danger and degradation.

On Tuesday morning, November 9, Piarroux met with Minister of Health Alex Larsen, whose office had been moved from the ministry building—like the National Palace, it had been destroyed by the earthquake—to one of several prefabricated buildings on the grounds. Over coffee, in an open and cordial meeting, Larsen turned quickly to the cholera issue and outlined his expectations of Piarroux. Most important, he wanted Piarroux to help Haitian authorities better understand the epidemic, explain where it came from, and predict its likely evolution. Larsen insisted on writing a letter of introduction to Dr. Roc Magloire, the director of the DELR, located in the Laboratoire National de Santé Publique (LSNP, or National Laboratory of Public Health). Magloire also served as Haiti's chief epidemiologist. Piarroux was to help DELR improve the epidemic monitoring system, and Larsen wanted to ensure Magloire's full cooperation.

That Tuesday was a day of meetings. Next was lunch with a group from the French embassy, hosted by Ambassador Didier Le Bret at his official residence in the gentle hills of suburban Canapé-Vert. Le Bret had served in his post since September 2009, but Piarroux knew him from years earlier when they had met in Paris to discuss cholera research in the DR Congo. The ambassador struck Piarroux as a relaxed man, very polite but ever careful in conversation. His reputation was as a dynamic and courageous diplomat but one always concerned about his image in the press.

Piarroux discussed the origin of the epidemic with the group, including a rumor that attributed the importation of cholera to a Nepalese contingent of MINUSTAH peacekeeping troops. He had first learned of the possible Nepalese connection in the days before his arrival in Haiti, in an article by Jonathan Katz in the online version of *La Presse*, a French-language newspaper published in Montreal, Canada.[11] Katz wrote of a cholera outbreak in Nepal that had occurred shortly before the troops left for Haiti and of sanitary problems at a Nepalese UN base near the town of Mirebalais in central Haiti. Piarroux raised the matter with Le Bret. The ambassador betrayed no visible surprise when Piarroux said it was a plausible hypothesis that needed to be explored, and he acknowledged having heard the rumors. Piarroux could not help but wonder whether Le Bret knew more than he was saying.

As the discussion continued, Piarroux learned more about another widely circulating rumor that had also been mentioned in the Katz article. The UN had contracted Sanco Enterprise SA, a waste management company based in Port-au-Prince, to empty septic tanks at the MINUSTAH camps. According to the rumor, Sanco employees had spilled the contents of a septic tank into a river. This rumor was amplified by tensions over significant payment delays.

Rumors are rampant in Haiti and are sometimes used as a means of control. Originating from the streets and neighborhoods, they can become tools for exercising power and used as weapons of resistance[12]—including against MINUSTAH, Haiti's most powerful group. For instance, in early 2009—five years after MINUSTAH first came Haiti—a rumor about UN troops stealing goats led to a confrontation at a Port-au-Prince art institute.[13] What began as a minor street scuffle between soldiers and a student soon escalated until an angry crowd congregated and began to bleat at the soldiers like goats—*bê, bê, bê*. The agitated UN soldiers grew angrier and angrier. Fortunately, school faculty managed to calm the situation, and the protest ended peacefully.

The goat rumor had originated on the northern coast a year or two after the 2004 arrival of MINUSTAH. Local farmers noticed their droves were disappearing, and suspected that UN peacekeepers at a nearby camp were slaughtering and eating the goats. They called the troops *vole kabrit* ("goat stealer" in Haitian Creole). As the rumor spread, another element was added—that soldiers had sex with the goats before killing them. Soon the rumor became a common anti-MINUSTAH theme, and goat bleating and signs and chants of *vole kabrit* became symbols in antitroop street protests.

The goat rumor was never confirmed. And so far, no one had said anything definitive about peacekeepers or Sanco rumors. There was no written or photographic evidence to add substance to the passing tales. Piarroux sensed that the UN might just be doing a poor job of getting rid of soldiers' excreta. But could one or even a few asymptomatic soldiers carrying cholera ignite a large, quick-moving, and far-reaching outbreak? Piarroux was skeptical and said so. He asked whether Ambassador Le Bret or any of the others had heard specifically of a cholera outbreak in the Nepalese UN camp. No one had.

Le Bret seemed visibly uneasy with Piarroux's questions, which Piarroux took as a warning to be vigilant about what he might say. The ambassador suggested Piarroux discuss the issue with Edmond Mulet, the UN secretary general's special representative in Haiti. As head of MINUSTAH, Mulet wielded considerable political and military power in the country. Many thought his power eclipsed even that of President Préval.

Piarroux's day ended with a visit to the local headquarters of the World Health Organization, now located in bungalows on the grounds of the UN logistics base near the international airport, far from downtown Port-au-Prince. A nightmarish traffic jam—a daily feature of life around Port-au-Prince—made for a two-hour trip as cars attempted to pass on both sides, horns honked incessantly, and vehicles spewed black smoke through which there was little visibility. The traffic was made worse by the narrow, winding, and often bumpy streets that wend their way through the city's steep hills. Small motorcycles—some carrying as many as four people—vied with cars and pedestrians for space. Everyone's life seemed endangered. Added to the mix were the *tap taps*, colorful, ornately decorated minibuses that serve as share taxis. Most of the tap taps Piarroux saw were anointed with religious-oriented names: *à la grâce de Dieu* (By the Grace of God); *Jésus-Christ est mon Seigneur* (Jesus Christ Is My Lord); *Don de Dieu* (Gift of God).

By the time Piarroux arrived at WHO headquarters, the top officials were gone, so he engaged several others working in small offices. No one had a clear idea of the epidemiology of cholera in Haiti or could offer management support for Piarroux's investigation.

How, Piarroux wondered on the way back to the hotel, could WHO personnel keep up their relationship with their downtown Haitian counterparts? Just the time it took to drive to and from government offices in the city center would be enough to discourage regular cooperation.

Piarroux had one more day of introductory meetings before he could do what he really wanted—fieldwork. On Wednesday morning, November 10, he met quickly with representatives of Médecins Sans Frontières. The local coordinator had been called away for an emergency, but deputies received him at the MSF offices. Piarroux stressed the importance of working together and sharing epidemiological information—a message of cooperation he felt was well received. Unfortunately, the MSF epidemiologist specifically responsible for supporting field activities was unavailable.

From MSF, Piarroux went with Faucher to the UNICEF office to meet with Françoise Gruloos-Ackermans, the organization's representative in Haiti who was known as "Mama UNICEF" for her strong commitment to children. Piarroux and Gruloos-Ackermans had crossed paths twelve years earlier during a cholera epidemic in the Comoros Islands, when Piarroux was heading the cholera mission there for Médecins du Monde and Gruloos-Ackermans was the Comoros UNICEF representative.

Piarroux stressed to her the importance of implementing his planned epidemiological surveillance system, which would allow Haitian health authorities to anticipate the future development of the epidemic. Gruloos-Ackermans was particularly interested in keeping up on Piarroux's fieldwork, explaining that UNICEF and DINEPA were troubled by the lack of information on the epidemic's evolution.

The UNICEF project that brought Faucher to Haiti had fallen well short of getting enough qualified epidemiologists to volunteer. In fact, Faucher was the only medical recruit who showed up in Haiti. So, with that project scrapped, the three agreed that Faucher would serve as liaison between UNICEF and Piarroux's investigative team, remaining in Port-au-Prince to follow the cholera situation, especially in the large urban areas where most experts feared the epidemic would next appear.

Later that afternoon, Piarroux was finally able to go to the DELR to meet with Dr. Magloire and learn more about the quality and flow of cholera data. Magloire had published nearly twenty articles in international journals over the preceding three decades, including with CDC, and the bespectacled senior scientist with his receding halo of white curly hair was well known to public health professionals in Haiti and abroad.

Piarroux found Magloire in the situation room, a makeshift classroom with tables arranged in a U shape. Each Monday and Thursday morning, a team would convene there to discuss disease surveillance. Graphs and illustrations covered the walls, full of information on the many diseases DELR monitored.

Piarroux's first order of business was to learn how the existing epidemiological surveillance system worked. Each afternoon in Haiti's hundreds of health facilities, staff were required to telephone to the relevant département some daily numbers: how many suspected cholera patients, how many hospitalized patients with suspected cholera, how many deaths among cholera patients. They also reported the number of suspicious deaths in the population outside the hospital. The département epidemiological units would then tally and process the data and, at day's end, send them electronically to DELR in Port-au-Prince.

Director General Thimothé was in charge of distributing the final disease information. He personally validated all the data collected from the départements and then posted them on the Web as regularly updated reports. Validation typically took twenty-four hours but sometimes more if Thimothé was absent—in which case no one else was allowed access, not even ministry medical officers. Haiti's president and his MSPP director general were exercising very tight control over public information about the epidemic.

Why such caution? Piarroux understood it wasn't just about public health. There were political ramifications. A couple of weeks earlier, President Préval had raised the possibility of delaying the scheduled November 28 election for deputies, senators, and a new president to avoid cholera contagion at polling stations.[14] Now there were only three weeks left in the campaign. Préval was finishing up the second term and was ineligible for reelection. His younger protégé, Jude Célestin, was running as the candidate of Préval's Unity (INITE) Party.

Haitian voters were unhappy with the slow pace of postearthquake reconstruction; the persistent presence of MINUSTAH, which so many considered an occupying army; and, of course, cholera. Dissatisfaction with INITE in general and Célestin in particular ran high, and candidates of other parties were doing everything they could to keep this in voters' minds.

From Piarroux's perspective, though, the biggest problem was with data. The slow and erratic system was practically useless to guide cholera control efforts. There were communication problems. Data tended to be incomplete. Some facilities were left out of the reporting loop. And while health officials could still use incomplete data to draw epidemic curves comparing one département with another, doing so raised a crucial question: How accurate were the epidemic maps?

Piarroux's first three full days in Haiti were now over; he had introduced himself and held meetings with various officials. He was feeling anxious, wanting to get started on the core of his mission. That Wednesday night, he enjoyed a meal at the Café de l'Europe in his hotel. The pasta and red wine reminded him of home. After dinner, he wanted to take a long walk through the city to clarify his thoughts and get some exercise but had been told not to because of security concerns. So instead, he sat in the restaurant and planned the next day.

For Thursday, November 11, he set one important goal, a crucial step: to create daily maps of cholera since the beginning of the epidemic. These maps would let him study how the disease had originated and uncover the dynamics of the unfolding epidemic. Then he wanted to get into the field as quickly as possible. The epidemic had spread fast, becoming deadly in a very short time. Piarroux knew how essential it was to figure out why before the footprints began to fade.

The next morning, though, no car was available, and Piarroux could not return to DELR until midmorning. He missed the beginning of the epidemiological surveillance meeting already under way in the situation room, where epidemiologists, Haitian data capture operators, and representatives of organizations that deal with communicable diseases in Haiti—WHO, UNICEF, various nongovernmental organizations such as MSF and Medical Emergency Relief International (MERLIN), and members of the Brigada Médica Cubana (BMC), the Cuban medical brigade—had already begun their discussion.

A deputy, Dr. Donald Lafontant, was running the meeting in Dr. Magloire's absence. He asked Piarroux to introduce himself and give a brief overview of his plans. The Frenchman reiterated his desire to work with Haitian counterparts to unravel the mystery of the epidemic's extraordinary impact and develop a monitoring system to help guide appropriate responses. But when he learned that data capture operators were being transferred from DELR to other epidemiological units by specific request of President Préval, he grew worried. Their skilled work would be critical to creating the epidemic tracking maps that would tell the daily story of the disease and, he hoped, offer clues to how the epidemic had begun.

Piarroux surveyed the group. He sensed some already knew the true story of cholera's first days in Haiti. Maps or no maps, were they willing to reveal all their secrets to a stranger?

As the meeting continued, the conversation shifted to the Brigada Médica Cubana. The Cubans occupied a prominent place in the Haiti cholera fight. Hundreds of Cuban-trained doctors and nurses were operating and supporting medical care facilities throughout the country, and the Cubans had mobile clinics that crisscrossed Haiti in search of diarrhea outbreaks not previously detected with the existing monitoring system.

Piarroux learned that Brigada physicians assigned to a hospital in the town of Mirebalais—in Centre département in the central region of Haiti known as *bas plateau*—had reported the first occurrence of suspected cholera cases some three weeks earlier. The Cubans' initial communiqué reached DELR on Monday, October 18, and told of sixty-one severe diarrhea cases, including one fatality the previous day. The severity of signs and symptoms led the Cuban brigade physicians to suspect something that had never existed before in Haiti—cholera. Data from two days later told Piarroux that a much larger outbreak had burst forth many miles away, in Artibonite département. This information further convinced him that field investigation was crucial.

Most of the foreigners left at the end of the meeting, but Piarroux stayed behind to speak informally with his Haitian colleagues. They became more forthcoming. He learned that the first cholera cases were believed to have occurred in the immediate vicinity of the UN peacekeeper camp in the small village of Mèyé (some locals refer to the village as Meille, its French name), not far from Mirebalais. Every one of Haiti's powerful foreign partners—from PAHO to WHO to the United Nations Office for the Coordination of Humanitarian Affairs (OCHA)—considered this a completely unfounded rumor. Even more disturbing, the same organizations were advising strongly against any investigation of the disease's origin. Many other care groups in Haiti were arguing that cholera prevention and care didn't require knowing how the epidemic got started. Poor-quality water and sanitation could be the source. Or perhaps it was simply fated in a country used to bad luck and just happened to come in the midst of nationwide efforts to recover from the devastating earthquake.

Piarroux had a different view. Impoverished countries with poor access to clean water are not generally subject to such explosive cholera outbreaks. More than eight thousand hospitalized cholera cases and five hundred deaths in the first three weeks of an outbreak—that was unique to Haiti. The closest parallel he knew of was something he had experienced himself during 1994 in Goma. The million or so refugees from neighboring Rwanda scooped up buckets of water from nearby Lake Kivu and neighboring ponds for household use. Then cholera appeared in the camps and in lake and pond waters, adding to the misery. Soon hundreds of corpses were piled up each day on the roadside. Foreign Legionnaires loaded them into trucks as if they were collecting garbage. Piarroux had never witnessed such devastation from a disease, and he remains haunted by the experience.

In some respects, conditions in Port-au-Prince immediately following the January earthquake seemed similar to what Piarroux had seen in Goma. But in Goma, cholera appeared within days of the humanitarian crisis. Cholera did not come to Haiti until nine months after the earthquake crisis. By the time the outbreak began in October, most refugee camps were already well managed. Furthermore, the earthquake had caused almost no damage in the regions most affected by cholera. Why, Piarroux wondered, would so different an epidemic be just as explosive and deadly as in Goma?

These thoughts brought Piarroux back to the question of cholera's origin. No one had yet attempted to explain the particularly violent nature of the October outbreak or how it began. On the contrary, there was an active effort to suppress any search for the origin. It would be too elusive, various experts suggested. Investigating the possible source near Mirebalais was not a priority. Dr. Claire-Lise Chaignat, coordinator of the WHO Global Task Force on Cholera Control, had been widely quoted in Haiti about the source: "I don't know if we are going to get an answer."[15] Still other international experts argued that uncovering the outbreak's source could endanger Haiti's security and stability, particularly if that knowledge were exploited for political purposes.

Security and stability were the watchwords when the international community spoke of Haiti; they showed up in nearly every statement by every diplomat from every other country who spoke of the island nation. Just a few months earlier, China's permanent representative to the United Nations, Li Baodong, had made a statement that could have come from any one of dozens of international political figures. "We are in favor," he said, "of strengthening the capacity of MINUSTAH so that it can better perform its current mandate." As MINUSTAH is a peace-keeping mission, "its core function is to safeguard security and stability of Haiti."[16]

Yes, security and stability. In late October, when the rumor had compelled hundreds of protesters to march on the military base near Mirebalais demanding that Nepal's UN soldiers leave Haiti,[17] there had been real concern over violence, which threatened security and stability. Sure, those protesters hadn't rioted, but what about the next group?

CDC officials were voicing similar thoughts about not searching for the source. First, the CDC spokesman David Daigle issued an explicit statement: "CDC is not directly investigating the [UN] base [near Mirebalais]."[18] The next day, Joe Palca of National Public Radio asked Dr. Eric Mintz—a CDC epidemiologist and cholera expert assigned to Haiti—about UN soldiers bringing cholera from Nepal.[19] He said he had heard the rumor, but "we have no evidence at all to support it."

Mintz was quick to share other origin hypotheses. "It is certainly possible that cholera could have been introduced by a traveler from anywhere in the world, who may have had illness or may have been an asymptomatically infected person, someone with cholera but who had no symptoms, no diarrheal illness," Mintz told Palca. "It's also possible that it could have come here through the environment"—meaning "through water in the Caribbean Sea or perhaps through standing river water that may have had a small reservoir of *vibrios*." In other words, Mintz concluded, the small reservoir might have, "for environmental reasons we don't understand . . . bloomed, someone became ill, and started the cycle of increasing water contamination." Piarroux was highly skeptical about the science behind Mintz's explanation.

President Préval had also voiced a strong opinion about searching for the source. Visiting Mirebalais two days after cholera was officially reported, accompanied by Minister of Health Alex Larsen and several other officials, he told a radio interviewer that the epidemic was imported but that he did not want its origin investigated.[20] It would be "irresponsible and dangerous" to identify a country as the source of the epidemic, he said—choosing words that surprised DELR epidemiologists and likely others.

Piarroux did not learn about Préval's radio interview until much later. The group at DELR feared that knowing the president's view might discourage him from carrying out his investigation.

By Thursday's end, things were looking up for getting into the field. Dr. Magloire had returned, along with the data capture operator Fanor and the medical epidemiologist Patrick Dely—who had been busy reconstructing the first weeks of the epidemic. They had phoned each département epidemiologist to get daily commune-specific information on cholera cases and deaths. The work was laborious, but considerable progress had been made.

While pleased with the effort, Piarroux knew his mission would require much more data. He needed to know the epidemic's entire history. Then he wanted to visit the affected sites, investigate, and reconstruct the epidemic puzzle. That's the job of an epidemiologist. Where local health officials were blindly fighting the disease, he wanted to offer insight and light.

Friday morning brought a car and driver, courtesy of the French embassy, to take Piarroux into the field. He especially wanted to meet the département epidemiologists who collected and transmitted each day's commune-specific data. First, though, he needed to review data gathered the day before by Fanor and Dely. Only a few départements had responded, and even then, some information was incomplete. No data had been transmitted recently from Ouest département, which includes Port-au-Prince. Sensing problems so close to where he was, Piarroux decided that was a good place to start.

4

STEALTH

Haiti is not a large country, only about the size of Maryland. So much can be seen in just a few days.

Piarroux had made his introductions in the capital and completed his initial meetings. It was Friday, November 12. Cholera in Haiti was in its fourth week.

Over breakfast, *petit déjeuner*, Piarroux pored over data gathered by Fanor and Dely from DELR. It was as incomplete as his meal. Piarroux had settled for some soft bread and margarine, hardly French. He had already endured pancakes and an omelet other mornings and longed for a taste of home.

Ouest département's data were missing—why so? For answers he decided to visit the département medical director and epidemiologist in their Port-au-Prince office.

The département's main office is across town from the hotel where Piarroux was staying. He went there with Fanor and Dely to discuss his concerns about the lack of current cholera information. In what data he did have, Piarroux had noticed a particularly alarming situation in Arcahaie and Cabaret, two of the département's coastal *arrondissements*—the administrative level between a département and a commune—in the north near Saint-Marc and the plains of the Artibonite River valley. Both arrondissements were affected very early, likely on October 22. Piarroux theorized that early-infected persons might have come across the hills from communities near the river. The data suggested cholera had first appeared in Arcahaie's coastal communities and then spread south to Cabaret, after which the disease continued to increase in both arrondissements as the epidemic expanded south.

Piarroux was told that Port-au-Prince's northern suburbs had recently been affected. The département medical director pointed to Cité Soleil, on the metropolitan area's Bay of Port-au-Prince, as an emerging cholera hot spot. Piarroux and his colleagues decided to head there.

Cité Soleil had begun as a shantytown but had grown to be a commune of several hundred thousand persons. Until 2007, competing gangs ruled the area, until MINUSTAH finally established governmental control after a request from the Haitian government. That required the use of force and cost some lives. Yet even with order nominally restored, Cité Soleil was still considered one of Haiti's most dangerous slums, with a terrible reputation. Piarroux felt quite uncomfortable even during a short walk around to get a sense of the place.

The group began with a visit to the MSF-supported Hôpital Sainte-Catherine, Saint Catherine's Hospital. For the people of Cité Soleil, the hospital's rehydration center was especially important. By the time Piarroux arrived, the cumulative number of cases treated at the hospital had already surpassed six hundred. Patients were everywhere, some perfused and others not. Many were receiving intravenous fluids. The hubbub was like a beehive.

High patient volume meant staff had no time to fill out cholera report forms for the Health Ministry, rendering official statistics incomplete. Even local data were questionable. Most of the six hundred-plus cases were not considered cholera; those were limited to cases requiring transfer to cholera treatment centers in Port-au-Prince. Since Saint Catherine's was closed at night, treatment was confined to daytime hours, which helped fuel the underestimation of the number of cases in Cité Soleil.

Next, Piarroux and his colleagues reviewed the commune's water system, the main transmission vehicle for cholera. Cité Soleil had a reservoir and, near the entrance to its most impoverished areas, water towers. Water was fed to individual distributors through a network of pipes; some distributors also bought water from companies using tanker trucks. Typically, water was sold by the bucket, which distributors filled in holding areas. So much handling of water created multiple opportunities to spread cholera. And like water in many areas of Port-au-Prince, water in Cité Soleil was treated by reverse osmosis—a water purification technology that uses a semipermeable membrane to remove impurities—rather than chlorination, which has been the standard for purifying water for human consumption in most of the developed world since the early 1900s. Without chlorine in the water, Piarroux wondered, what would kill any contaminant organisms that got into the supply during storage or distribution?

The group continued on to Camp Sartre, a group shelter in Cité Soleil that houses victims of the earthquake and was still largely unaffected by cholera. How could this be possible, Piarroux asked, since the disease was so frequent in the surrounding neighborhoods? Again, the answer was water. DINEPA provided water to the camp that was chlorinated on a regular basis, killing the cholera organism. The camp distribution system used multiple hand faucets for this water, each serving one hundred or more families. Latrines were provided and maintained by World Vision, a United States-based NGO, and were cleaned regularly by the local Red Cross or residents themselves. Local water and waste sanitation services seemed effective.

As the visit to Cité Soleil came to an end, Piarroux reflected on what he had learned so far. He had met many of the key players in the ongoing cholera drama. Officials were receptive and certainly welcomed the presence of a committed epidemiologist. The trip into Ouest département, Haiti's most populous, had provided a better sense of that area's situation. But it was apparent that the problem in Haiti involved more than figuring out how best to track the epidemic's origin and course. His many meetings had given Piarroux the feeling that few if any had a clear picture of the epidemic, nationally or locally. Everyone recognized they were dealing with a major health crisis, but where were insights on transmission risk factors? Absent the full picture, public health officials were having trouble understanding the intricacies of the epidemic, which was necessary for prioritizing local control actions.

In Piarroux's experience, the more acute a crisis, the more people who show up to advise. That often added to the confusion. Haitian public health officials were not familiar with cholera. No one in Haiti had ever had any reason to expect such a violent outbreak. Cholera cases and deaths had exploded in the country in mid-October, stretching national and international care providers to their limits almost immediately. They struggled to keep up. Perhaps it was the mounting cases, treatment priority, and limited resources that explained the pushback over searching for the disease's origin.

Toward the end of October, though, the occurrence of cholera had mysteriously decreased. The reprieve was short-lived—cases rose again in the early days of November. What could explain this variation?

Some experts were attributing the November upturn to Hurricane Tomas. Had the storm stirred up dormant cholera in the tidal estuaries? Again, Piarroux was skeptical. After all, the early-November outbreaks had hit mountainous areas as well as flood zones. Cholera was found in both rural and urban areas and not just in communities near coastal or tidal waters.

It was apparent to Piarroux that the tools in place to monitor the epidemic were largely inoperative. He wondered about the few maps he had seen, with data aggregated and displayed at the too-large département level and in overly long weekly periods. What conclusion could anyone draw from such maps other than that the situation was serious? In three weeks, the outbreak had already hit about half the country and had clearly become a major epidemic. Haitian health authorities needed more detailed maps to understand what was happening, and Piarroux was determined to provide them.

It was Saturday, November 13, and Piarroux was finally ready to explore the situation in central and northern Haiti, beginning in Centre département. He knew a trip to Mirebalais, Centre's largest town, was pivotal. If the rumors were true, the first cholera cases might well have come from a small village a few miles south of Mirebalais. The coming weekend trip would mean plenty of mud and dust but also might tell the story of the epidemic's origin.

Before leaving, Piarroux sent a short note to the French embassy about an epidemic "growing faster than expected and becoming exceptionally large" because of what he characterized as an unusual beginning. He urgently requested a meeting with President Préval and other top officials immediately upon his return from the countryside. He needed to explain what was occurring. "The main weapon to fight back cholera," he wrote, "will be chlorine."

The driver arrived early that Saturday morning. Piarroux was to travel with two Haitians, the statistician Fanor and the epidemiologist Robert Barrais.

Piarroux and Barrais had much in common. They were both physicians, about the same age, and married, with three children. Barrais had been a science teacher but in midlife had turned to medicine. As he got to know Barrais, Piarroux grew to appreciate in particular his easygoing and insightful manner, which served him so well when interviewing people about disease-related events and as he tried to uncover patterns in epidemiological puzzles.

The trip's purpose was to investigate how cholera might have originated and to assess how the disease had spread so quickly into the country's north. They headed first for the village of Mèyé in the Centre département, just south of Mirebalais. Dr. Magloire had determined from data that this was where cholera had first been reported.

Piarroux wondered whether Mèyé would live up to its name. The Creole word *mèyé* translates to *meilleur* in French, or "best" in English. This, to Piarroux, implied a good place to visit. By either name, the village—a few kilometers south of Mirebalais, across the highway from the UN camp housing Nepalese peacekeeping troops—was small enough to be ignored on most maps.

Mirebalais itself is a nearly sixty-kilometer drive northeast of Port-au-Prince on a major highway. The road passes first through a small plain, plaine du Cul-de-Sac, and then goes up into the Chaîne des Matheux mountains. After the earthquake, refugee camps were built on the lower slopes of the mountains, and in the distance Piarroux could see the blue plastic sheets of temporary shelters supplied by various humanitarian organizations. The vegetation surrounding the camps was sparse, with no trees or shrubs to stem damage from erosion. There were no villages or towns nearby, and the land seemed unsuitable for crops. Piarroux couldn't help but question the decision to put the camps in such a hostile environment. How did people find work or get provisions?

Barrais explained that the lakes in the plaine du Cul-de-Sac visible from the road were brackish lakes with alkaline water. Not many people lived near them, but Piarroux knew that if cholera appeared, it would be troublesome for the local populace. *Vibrio cholera* is known to be fond of alkaline water.

They continued their journey, bouncing over the bumpy highway, working out the next steps of their investigation, and sometimes discussing politics. Barrais was concerned with issues of social inequity and the everyday problems Haitians face. He spoke of his country's growing gang problem. Piarroux engaged but never without keeping his eyes fixed on the road, worried about the driving while trying to notice the surrounding landscape.

After passing through mountain valleys with farming communities, they left Ouest dépertement behind, entered Centre dépertement, and soon passed a small MINUSTAH camp near the village of Terre Rouge. The front gate sign announced that the camp housed a platoon of Nepalese peacekeeping troops—typically, one officer and about twenty-five to forty soldiers. It was clearly much smaller than the major MINUSTAH camp farther along the road near Mirebalais.

As they left the camp, the road crossed over a pass and then descended to a lower plateau that extended toward Mirebalais. On the left, a few kilometers before Mirebalais, they passed the guarded entrance of the much larger UN camp: Annapurna Camp, named for the peaks of the Himalaya Mountains in north-central Nepal, famous for their stark beauty and dangerous, often deadly, climbs. Inside the camp, established in early 2005, was a UN-sponsored battalion from Nepal, serving in Haiti as members of MINUSTAH. Battalions are typically three hundred to one thousand troops, with either a lieutenant colonel or a colonel in charge.

MINUSTAH had been a dominating presence in Haiti since its arrival in 2004. Some praised the troops for maintaining law and order; many others saw them as an affront to national pride, an outside force with no business in a free republic. Loud voices throughout Haiti called for expelling the "occupiers."

Cholera rumors involving MINUSTAH, on top of ongoing tensions, added more unwelcome flavor to the political broth. UN troops were well aware that Annapurna Camp had been blamed for the epidemic. These troops might be suspicious of strangers, surmised Piarroux, especially those from foreign countries. So he decided stealth was the best course. Be discreet. Stay out of sight. He hadn't

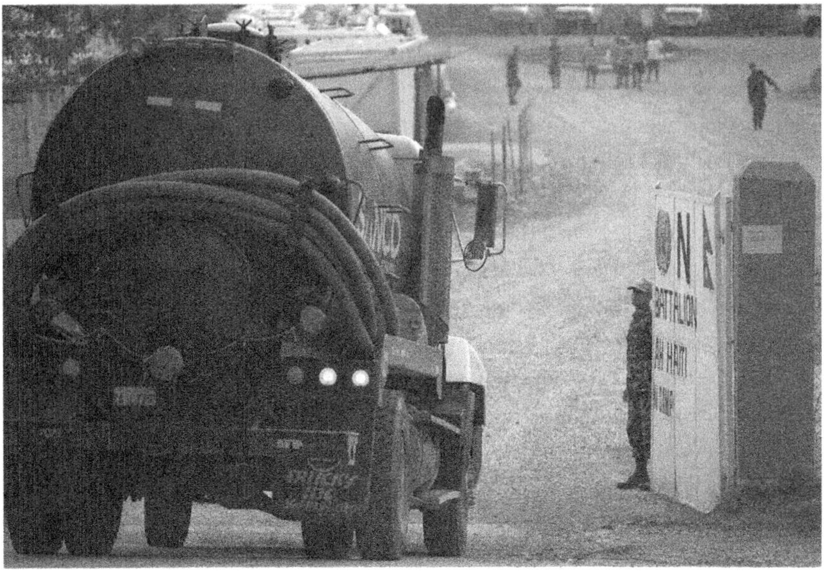

FIGURE 4.1. Sanitation truck entering Nepalese MINUSTAH camp at Mèyé, Haiti. AP Images, Ramon Espinosa, Associated Press, October 27, 2010.

asked permission to investigate the camp, doubting it would have been granted. Barrais had told him that even doctors from Haiti's Health Ministry had been denied entry.

Directly across from the MINUSTAH camp, they passed Mèyé and its few dozen houses. Piarroux and his team crossed a bridge over the creek that went by the hamlet. Part of the Mèyé tributary system that continues four kilometers north to the Artibonite River, the creek flowed strongly. The rainy season had just ended.

A short ways north of Annapurna Camp, they pulled to the side of the road. Piarroux remained in the car, inconspicuous, while Barrais and Fanor doubled back toward the camp on foot. For twenty minutes they explored the scene, spoke with a few local residents, and took photographs. When they returned, they said villagers had told them the first cases of profuse watery diarrhea had begun in mid-October. Several patients were admitted to the hospital in Mirebalais, and on October 17 one of them—a twenty-year-old man—had died.

They also learned that villagers had no access to safe drinking water but instead filled buckets from the stream across the highway that flowed past the MINUSTAH base. Around the time when the epidemic began, they had observed pipes coming from the base that dumped foul-smelling liquid directly into the

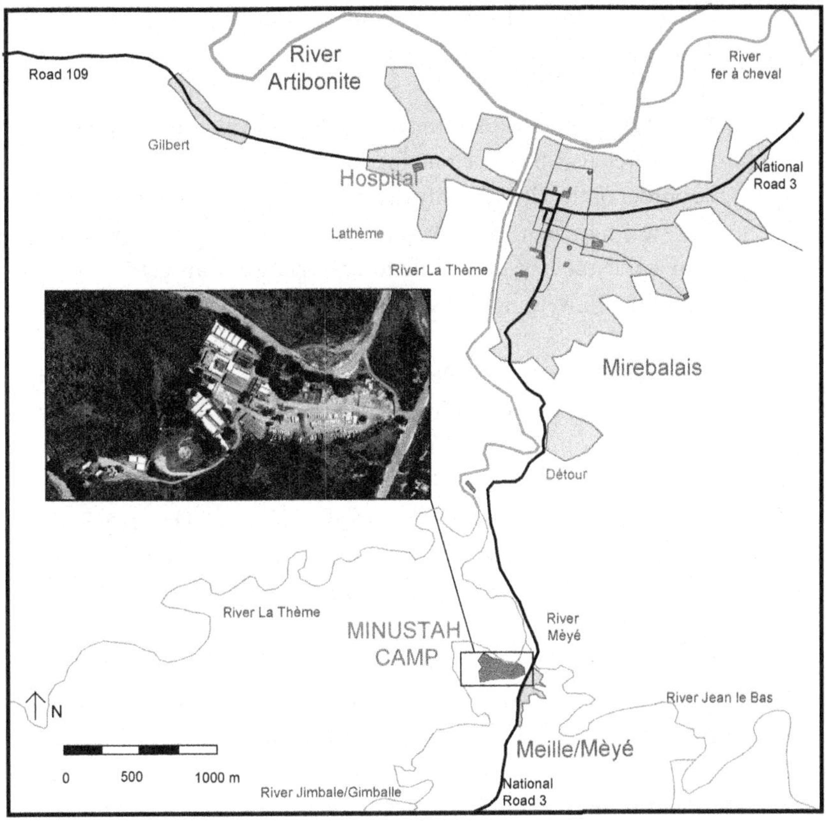

FIGURE 4.2. Meille/Mèyé, MINUSTAH camp, and Mirebalais in Centre département. Created by Martine Piarroux.

stream. Neither Barrais nor Fanor saw these pipes; the villagers said they'd been removed by the troops shortly after the cholera cases appeared.

These people had a lot to say, Barrais told Piarroux, but seemed fearful their answers might lead to reprisals from the MINUSTAH soldiers. Whether or not these fears were justified, Barrais insisted they were very real.

Barrais also shared another tidbit of information. Villagers said that the three researchers were not the first to come around asking about cholera. In the early days of the outbreak, government officials had shown up in the village to do a field investigation. They knew no details, and later, back in Port-au-Prince, Barrais could find no report.

With new and important epidemiological clues in hand, Piarroux and his colleagues moved on to Mirebalais. Any more digging around in Mèyé might stir up too much local excitement and attention, potentially jeopardizing further investigation. It had been a very productive first stop.

The river from Mèyé merges with a stream from the surrounding hills and then passes through Mirebalais before emptying into the Artibonite River, a natural barrier at the border of the city of eighty thousand inhabitants several kilometers to the north. It was here that Piarroux and his team would uncover their next field clues. The epidemic had done little to keep people from gathering in the shallow waters of the converging rivers, with women doing laundry and children playing.

The city's water system was under repair. Open trenches made driving a challenge. Piarroux, Barrais, and Fanor headed to *l'hôpital communautaire*, the community hospital in the northwest section of Mirebalais, about eight hundred meters from where the Artibonite River and the river from Mèyé merge. In the hospital parking lot, they were surprised to meet Dr. Jean-François Schemann, a physician from the French embassy, and Professor Henrys from Préval's presidential advisory group. The two men had come on their own to assess the situation.

They all went in to meet the medical staff: a Haitian team and some members of the Brigada Médica Cubana, which would soon grow to 1,200 and, by year's end, treat more than thirty thousand cholera patients in forty centers across Haiti.[1] The BMCers showed them the cholera treatment center behind the hospital, opened a few days earlier after it became impossible to treat the growing influx of patients in one of the hospital's regular wings.

Piarroux had visited numerous cholera treatment centers in other countries and could tell that the BMC doctors were doing a very good job under difficult circumstances. Triage sorted patients according to clinical condition. In a large tent that could accommodate dozens of patients, those most dehydrated were treated immediately with intravenous infusions. The worst cases were typically given antibiotics and zinc supplementation. In another tent, those with milder symptoms were given oral rehydration solutions; they were reported as "suspected cholera cases, seen externally" and not hospitalized. If their health improved after a few hours, they were sent home with oral rehydration salts. If they got worse, they would join patients in the larger tent.

Piarroux was anxious to hear from the BMC physicians about the early cholera cases while memories were still fresh. Beginning in mid-October, they had noted and recorded an abnormal number of patients with watery diarrhea, the intensity of which—coupled with the extent of dehydration—put the idea of cholera in their minds. Yes, they knew cholera had never been recorded in

Haiti, but they couldn't deny what they saw with their own eyes. As the abnormal diarrhea cases increased, they consulted their medical textbooks but soon realized they needed more information on cholera diagnosis, medical management, and care.

Their superiors went to DELR in Port-au-Prince on Monday morning, October 18, to report this unusual outbreak of severe watery diarrhea to public health officials. That afternoon, government officials quickly assembled a Haitian medical team to travel to Mirebalais, where they learned that the first patients had come from Mèyé, after which cholera cases began to show up in districts south and west of Mirebalais—all places bordering the river tributary system that flows north from Mèyé toward the Mirebalais convergence with the Artibonite River. Once cholera reached Mirebalais, it spread quickly through neighborhoods. The BMC doctors treated nearly fifty cases on Sunday, October 17; by the next day, the number had swelled to more than three hundred. In the days following, cases were identified in other communes of Centre département, particularly one to the east and another to the north of Mirebalais.

In those first days the BMC physicians had kept good computer records of their work—cholera cases, inpatients, and deaths. Between October 16 and 31, they identified more than four thousand suspected cholera cases. Nearly half those patients were hospitalized. Of those, only ten died, but that death count was incomplete. Numerous cholera deaths occurred at home and were never included in official statistics.

As he toured the facility, it was obvious to Piarroux why the Brigada Médica Cubana doctors had gotten such good results confronting a disease they had never before seen. Their quick provision of care proffered a huge benefit to patients from Mirebalais and the surrounding area. He was also impressed by how the doctors had reached out immediately to collaborate with Haitian officials.

Later, it was confirmed that the suspicious outbreak had begun days earlier.[2] While the time at which patients are admitted to a care facility is important to clinicians, disease detectives look for the "onset time"—when people first become infected. "The first hospitalized case with severe watery diarrhea and dehydration was admitted to the [Mirebalais community] hospital on 16 October," wrote BMCers. "Clinical manifestations began 12 to 24 hours before clinical admission of these patients to the hospital."[3]

It turns out, though, that the first confirmed cholera case in Haiti was never admitted to the hospital. He was identified at home by Haitian epidemiologists on October 19 during their initial field investigation. His diarrhea had started on October 14—making him the earliest cholera case with a positive stool culture. This information didn't come to Piarroux until the very end of his stay in Haiti.

From Mirebalais, Piarroux's group drove along the south bank of the Artibonite River, eyeing the changing terrain. The river lies in a narrow valley between two mountain ranges, the Montagnes Noires to the northeast and the Chaîne des Matheux to the southwest, meandering for about fifty kilometers through a sparsely populated agricultural area before coming to the larger fertile region of the Artibonite valley. Along the way, they passed by Saut d'Eau, a commune south of the river in the hills overlooking Mirebalais. On the north side of the river was the foothills commune of Boucan Carré. Both had few residents living near the river and both had been spared from cholera, at least in the epidemic's early weeks.

For the first twenty-four kilometers, the road passed only a few scattered houses and small hamlets. Then they entered Artibonite département and arrived at La Chapelle, the main town of another commune situated some distance from the river. La Chappelle, too, had remained mostly free of early cholera. All three communes got their water from numerous small streams that descended from mountains and not from the river.

After another twenty-four kilometers, they reached Verrettes, where the landscape begins to change. The valley widens on both sides of the river, and the mountains give way to an alluvial plain irrigated by a network of canals fed by the Artibonite. This alteration of terrain coincided with a troubling change in the epidemiological pattern of cholera. Verrettes and the municipalities bordering the coastal plain were still experiencing the epidemic as Piarroux arrived.

Cholera had erupted abruptly in Verrettes. There had also been a sudden influx of patients with gastrointestinal disease at Albert Schweitzer Hospital in the nearby town of Deschapelles. Ian Rawson had blogged on October 20 that thirty patients with similar gastrointestinal symptoms had been admitted late Tuesday and through Wednesday, many having drank from the Artibonite River. Piarroux's impression was that the cholera epidemic here had begun on October 19–20. But why had it occurred in Verrettes and Deschapelles a mere day after the dramatic increase of about three hundred treated patients in Mirebalais? The question intrigued Piarroux. Verrettes and Deschapelles are about fifty to fifty-five kilometers downriver from Mirebalais. Human movement by road couldn't explain such a sudden, dramatic spread of the epidemic. Could the river itself provide the answer?

Piarroux and his colleagues decided to take a closer look at the Artibonite where it flowed along Verrettes' eastern edge. They headed to the river a few kilometers upstream of the *barrage de Canneau*, the Canneau Dam, which diverts water into two major irrigation canals branching into ditches that feed the thirsty rice fields before reentering the river farther along. The south channel takes about four times the water of the north channel.

To reach Verrettes from Mirebalais, cholera microbes would have to flow fifty-plus kilometers along the river's tortuous path in about a day. The group had

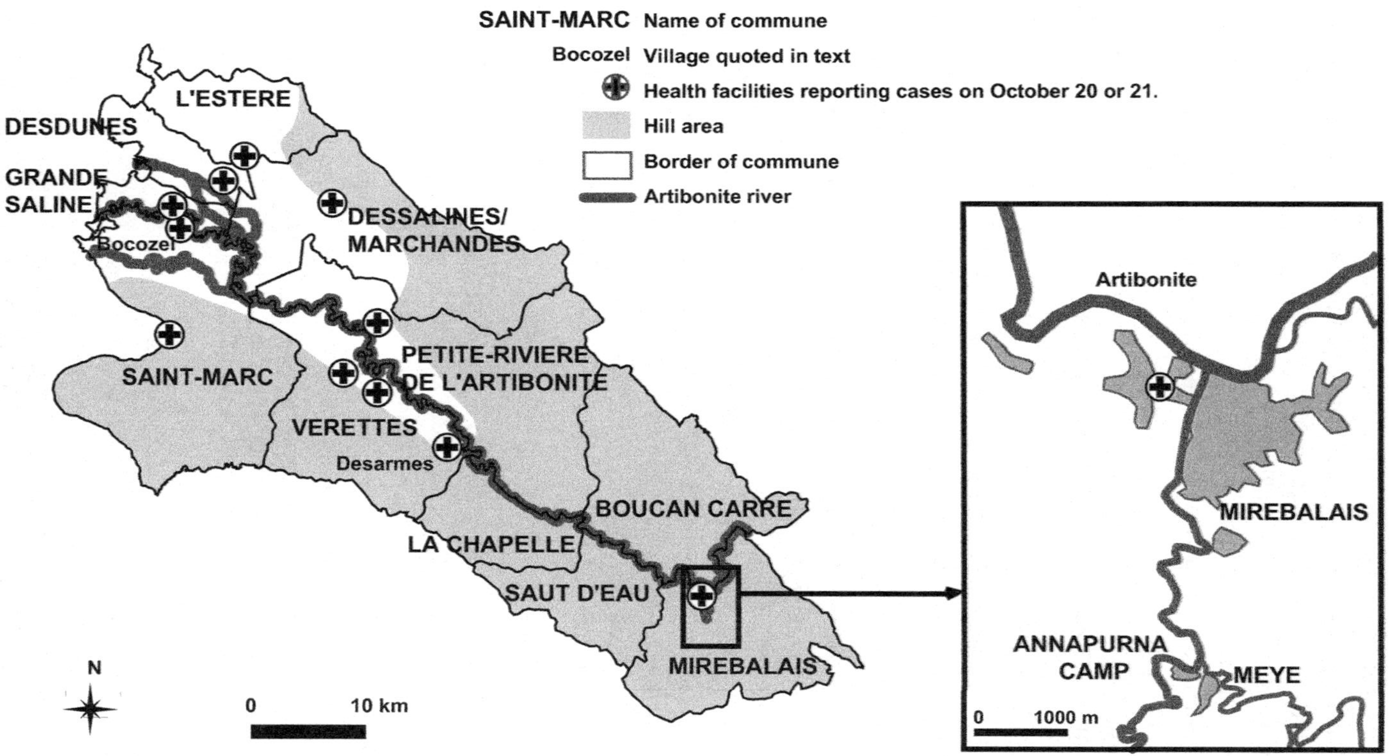

FIGURE 4.3. Health facilities reporting cholera cases on October 20 or 21 in communes near the Artibonite River. Based on Piarroux et al., "Understanding the Cholera Epidemic," 1163.

brought no scientific instruments, so Piarroux snapped into action to measure the river's flow using a time-honored method: he threw a tree branch into the middle of the river and estimated the midriver current with the second hand of his watch. It was about eight to ten kilometers per hour.

Piarroux considered the impact of river flow on the speed of travel of cholera and river volume on the concentration of cholera. If the river was indeed the gateway to the epidemic in the coastal plain, its high volume suggested a massive number of cholera organisms would have to be introduced to cause such an explosion of cases. How many bacteria were necessary to reach, even if only for a few hours, a sufficient concentration in the river and downstream channels to infect thousands and kill hundreds? Piarroux made a mental note to check later for answers in the medical literature.

There were more questions. Why had the cholera outbreak occurred in downriver Verrettes but not upriver La Chapelle? The two communities, separated by twenty-four kilometers, both lie within two kilometers of the Artibonite River. They share similar cropping systems: beans from January to March and maize or sweet potatoes from April to May. Verrettes also has rice from June to December.[4] The low-cholera commune of La Chapelle in the narrow part of the valley had fields and households fed not by the river but by streams from the Chaîne des Matheux. The high-cholera commune of Verrettes in the widening valley had some fields irrigated by mountain water but more by Artibonite River water, the same source from which most people in town drew their water. These differences told Piarroux that the Artibonite River held the important clues.

Piarroux and his group left Verrettes and headed west, then drove southwest at the next major junction to the coastal city of Saint-Marc. The trip from Mirebalais through Verrettes to Saint-Marc was about seventy kilometers.

Saint-Marc lies in a coastal enclave, surrounded by the Chaîne des Matheux. The commune, the Artibonite valley's most populated region with nearly a quarter-million inhabitants, includes a rural section in the delta area of the river. The city, while not itself in the Artibonite watershed, is close enough for patients to come easily for medical care the villages couldn't handle—such as treatment for severe cholera.

Piarroux had two objectives in Saint-Marc: check when the outbreak began in the city and identify the probable source of the first cases. DELR data showed that nearly two thousand suspected cholera cases had been recorded in Saint-Marc in just three days, October 20–22, and *l'hôpital de Saint Nicolas*, Saint Nicolas Hospital, had the dubious distinction of having the first laboratory-confirmed cholera cases in Haiti. Many experts thought Saint-Marc was the starting place of the epidemic. Piarroux questioned this thinking—cholera cases had occurred in Mirebalais in mid-October—but he still wanted to take a closer look.

What could have brought cholera to Saint-Marc? Most obvious, Saint-Marc is a major port, receiving ships from around the world. Could passengers, crew members, or even bilge water in a ship's bottom hull have brought the disease? Probably not, since cholera would first have appeared by the city's docks and then spread to the surrounding countryside.

Another hypothesis was environmental. Perhaps cholera had existed for a long time in the indigenous environment, settling in the brackish waters of the estuary region where the Artibonite River meets the Caribbean Sea. But even then, thought Piarroux, Haiti's first cholera cases would have come from the rural regions of Saint-Marc commune, close to the river's estuaries—not from near Annapurna Camp in Centre département.

Then there was the timing. Neither hypothesis could explain how, if the epidemic had begun in Saint-Marc on October 20–22, cases could have been reported several days earlier in the distant hamlet of Mèyé or in Mirebalais. And either explanation required *Vibrio cholerae* to have been brought about seventy kilometers upriver to Mirebalais from the Saint-Marc commune. This seemed to defy logic.

Saint Nicolas Hospital in Saint-Marc was already famous for cholera. A few weeks earlier, BBC News had broadcast, "At one point on Thursday [October 21], hundreds of people were laid out in the [hospital's] car park . . . with intravenous drips in their arms to treat dehydration, until it began to rain and they were rushed inside."[5]

By the time Piarroux and his colleagues arrived, each day was bringing nearly two hundred new cholera cases to the hospital, which had carved out space among its buildings to treat patients. Many were under observation, receiving oral rehydration solutions, while others were being infused with intravenous liquids. The epidemic was in full swing, just as in Mirebalais and Cité Soleil. Médecins Sans Frontières was assisting the Haitian staff.

Screening case records, Piarroux's group noted two waves of the epidemic in Saint-Marc. The first was particularly explosive, with more than 400 suspected cases reported on October 20 and nearly a thousand the following day. The hospital director confirmed that nothing unusual had happened before October 19, not even a hint of cholera: no abnormal increase in diarrhea cases and no unexplained deaths. After only two days, the number of cases declined just as suddenly as the first cholera patients had appeared: from the peak on October 21, the number reached a low of 120 on October 28. Then there was a second wave:

a gradual increase in the number of cases to about 200 each day. Notably, in the sudden rise and nearly as sudden decline, most patients were from rural areas in the Artibonite delta. In the second wave of gradual increase, more patients were coming from the city of Saint-Marc.

Space and time are vital clues for disease detectives. Epidemiologists know that infectious disease outbreaks often tell their story when new cases are observed in geographic *space* and occurrence *time*. In the Saint-Marc region, the space for the early cholera cases was the rural areas near the Artibonite River and not the urban area by the port. To Piarroux and Barrais, this space observation supported the hypothesis that cholera had come from the river and its canal offshoots. The time dimension pointed to the same water sources.

A plot of the case onset times for the first wave of the cholera outbreak looked like a child's playground slide, sloping up sharply like the ladder and then down at a wider angle. Two concepts, a common source of infection and the incubation period, provided the likely explanation. Cases arising explosively near the Artibonite River during the first wave suggested a common-source outbreak, caused perhaps by a cholera-contaminated sewage plume streaming down the river.[6] As the plume flowed by, cholera microbes would infect those who drank the water. After an incubation period—for cholera, this is typically a day or two, but it may range from a few hours to six days—the number of new cases would rise quickly to a peak in the first day or two and then gradually decline during subsequent days. Having the first wave of cases arise from a common source, undergo an incubation period, and then fall explained the up-and-down appearance of the wave.

The first wave of cases became the source for the second wave. Patients contaminated by river water in the early days probably went home, or elsewhere, and infected others through their feces or vomitus; home and elsewhere likely included Saint-Marc and the surrounding urban area. This broadened the geographic distribution of cases away from the river—an important characteristic of the second wave.

In Saint-Marc, Piarroux noticed a shop with a sign in the window advertising ice cream "guaranteed" to be cholera-free. It was a sad reminder of the horror of epidemics. He was by now experiencing the emotional pain that comes with seeing human misery. Haitians stricken by the cholera epidemic faced awful conditions. Patients received care, but seeing people assembled by the hundreds, bed against bed, with vomiting, diarrhea, and no space to preserve personal dignity reminded Piarroux of Jean Giono's novel *Le Hussard sur le Toit—The Horseman on the Roof.*[7] Giono was one of the twentieth century's most celebrated novelists from the French province of Provence; Piarroux's Marseille is Provence's capital.

In the novel, set in 1832, an idealistic young Piedmontese freedom fighter and cavalry officer named Angelo Pardo makes his way from exile in Provence to join his best friend in Manosque—but a cholera epidemic breaks out and transforms everything. The young traveling horseman comes upon town after town in ruins.

At every juncture, as had Pardo, Piarroux and his team came upon new horrors. Saturday was passing quickly, and they still needed to travel forty kilometers up the coast to Gonaïves. What would be the next horror?

When they arrived late Saturday afternoon in Gonaïves, capital of Artibonite département, Piarroux and his colleagues learned from the département's epidemiology team that the first alert had come on October 19, late afternoon, from the village of Bocozel, near the Artibonite River: three schoolchildren with severe acute diarrhea, dehydration, and vomiting had died near their classrooms. Two of them were the schoolboys mentioned in chapter 1. That same day, the coordinator of the clinic at L'Estere, another Artibonite delta town, reported cases of particularly severe diarrhea and vomiting. Patients were taken to the hospital in nearby Dessalines; people in town with the same symptoms had died.

By the next day, there were simultaneous alerts at two major hospitals in Saint-Marc as well as at health centers in Grande Saline, Desdunes, and Petite Rivière de l'Artibonite, the hospital and a health center in Verrettes, and the Albert Schweitzer Hospital in Deschapelles.

Initially, Gonaïves—the city on the coast just north of the region shown in figure 4.3—had been largely spared, with only one suspected case admitted to a local clinic on October 20. That patient, though, came from a village near Dessalines. Piarroux was not surprised. After all, Gonaïves got its water from various northern rivers, not from the Artibonite.

Valuable clues about space and time were compounding. The département epidemiologists had described an explosive epidemic that caused near-simultaneous cholera in a wide swath of the Artibonite valley either in the afternoon of October 19 or the morning of October 20. By the noon government reporting time on October 20, département staff had tallied more than one thousand suspected cases. Half had been hospitalized; about sixty had died. Another two thousand-plus cases were reported the next day; 60 percent were hospitalized. The daily number of deaths, however, remained close to seventy. By the third day, the epidemic seemed to have peaked, and then it began to decline. By October's end, daily totals had fallen to a more constant lower level of cases, hospitalizations, and deaths. This space-time pattern for the communities of Artibonite département was similar to the three phases of the outbreak in Saint-Marc.

Over eight days, Artibonite département had seen at least twelve thousand cholera cases. Their geographic distribution again pointed to the Artibonite

River as the source. The communities most affected were on the banks of the river, downstream from Mirebalais. Only three communes along the upper Artibonite River, all of which drew their water from mountain streams, had been spared.

The source of cholera was becoming clearer, but a mystery remained. How had cholera organisms overcome the diluting effects of Haiti's largest river? How were those organisms able, so quickly, to cause deadly outbreaks in so many communities? Piarroux and Barrais reasoned that cholera had probably come from the Mirebalais region where the first cases occurred. They theorized that a large number of *Vibrio cholerae* must have made their way into the river at about the same time and then flowed during the next day or two to valley communities. How could such a large number of organisms have entered the river either all at once or in rapid succession? There were only two explanations that made sense. One was that a very large number of cholera patients had simultaneously defecated into the river—a likelihood that defied logic. The other was a major sewage spill or persistent discharge.

The team didn't yet have all the evidence, but Piarroux was quite certain that Mirebalais, the village of Mèyé, and the MINUSTAH camp all had more tales to tell.

5

HYPOTHESES

With only about twenty American dollars between them, Piarroux and Barrais checked into a small, shabby, and overcrowded hotel in Gonaïves. They met for a dinner of rice and some dressing with only traces of meat and vegetables. Each enjoyed the luxury of a glass of beer.

The epidemic was their dinner conversation. The two epidemiologists now understood, if only tentatively, how the first wave of cholera had affected Mirebalais and the lower Artibonite valley. But Piarroux wanted to learn more about the spread of the disease throughout the northern part of Haiti. So the plan was to rise early the next morning, Sunday, November 14, and continue toward the country's northern coast and the city of Cap-Haïtien.

The highway north from Gonaïves, which followed a valley, was difficult. In places, it had collapsed because of an earlier flood. The road climbed upward into the Massif Du Nord mountains, through eucalyptus, mango, and some pine trees, past steep gardens and banana trees. It crossed a first pass before descending abruptly into a valley. Here and there, the travelers could see shacks clinging to the mountainside, poking through the dense vegetation and accessible only by small paths along the green slopes.

Piarroux had traveled to many places in the world. Haiti, he thought, really is beautiful—despite all the disasters.

The first stop on Sunday was Plaisance, on the main road linking the Artibonite plain and Haiti's northern coast. It was Fanor's hometown, and so they paid a visit to his family. The discussion turned quickly to cholera, and Piarroux learned the disease had arrived only two days after the explosive epidemic in the Artibonite coastal plain. Many of the cases were local people working in the plain who were in the prime of their lives. Some died within hours; others were fortunate enough to recover at the local hospital.

Workers were terrified, and many had fled from the devastation in the Artibonite plain. Of course, thought Piarroux, who wouldn't be tremendously fearful given the circumstances? Confronted with sudden calamity—what at first was unknown and unnamed but came to be known widely as *kolera*—no one wanted to continue working in the Artibonite rice fields or salt marshes. Workers couldn't help but think that their families in Plaisance and other communities, safe havens in the mountains away from the local scourge, must be safer. And so they rushed home by bus and by truck and then on foot to even the smallest hamlets.

Of course, the deadly disease—invisible to the eye—soon caught up to them. How could these sick individuals know that cholera was in their fecal debris, just waiting to contaminate their families' food and water? How could they know that the organisms were gradually defiling the physical environment around them? What did they know of cholera? Their country had never before been befouled by the scourge of this disease.

Meanwhile, shared food and water propelled the organisms from one household to another. New cases appeared. Sometimes a village well would be contaminated, resulting in dozens of new victims.

The epidemiologists left Plaisance, climbing a new pass before journeying along the Limbe River and following the valley to the northern coast. Cholera in the Limbe valley first appeared upstream on October 22, followed in time by occasional downstream cases. Despite the fact that the Limbe passes by well-populated villages, there was no explosive outbreak downstream, as had occurred with the Artibonite. Piarroux and Barrais sensed another mystery.

After flowing by the town of Limbe, the river twists and turns for fifteen kilometers, passing Bas Limbe shortly before reaching the Atlantic Ocean. Despite the short distance, Bas Limbe remained untouched by the cholera outbreak until November 3, or nearly two weeks later. Again, the detectives gathered time and space evidence, which presented a picture much different than the one-day span between the outbreak in Mirebalais and the explosive and simultaneous outbreaks in downriver communities of the Artibonite valley. Later Piarroux would learn that the Bas Limbe outbreak persisted for some time and did not peak until early December, a situation that was also quite different from the explosive form of outbreak elsewhere.

What accounted for these different disease patterns? As the Limbe River flowed by the upriver town that bore its name, the local populace, including anyone who might have cholera, used its water for washing clothes. Also, on rainy days, runoff from surrounding homes flowed directly into the river. Residents of downriver Bas Limbe, then, should have been exposed to cholera bacteria carried by the river, just as had happened in the Artibonite valley. But this did not provoke an outbreak, at least not for nearly two weeks.

For Piarroux, the likely explanation was that cholera concentration was never as high in the Limbe River as it had been in the Artibonite. Since the Artibonite water volume is much greater than that of the Limbe River, the Artibonite must have contained a very high volume of vibrios that overcame water dilution, perhaps arising from the major sewage spill Piarroux already suspected. In the Limbe valley, where cholera had entered the river, the concentration was too low for major transmission. Piarroux hypothesized that the probable source of cholera cases in Bas Limbe was infected people moving along the valley roads at a pace considerably slower than the rapid flow of the cholera-diluting river.

The trip from Bas Limbe to Cap-Haïtien took Piarroux and his colleagues along the coastline, around a bay, and past rice fields and irrigated crops. Cap-Haïtien is Haiti's second-largest city after Port-au-Prince and is the capital of Nord département. By the time they reached the city, they had traveled some hundred kilometers from Gonaïves.

They headed immediately to the government office, where the regional epidemiologist and département medical director awaited. They learned that cholera had arrived in Nord département on October 22, starting in Plaisance and then on October 24 reaching the mountain community of Pilate, where victims had worked on road construction in the Artibonite plain and fled home in fright as the epidemic spread. One such sick worker was treated by his family but quickly died. Within three days, his entire family was stricken. From their house, the epidemic spread through the community. A similar scenario had taken place in Limbe and in Limonade, south of Cap-Haïtien.

Cholera spread to Cap-Haïtien on October 26. Water problems helped explain why. City water service from Cap-Haïtien's leading provider was often irregular, and so people resorted to storing water—which, if contaminated by *Vibrio cholerae*, would transmit the disease to every member of the household. There were also neighborhoods where residents used wells, some of which were nothing more than holes dug near rivers or streams. Still other residents got their water from traveling tankers. The regional epidemiologist had learned that some unscrupulous water sellers in Cap-Haïtien had pumped water into the tankers directly from unprotected sources and then pretended they were delivering treated water.

There were other water problems too. The regional epidemiologist explained the local practice for handling the deceased. Before burial, family members would routinely wash cholera-ridden corpses and—of course—would end up contaminating their hands, damp clothing, and household water. Piarroux had seen this phenomenon wreak havoc elsewhere. The traveling microbes would cause more cholera deaths.

Funeral ceremonies are a common problem in cholera epidemics. Often, when cholera arrives in a new area, the disease is detected after a burial, when many people are contaminated at once. In Comoros during the 1998 cholera epidemic, Piarroux and his team soon realized that funeral ceremonies were causing secondary cases of the disease. The Comorian tradition was to wash the dead and empty their intestines by applying pressure on the abdomen. After the burial ceremony a meal was shared, typically involving dozens of guests. If people who had handled the body and then not washed their hands happened to prepare that meal, their actions could lead to food contamination and cholera among the guests.

In Comoros, this problem was so prevalent that the team had to turn to community and religious leaders for help. Ultimately, persons trained and equipped so they wouldn't contaminate themselves were assigned responsibility for washing the dead.

Experiences like these taught Piarroux to observe local customs and intervene accordingly.

The next stop would be Fougerolles but only after a quick bite to eat at a local fast-food restaurant. Piarroux was struck by the public service announcements blaring from the restaurant's radio that encouraged hand washing to fight cholera. Everyone in the restaurant was wearing gloves.

The regional epidemiologist had suggested visiting Fougerolles, a neighborhood in the heart of Cap-Haïtien near the ocean shore not serviced with city water. The team spoke with two of the three hundred or so dealers people relied on to distribute drinking water from large tank trucks.

Piarroux saw water stored in concrete basins that supposedly had been chlorinated to kill various microbes, including cholera. Dealers would sometimes dip buckets into these basins, fill them, and hand them directly to their customers. For customers who lived too far from the basins, the dealers would also distribute water from the tanker hose directly into customer buckets at several locations. It was nearly impossible to avoid contamination of the water by dirty hands. And though the dealers insisted their basins were chlorinated, none could offer verification.

Several Fougerolles community leaders wanted to show Piarroux and his colleagues a so-called colonial well along the main road, the old style that provided access to groundwater about two meters below the surface. The well was poorly protected from street water runoff, if at all. And yet it was the sole source of free water for the neighborhood's poorest inhabitants. One resident told Piarroux the water tasted brackish and she used it only for washing, bathing, and cleaning dishes. But dishes "washed" with contaminated water are still a ready source of cholera.

Water wasn't the only serious problem. Sanitation was even worse in Fougerolles than in the equally impoverished Cité Soleil district in Port-au-Prince. Most neighborhood dwellings lacked latrines. Residents were encouraged to use one of the many communal latrines on stilts by the ocean, from which feces fell directly into the sea or banks during low tide. It was impossible to walk through the area without soiling feet or shoes and spreading fecal waste.

Finally, there was the matter of fish. Though they were cooked before eating, there's more to avoiding contamination than killing microbes with heat. Fishermen could transmit cholera from their hands. Vendors, too, handled all the damp fish they sold. Contaminated fish touched kitchen counters, where the cooked fish was returned to be soiled again.

Cholera had already appeared in Fougerolles. There were colorful posters everywhere explaining what to do when a person had diarrhea and was vomiting and how to keep from getting the disease. Leaflets explaining transmission and how to identify cholera had been distributed throughout the neighborhood. But cholera awareness had paled in comparison with what safe drinking water or decent toilets would have meant. Fougerolles residents soon believed that without water and sanitation very little could be done to quell cholera's spread.

People raised their voices in anger at the Haitian government, but their anger against MINUSTAH was even greater. Two months earlier, in September 2010, Haitians had clogged the streets of Cap-Haïtien to protest the death of a sixteen-year-old boy, Gérard Jean-Gilles, who had been found hanging from a tree in a local base housing MINUSTAH peacekeeping troops from Nepal. UN officials classified the death a suicide, stating that the boy had hanged himself—a finding friends and relatives disputed. They pointed out that he was regularly welcomed on the base, providing services for the soldiers in exchange for money or food. They surmised that he might have stolen some money and, caught by the troops, might have been tortured and suffocated to death.

It took a full seventy-two hours before MINUSTAH officials released the young man's body for autopsy. While the findings were inconclusive, suicide by hanging was ruled out since no cervical vertebrae were damaged. There was no further investigation by MINUSTAH[1]—which only fueled the protests. So when the rumor reached the city that UN peacekeepers might be responsible for the cholera outbreak, demonstrators again took to the streets.

Fortunately, Piarroux and his team of epidemiologists were not trapped by the November 15 riots that occurred in Cap-Haïtien, having returned to

Port-au-Prince as soon as their field investigation finished, arriving late that night. The long journey back to the capital gave them an opportunity to summarize their findings and elaborate on their hypotheses.

Nothing satisfies an infectious disease epidemiologist more than finding the source of an outbreak, learning exactly how the disease began. In Haiti, solving the source mystery provided Piarroux and Barrais a unique opportunity to consider and understand the devastating impact of nature or of neglected prevention policies. Once the source was tentatively understood, though, their work was far from over. They continued to investigate for details and confirmation. They assessed factors that had likely permitted and encouraged cholera to move from one community to another until the entire country had been affected. Such detective work takes time, hard work, and insight in the field and laboratory. All is prelude to testing and confirming hypotheses, providing sufficient evidence to convince fellow scientists and others. As lawyers know, facts and figures alone do not sway judges and juries. You need to present your information well and win your audience's trust.

Like police detectives and prosecutors, who often begin their work from multiple theories of the case, epidemiologists typically have several hypotheses in mind, based on knowledge of the agent and recent reported cases or deaths. As noted earlier, in Haiti, most hypotheses put forward for how *Vibrio cholerae* had arrived in the country were in one of two categories: environmental or human activity—long points of contention among the world's leading cholera investigators.

The environmental hypothesis assumes the *Vibrio cholerae* organism lies dormant in coastal waters for many years until some event disturbs the local environment, leading to an outbreak.[2] That event might be a storm. It might be an earthquake, like the one that struck Haiti in mid-January 2010, nine months before the cholera outbreak first appeared.

Nonscientists had reason to associate cholera with the earthquake—or at least with its aftermath. A month after the quake, the *New York Times* wrote, "Public health officials warn that waste accumulation is creating conditions for major disease outbreaks, including cholera, which could further stress the ravaged health system."[3] Several weeks later, Bill Clinton, now serving as UN special envoy to Haiti, voiced similar concerns. He told a reporter that the feces of children forced to defecate outdoors "may be contaminating every piece of standing water, and that could lead to diarrhea, dysentery, cholera and tetanus, and we could have a huge second wave of casualties."[4] People reading such things wouldn't have been surprised when nine months later cholera actually did arrive in quake-stricken Haiti.

Beyond the musings of reporters and politicians, though, the environmental hypothesis is a scientific one—according to which the cholera organism must have been residing in or near Haitian waters, waiting to be awakened by the earthquake. Recognizing that the microbe can live in water, some scientists focused on the role of the many environmental strains of *Vibrio cholerae* that are different from the two types that cause epidemic cholera.[5] Supporters of the environmental hypothesis reasoned that after the earthquake these nonpathogenic cholera bacteria, normal in Gulf of Mexico waters, traveled by ocean currents to Haiti. There the microbes altered their form to a disease-causing strain, were consumed in food or water, and became the epidemic's source.

Others thought cholera organisms had long been present in Haiti's estuarine zones,[6] at the coastal border between the Caribbean Sea and the Artibonite River. Such zones occur where the freshwater Artibonite flows into the saltwater Caribbean, moving through an estuary in which shrimp-like copepods and other shellfish reside. Earlier studies in South Asia showed that *Vibrio cholerae* can live on the surface of copepods in a manner that may benefit both,[7] often for years.[8]

Adding fuel to the environmental hypothesis was the early report of cholera cases in the port city of Saint-Marc, on an ocean bay just south of an estuarine zone. People living in or near the city could have become infected when consuming copepods with *Vibrio cholerae* attached. In faraway Bangladesh, a country that suffers from endemic cholera, removing copepods by filtering the drinking water in villages reduced cases significantly, suggesting a causal relationship.[9]

Piarroux wasn't buying the argument. He accepted that *Vibrio cholerae* might have existed in the aquatic environment long before the epidemic occurred but not that it was the toxigenic form that causes disease in humans. If that were so, wouldn't Haiti's first cholera cases have come from Saint-Marc commune's rural regions, close to the estuary region of the Artibonite River, and not from near MINUSTAH's Annapurna Camp? No, Piarroux believed he was going to have to slay a different dragon.

Still, the experts on the environmental hypothesis side of the scientific divide seemed sure that the answer was in the climate-water connection. In late October 2010, Professor David Sack of the Johns Hopkins University School of Public Health told National Public Radio, "Cholera is an environmental bacterium" that "can persist in the environment for many, many years without any human infection."[10]

"The most likely explanation [for the Haiti cholera outbreak] is a rise in temperature and salinity in the river estuaries around the Bay of Saint-Marc in the Artibonite Department of Haiti," Sack insisted, "That area, seventy miles northwest of Port-au-Prince, is the epicenter of the current cholera epidemic."

Three weeks later, Rita Colwell offered further support—and when she spoke, people listened. Hers had long been an extremely influential voice for the environmental theory. A former president of the National Science Foundation,

Colwell—Distinguished Professor at both University of Maryland and Johns Hopkins—in 2010 was named Science Envoy of the United States, a new international leadership program established by the U.S. government.[11]

"They have been fortunate in Haiti that for 50 years the conditions have been such that they haven't had an intense increase in cholera bacterial populations," Colwell declared. "But they've had an earthquake, they've had destruction, they've had a hurricane. So the conditions would lead to a very high probability of an outbreak."

Perhaps taking note of the rumors swirling around MINUSTAH troops, Colwell continued, "I think it's very unfortunate to look for a scapegoat. It is an environmental phenomenon that is involved. The reason we don't know [the catalyst] is because the medical community is not receptive to climactic causation or correlation."[12]

Despite Colwell's credentials, not all epidemiologists are of a similar mind. The human activity hypothesis sits at the other side of the scientific divide. It assumes that cholera is brought by the actions of people. For instance, the cholera microbe could have accompanied persons traveling to Haiti, either in the travelers themselves, in contaminated foods, or even in polluted bilge water in ships. Travelers could be anyone, including people working for one of the thousands of NGOs doing relief work in the aftermath of the earthquake.[13] Their risk of harboring communicable agents depends on where they traveled from, how long they spent there, their vaccination and treatment history, and the conditions of their stay. Such information, though, is rarely available.[14]

Fortunately for Haiti, most NGOs working there are based in Europe or the Americas—regions with no cholera. However, NGO staffs often include people who've done similar work in other parts of the world where sanitation is poor and infectious diseases common.

Might cholera have come to Haiti from some other human activity? For instance, travelers could have brought cholera-infected food, a well-documented potential source of origin.[15] Once in Haiti, the cholera microbe could have survived and multiplied in a variety of moist foods.

Or was it from sailors? Saint-Marc, where most consumer goods from other countries arrive in Haiti, seemed a candidate as the disease's port of entry. Perhaps a ship with infected crew members had docked in Saint-Marc. Diarrhea can be embarrassing, so perhaps the infected sailors went quietly below during their journey and defecated in the bilge area. Over the course of a long trip on the sea, the water that normally accumulated there would mix with infected feces to create a toxic brew. Then, when the ship entered Saint-Marc's harbor, the bilge water might have been dumped into the sea, contaminating the coastal area and the habitats of copepods and shellfish.

Piarroux dismissed this explanation too. He had just come from Saint-Marc, and if its piers were the origin point, wouldn't the first appearance of cholera in Haiti have been in that section of the city? Wouldn't it have spread from there to the countryside, not the other way around?

There remained one looming possibility as part of the human activity hypothesis. Could the rumors swirling around Haiti that MINUSTAH troops were the source of the deadly cholera epidemic be true?

For a century after the French left Haiti in 1803, the country had been free of foreign troops. Then, on July 28, 1915—after a four-year period of great political instability, with one after another political assassination, six changes in the Haitian presidency, and a series of coup d'états—President Woodrow Wilson sent the *USS Washington*, a military vessel with "20 cannons and a complement of nearly 900 men," to establish stability and order. He had concerns that the United States did not have "the legal authority to do what we apparently ought to do" but concluded that it was "necessary to take the bull by the horns and restore order."[16]

United States troops occupied Haiti for nineteen years, until President Franklin Roosevelt transferred power back to the Haitian government in 1934. No cholera was discovered in Haiti during those nearly two decades, and it is very unlikely that American troops were infected with the disease.

The next foreign troops arrived in 2004, but this time they were sponsored by the United Nations. Justification for the UN action centered on turmoil surrounding deposed President Jean-Bertrand Aristide. After years of repression and instability associated with the Duvalier family dictatorship and a succession of military rulers, the Haitian people had elected Aristide, an activist and liberation theologian, as president. He served three times as Haiti's democratically elected leader. His first term lasted a mere seven months before the Haitian Army overthrew his government in September 1991. Under pressure from the UN, among others, the Clinton administration deployed U.S. troops to the country and reinstated Aristide in October 1994; he completed that first term in office in 1996.

Four years later, in 2000, Aristide was again elected president. In February 2004, as before, a coup ended his term. On the last Sunday in February, he and his wife were whisked away from their home, purportedly by U.S. Special Forces soldiers, and flown to exile in the landlocked and sparsely populated nation of Central African Republic.[17] Some argue he fled, while others believe he was kidnapped. Whatever the reason, the presidency of Aristide—who had been freely elected by the people of Haiti—was over.[18]

Also that fateful Sunday, the chief justice of the supreme court was sworn in as interim president and immediately "requested international assistance from the United Nations and authorized troops to enter the country."[19] Shortly thereafter, a new United Nations peacekeeping program was established in Haiti, MINUSTAH.[20] The UN's aim was to reduce the threat Haitian instability posed to regional peace and security, and the program involved thousands of international troops and police—many from less developed countries in Africa and South Asia where cholera was present.

After the mass destruction wrought by the January 2010 earthquake, MINUSTAH's mandate was extended until October 2011.[21] Complicating the situation was a heated political campaign for Haiti's presidency and parliament that lasted from June 2010 to May 2011. At the campaign's beginning, MINUSTAH was authorized to expand its military personnel to a new level of nearly nine thousand and its police to more than four thousand personnel.

Many Haitians to this day (at this writing, the UN presence continues) see MINUSTAH as occupiers. And so, as the cholera epidemic expanded during October 2010 in Centre and Artibonite départements and Haitians began to question the disease's origin but got no satisfactory answers, and as many Haitian government and international officials focused only on stopping the spread while openly discouraging any effort to find the epidemic's origin, it came as little surprise that popular attention turned to MINUSTAH. The rumor mill began to churn throughout Haiti, telling of a MINUSTAH camp in upriver Centre département, near Mirebalais, that was somehow involved with cholera.

When the rumor became widespread, many officials—especially foreign ones—were quick to jump to MINUSTAH's defense. The standard pushback was that the rumor was politically motivated in the midst of the election campaign. Officials rejected any possibility that peacekeepers could be the explanation for how cholera had come to Haiti.

On October 26, the MINUSTAH spokesman Vincenzo Pugliese hastily called together the press in Port-au-Prince to issue a statement. He acknowledged the rumors. Asked to confirm that MINUSTAH employed good sanitation at the incriminated camp in Mèyé and that there was no cholera present in the troops, Pugliese insisted the septic tanks there met "the construction standards of the [U.S.] agency for environmental protection."

"These septic tanks are emptied each week [into a landfill site] by four trucks from a privately contracted company," he explained. "Permission was obtained from the Mayor of Mirebalais to use the landfill site. It is 250 meters from the river by [the village of] Mèyé, which is more than 20 times the distance required at the international level." Pugliese added that a new contingent of MINUSTAH soldiers had arrived at the Mèyé camp on October 15, 2010 and that "no member . . . has symptoms related to cholera or any other disease."[22]

The rumor wasn't going away. It continued to swirl. But MINUSTAH was not through pushing back. On Wednesday, October 27, in a follow-up story in the Haitian newspaper *Le Nouvelliste*, local UN officials expanded the scope of their defense.[23] During Piarroux's field investigation, villagers had told Barrais and Fanor about the pipes they had seen coming from the UN base that dumped foul-smelling liquid directly into the stream from which they drew their drinking water. UN troops had removed those pipes right after cholera appeared. Hinting at the matter of the pipes, the UN insisted MINUSTAH in Mirebalais did not throw human organic material into the river but rather "actually uses seven septic tanks" located near the river.

Le Nouvelliste is widely read in Haiti, including by some foreign journalists in the country. That same Wednesday, Sebastian Walker, the Al Jazeera English reporter assigned to Haiti, traveled to the MINUSTAH camp south of Mirebalais and televised what he found—which contradicted UN statements.[24] Walker had gone to Mèyé to explore whether there was anything to the rumor. He observed Nepalese peacekeepers at the camp "working furiously to contain what looks like a sewage spill" and explained, "The disease is waterborne and untreated waste running into the river is a big danger, and that's exactly what we found."

The report showed UN soldiers digging near a row of toilets by the camp fence. "It certainly smells like sewage and there are toilets right there, and the liquid seems to be draining into this river just a few meters away, which flows into the nearby town of Mirebalais," Walker said. "Local residents had said that they had frequently seen sewage from the base leak into the river, and that families in the area had recently become ill."

A translator spoke to a local woman in Walker's broadcast. "Only people downriver have been infected," she said. "A child close to here died. Another family had three kids get diarrhea, and one died the same day."

Then Walker introduced Nigel Fisher, MINUSTAH's temporary deputy special representative, who said, "There has been a rumor that the Nepalese in Mirebalais are a source of cholera. We have taken samples from the river and they have been confirmed by the National Laboratory to be negative."

Walker challenged Fisher's statement. "But downriver from the Nepalese base there are certainly cases of cholera. Fifty cases have been confirmed in the local prison and the river runs on into Artibonite [*département*], the worst affected region."

Then there was what seemed like a smoking gun. "The Nepalese contingent wouldn't tell us when they arrived here, but UN headquarters confirmed it was mid-October, just weeks after a cholera outbreak in Kathmandu [the capital city of Nepal]." The news came from a September 23, 2010, article in the *Himalayan Times* describing a local cholera outbreak in Kathmandu shortly before the Nepalese troops left the city for Haiti.[25] At that time, however, neither the World

Health Organization nor any other reliable medical source reported cholera being present in Nepal. Some dismissed the article as unsubstantiated.

Walker's video report went worldwide to people who were mostly learning for the first time that UN peacekeeping troops from Nepal might be involved in the cholera epidemic in Haiti, or that there might have been a cholera outbreak in Kathmandu.

Jonathan M. Katz was the sole full-time Associated Press (AP) reporter assigned to Haiti. He had been working on the cholera story and, like Walker, wanted to get a firsthand look at the situation in Mèyé after reading what Pugliese had said. He saw the same conditions as Walker and by late evening filed a major story on potential UN troop involvement with the cholera epidemic. It appeared that evening on the Internet and in English-language newspapers throughout the world the next morning.[26] It was his article that Piarroux had read in the French language *La Presse* before arriving in Haiti.

Katz saw something quite different from what MINUSTAH had been claiming: a buried septic tank overflowing with black liquid inside the base's fence, and broken pipes jutting out from the liquid. One pipe was just behind the camp's latrines, and the leaking liquid was making its way down to where people were bathing in the river. "[T]he stench of excrement wafted in the air," he reported.

Across the highway from the UN camp, Katz found the "safe" landfill site: open pits situated uphill from local homes, next to a steep slope heading directly to the river, with pools of runoff that attracted ducks and pigs. He could see clearly where water from the pits had flowed downhill during recent heavy rains. Local residents told the reporter that the septic tank on the base side of the fence, as well as the uphill pits, overflowed again and again into the river "where they bathe, drink and wash clothes."

Before filing his story, Katz interviewed Pugliese and asked about the waste samples being collected. Pugliese confirmed that a military team was testing specifically for cholera. It was, as Katz wrote, "the first public acknowledgment that the 12,000-member force is directly investigating allegations its base played a role in the outbreak." Investigators, Pugliese said, were testing only kitchen and shower liquids, and he denied that what Katz had seen spewing from the septic tank was human waste.

Asked about the jutting pipes, Pugliese said they had been exposed for the tests. He couldn't explain why the liquid coming from them was allowed to flow to the river. He insisted that samples from the base showed no sign of cholera. Additional tests, ordered by the MINUSTAH military force commander, aimed to confirm those earlier negative findings.

Finally, he told Katz that the new Nepalese contingent included not a single member with cholera. "The unit's commander declined to comment," Katz added.

A dramatic image ran with Katz's article in many news outlets. The caption read, "A tanker truck deposits excrements from the Nepali UN base in an area 400 meters away from the base in Mirebalais, Haiti, Wednesday, Oct. 27, 2010."[27]

Katz had observed a tanker truck arrive at the base to drain the septic tank. And he watched the flows behind the base come to a halt as the septic tank was emptied. He saw the same truck dumping into the pits across the highway.

The reporter contacted Marguerite Jean-Louis, chief executive officer of the waste management company Sanco Enterprises S.A. to ask about what he had seen. Like the unit commander, Katz wrote, "She declined to comment, citing her contract with the UN."[28]

The Walker and Katz stories created an uproar around the world. Over the next weeks, pundits and professionals in the United States, France, and elsewhere weighed in with opinions and scientific observations. This all fueled the ongoing scientific "debate" between the environmental and human activity theorists.

Haitians, of course, reacted immediately. Sanco demanded *Le Nouvelliste* print its official response to Katz's article. That happened on Thursday, October 28. Sanco officials "rejected out of hand the charges against their company that employees poured excrement into the river by Mèyé near Mirebalais," the article stated.[29] The company insisted that after first obtaining permission from the Mirebalais mayor it dug a septic pit "some 250 meters from the river" in which the waste from the truck was to be deposited, rather than trucking the liquid waste to a major dump site just outside faraway Port-au-Prince.

The AP photo was especially irritating to the Sanco spokeswoman, who had been in Mèyé with the CEO when it was taken. She reminded readers, "It's not in the river that the truck empties its cargo, but in an open septic pit."[30]

Months later, Piarroux wrote to Katz and asked about the AP photo. Katz confirmed that the Sanco official was correct—the liquid waste was being emptied into the septic pit. But Katz noted that villagers had told him that the shovel-dug septic and nearby landfill pits "overflow and run down into the river" when it rains.[31]

Meanwhile—as the Sanco officials were proclaiming their innocence—Haitians in the vicinity of Annapurna Camp were taking to the streets in protest. That Saturday's Al Jazeera News reported that the previous day demonstrators had been "waving tree branches and anti-UN banners," and chanting "like it or not, they must go" as they walked from Mirebalais to the UN camp at Mèyé.[32] The report also stated, "The troops [from Nepal] arrived in shifts starting on October 9, after the outbreak in their home country and shortly before the disease broke out in Haiti." That was six days earlier than the UN spokesman had told the *Le Nouvelliste* reporter.[33]

Dr. Claire-Lise Chaignat, head of the World Health Organization's cholera task force, told Al Jazeera that any speculation about the source of the outbreak was "premature," but then she offered her own—that "UN troops from Nepal having brought the disease to Haiti seems very unlikely." Her stated rationale? The amount of time it takes for troops to be transported from Nepal is "long enough" for the disease to have already "declared itself" during the trip, she said, and "troops and armies normally live in good sanitary conditions and are not exposed to conditions which are conducive to getting cholera."

Chaignat's counter to the swirling rumor also appeared in news outlets around the world. A major WHO official and cholera expert had declared MINUSTAH innocent. But Haitians remained unconvinced. They demanded a thorough investigation of the source of cholera in their country.

For a few weeks, all international officials, with no exceptions, adopted the same position, exonerating MINUSTAH soldiers.

6

MAPS

Maps are closely intertwined with epidemiology. They allow disease detectives to view illness or death patterns in space and time, showing gradual—or sometimes explosive—spread through a community, country, or even the world. If the mapmaker intends to focus on disease cases without taking into account the underlying population, spot maps are typically used. They show where each case resided or worked—suggesting a possible relation to a suspected source.

In 1854's Broad Street Pump outbreak in the Soho area of London, the epidemiologist John Snow used a spot map to focus on the neighborhood pump as the likely source of the cholera outbreak.[1] Snow's map—perhaps the world's most famous cholera map—did not offer *proof*, but it visually supported other written evidence that the pump was the most probable source.

Every July or August, the World Health Organization publishes a report on cholera from the prior year, along with a world map that most often shows case-fatality—the percentage of cholera cases that subsequently die from the disease—by country, or occasionally the number of cholera deaths by country. The map for 2009, the last year reported prior to the Haiti outbreak, shows countries with at least one cholera case, whether cholera cases were designated as imported, and—using shading—the percentage case-fatality.

Cholera in the Americas that year was imported to Canada and the United States. There were also five cases of confirmed cholera in landlocked Paraguay, mysteriously arising in an isolated Indian settlement in the western Chaco region. While the source was not determined, the outbreak was believed to be waterborne.[2]

Cholera was also evident in much of sub-Saharan Africa and regions of Asia, including Nepal. The countries with the highest case-fatalities were all in Africa, the region that also reported the highest number of cholera cases.

When the underlying population is known, maps are created that use colors, patterns, or shading to show varying levels of disease rates. Here the epidemiologist must first know the population of a geographic area—most often gathered from a recent census. The population is combined with the number of illness cases or deaths—usually obtained from health departments—to derive rates per time period when cases occurred. The colors, patterns, or shades are then assigned to the geographic areas of the map to tell stories of associations or possible causes.

Maps were used in a similar manner in Haiti. On the day after cholera was officially reported in the country, the map in figure 6.1—the first of many disease maps—was published in an Emergency Operations Center (EOC) report by the Haitian Ministry of Public Health and Population, in collaboration with PAHO.[3]

The map showed cholera in two départements, Artibonite and Centre. It focused attention on the Artibonite River, which made perfect sense given cholera's water-loving nature. The report emphasized that reported cases were "mainly coming from communities along the Artibonite river basin that runs through the mentioned departments."

Was the northwest-flowing Artibonite River the source of early transmission, or did cholera spread along roads with travelers or food and water products moving from one region to another? If cholera began in the coastal communities of Drouin and Saint Marc, how did the agent get to the interior town of Verrettes or even farther to the city of Mirebalais in Centre département? The map offered no answers but certainly posed interesting questions.

PAHO posted other disease maps regularly on its website; they showed cholera at the département level. These maps were a useful online tool for Piarroux, and when he first arrived in Haiti he took a series of screen-captures of the PAHO website.[4] Soon, though, he found a major flaw: the maps showed information for large areas—each of Haiti's ten départements—but not for smaller ones. What about the 140 communes in the ten départements? At the département level, the maps failed to draw any attention to local hot spots—information vital to community public health workers. Maps at the commune level, Piarroux knew, could be used to guide local control measures such as water purification with chlorine or targeted public education and awareness campaigns.

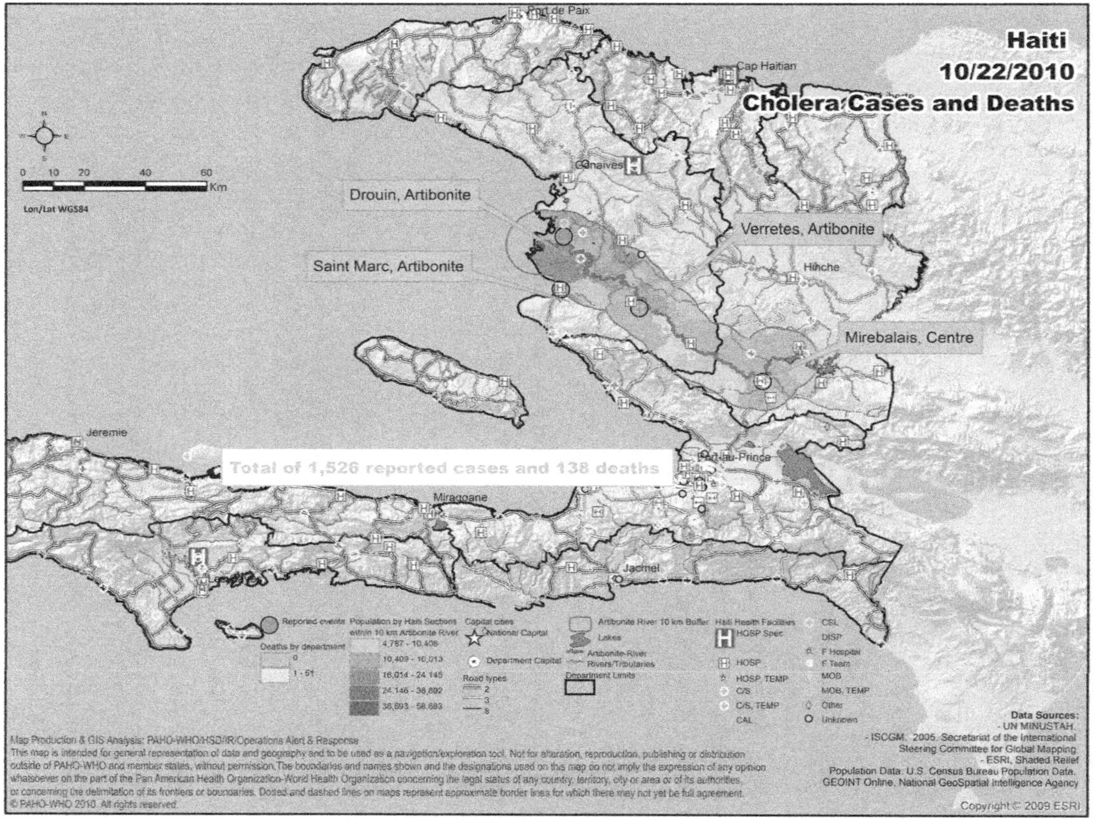

FIGURE 6.1. First EOC map of cholera epidemic in Haiti. Image from PAHO, "Cholera Outbreak in Haiti," *EOC Situation Report* no. 1, October 22, 2010.

Those who had made the PAHO website maps seemed unaware of local needs. Fortunately, though, more detailed maps soon became available. Shortly after the first EOC cholera map was published, the UN's Office for Coordination of Humanitarian Affairs (OCHA) began to issue a series of colored maps, sometimes in English and other times in French. They showed cholera by commune. For instance, the map in figure 6.2—one of the early OCHA maps—presents cumulative cholera deaths and hospitalized cholera cases from October 20 through 24.[5]

In the upper Artibonite River region, cholera appeared in two communes next to the river near Mirebalais, coded in light gray for places affected in Centre département. Moving downriver to the northwest there was a gap, with no cholera in the next two communes. Continuing toward the coast, cholera was evident in many communes by the river, coded in dark gray for outbreak areas in Artibonite département, as it flowed toward the ocean. By focusing on the communes in the two départements, the OCHA map provided a much more useful level of detail than the first EOC map.

Two days later, OCHA published another map, this time showing cumulative deaths and hospitalizations for October 20 through 26.[6] The map, this time in French, had a slight but notable change in its legend for cholera in the communes in Artibonite département near the river: what had been called an "outbreak" in English now was called an "epidemic" in French. Then on October 27 the two reporters, Walker and Katz, broke their stories about Nepalese peacekeepers.[7]

Another day passed before OCHA issued its next map (figure 6.3) the evening of October 28, again in French.[8] By then, the epidemic had continued to expand. The map presented the cumulative deaths and hospitalizations in Centre, Artibonite, and Nord-Ouest départements from October 20 through 27. The map looked similar to the earlier maps, but there was a major change to the legend, telling of the source: now the communes by the river in Artibonite département, in dark gray shading, were identified as the "zone where cholera began."

Light gray shading for communes affected by cholera—but not "where cholera began"—was used for the two communes in Centre département, near the MINUSTAH camp visited by the two reporters. The same light gray shade was also used for communes away from the river in Artibonite département and many in the Nord-Ouest département.

The OCHA maps continued to falsify where cholera began until November 10, 2010, when the last in the series was issued showing cumulative data from October 20 through November 8.[9] Each time, the OCHA map showed a dark gray

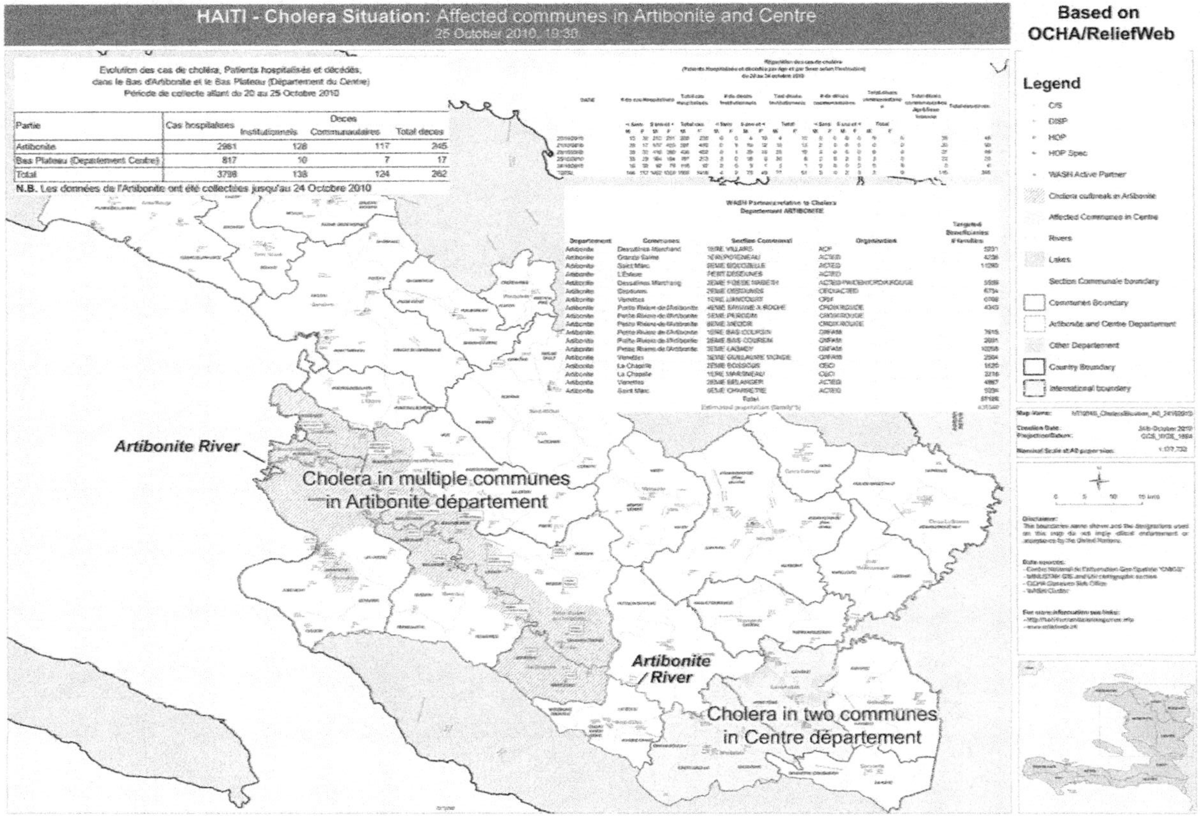

FIGURE 6.2. Early OCHA map of cholera epidemic in Artibonite and Centre départements. For clarity, the author has added the text and gray shading in the body of the map to the original colored maps. From OCHA, "Haiti—Cholera Situation," October 25, 2010.

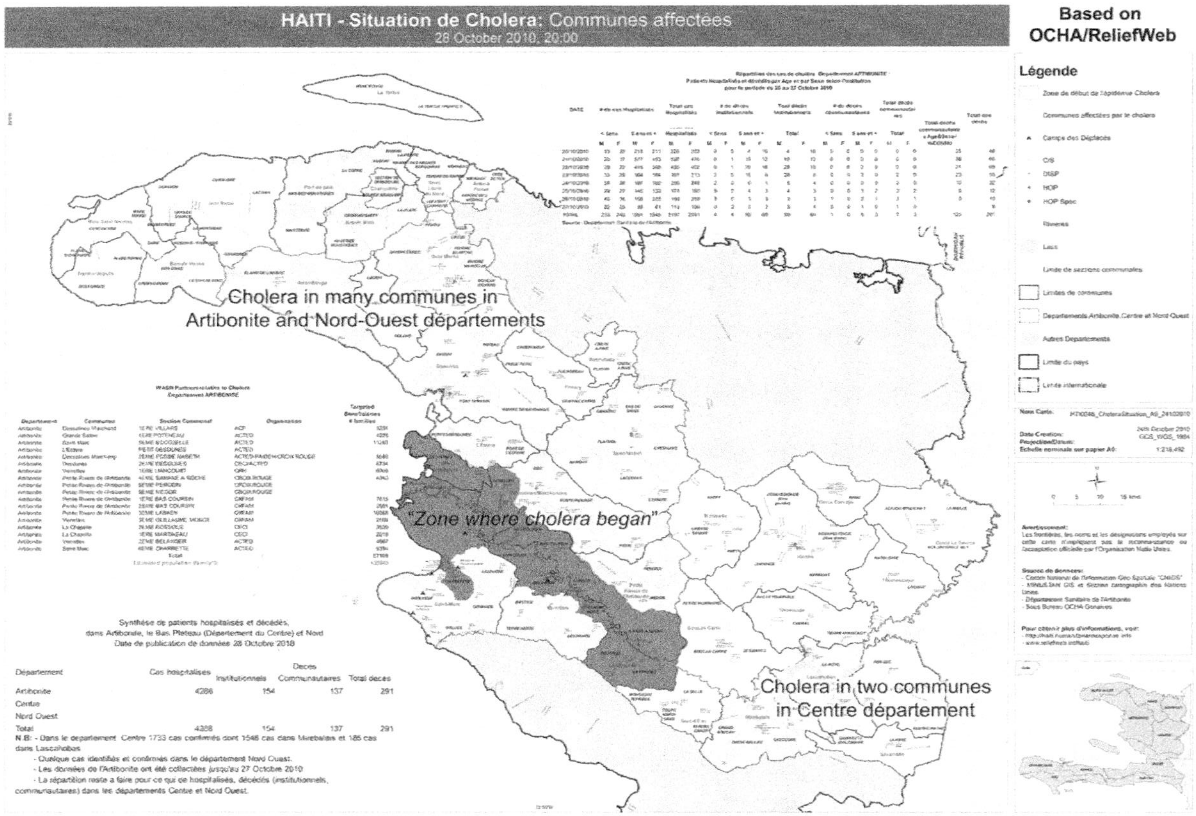

FIGURE 6.3. Later OCHA map of cholera epidemic in Artibonite, Centre, and Nord-Ouest départements. For clarity, the author has added the text and gray shading in the body of the map to the original colored maps. From OCHA, "Haiti—Situation de Cholera," October 28, 2010.

area in the lower Artibonite valley surrounding the Artibonite River as the region where the epidemic had its origin. Yet upriver in the Mirebalais commune, the map legends stated the area was merely "cholera affected."

With this erroneous legend, the maps of the UN agency skillfully shifted attention away from the human transmission hypothesis and the Nepalese peacekeepers as the source and toward the environmental hypothesis involving the coastal estuaries of the Artibonite River delta. Had reporters' dispatches influenced the OCHA mapmakers to change the legend? To Piarroux, it certainly seemed possible. It was not only epidemiological falsehood but also cartographic deception.

7

ALTERED REALITY

The head of the World Health Organization's cholera task force, Dr. Claire-Lise Chaignat, told reporters it was "premature" to be speculating about the source of Haiti's cholera outbreak but that the idea it had been Nepalese troops seemed "very unlikely." The UN's Office for Coordination of Humanitarian Affairs had issued a series of maps seemingly designed to focus attention away from the troops as the source—or any humans, for that matter—and toward an environmental origin.

A team from the U.S. Centers for Disease Control, however, had been working in the field since the outbreak's early days. Its first investigatory report was issued on October 28 on the Web. It came a day after Walker's Al Jazeera news video and on the same day as Katz's AP article.[1] Eight days later, CDC formally published the report in the *Morbidity and Mortality Weekly Report*, distributed for free to a worldwide clinical and public health audience.[2] It included early news of Haitian cholera cases and deaths: "A total of 4,722 cholera cases with onset during October 21–27 and 303 deaths had been reported in Haiti. Most cases have been reported from Artibonite Department, a rural but densely settled area with several small urban centers."

A PAHO report and map were CDC's source for the numbers.[3] The CDC authors reported correctly that most cases were in Artibonite dépertement (shown in the map as 3,612 cases and 273 deaths), but they made a notable omission in the map story that would give any reader a false impression of how the growing epidemic had unfolded.

The CDC report described clinical characteristics of the cholera outbreak and on the issue of origin stated, "The outbreak appears to have spread from an initial concentration of cases in Artibonite Department." There was no mention of cholera in upriver Centre département—despite the fact that the very PAHO map cited indicated that 1,079 cholera cases and 28 cholera deaths had occurred there. And the authors wrote not one word about the news accounts that revealed cases of earlier cholera in Nepal and subsequent sanitation problems at the Nepalese peacekeepers' camp, also in Centre département. *MMWR* articles often include editorial comments that add insight and perspective. But the *MMWR* editors were silent on these important omissions.

It seemed unlikely the omission of cholera in Centre département was accidental. Were CDC officials laying the groundwork for a different epidemiological finding that favored the environmental origin hypothesis? Was it a calculated political move to avoid human blame? Or both?

Adding to the intrigue, Dr. Jordan Tappero—an epidemiologist identified as a leader of the CDC's cholera response team in Haiti—made a direct and very well-publicized statement to a reporter. CDC's primary focus, he said, was "to save lives and control the spread of disease."[4] Asked how cholera came to Haiti, though, his response was far more calculated. "We realize that it's also important to understand how infectious agents move to new countries. However, we may never know the actual origin of this cholera strain."

What was Tappero up to? Was he simply trying to manage public expectations, given the epidemiological challenges of a search for the source of the disease? Or did he have a broader purpose?

Trouble was brewing at the French embassy just when Piarroux was leaving Port-au-Prince on his field trip.

Unbeknownst to the French epidemiologist, Ambassador Didier Le Bret was about to embroil Piarroux in an unwanted controversy—one he learned about only when he was back in France a month later. In a private diplomatic communiqué sent that Saturday to government officials and diplomatic colleagues in Port-au-Prince, Europe, and North America,[5] the ambassador wrote generally of the investigation but then stated, "According to initial findings of Professor Piarroux, the origin of the epidemic is clear: the Nepalese battalion of MINUSTAH has contaminated the Artibonite River. The speed of transmission also seems to confirm the massive nature of the burden of *vibrios*, injected into the very river." Although Piarroux's main hypothesis still needed to be confirmed by a field investigation, the ambassador suggested that he had reached a definitive conclusion.

Conflating Piarroux's work with other findings and local and international reports, the text continued, "The first cases [of cholera] appeared on October 13 on the outskirts of the city of Mirebalais (on the central plateau), in the immediate vicinity of a camp of MINUSTAH, not far from a tributary of the Artibonite River, four days after the arrival in the barracks of a new contingent of the Nepalese Army. It was also established that a cholera epidemic had broken out in Kathmandu two weeks before the departure of the soldiers from their country of origin and the *vibrio* present today in Haiti is of Asian origin."

Focusing on the Nepalese peacekeepers, the ambassador addressed the start of the epidemic. "Some of the Nepalese soldiers who had arrived on October 8 in Mirebalais were already infected with the *vibrio*. A veritable epidemic was then triggered in the camp. The soldiers involved were not only infected, they were sick." The medical staff, he wrote, had "long experience with acute diarrhea, and may not have sought to learn the origin of the condition." Even though infected with cholera, the soldiers were "young and strong," and as a result, "the troops were up in a few days, but their excreta, released into the wastewater treatment system in the camp, were overloaded with *vibrios*."

The ambassador then described how the infectious microbes had entered the river water. "The camp septic tanks were drained on October 18 by a Haitian company. For convenience, but out of negligence, the waste content was released directly into a tributary of the Artibonite River."

After attributing these findings to Piarroux, the ambassador made an unexpected and disturbing comment. He cited conversations with Alex Larsen, the Haitian minister of health, and suggested Piarroux needed to be reined in. Le Bret planned to tell Piarroux to "refrain from public comment and be limited, at this stage, only to returning his report to the health authorities of the country." The Haitian government, he wrote, "does not want to embarrass MINUSTAH on the eve of elections," and he added that the "risk of retaliation [against the UN] is real."

Le Bret then wrote a powerful and consummately *political* sentence. "The official position [of the embassy of France] therefore remains: cholera is of the Asian strain, but there is no evidence that it was introduced by elements of the Nepalese battalion." It was a complete distortion given his veritable endorsement of Piarroux's preliminary findings.

How the epidemic began had apparently been dropped as an official priority of the French embassy.

The only hint of a problem came when Piarroux and his team returned to the embassy on Monday morning, November 15. Piarroux had been counseled by the embassy to be especially careful in public presentations. This was reasonable, he thought, even if somewhat vague. He had seen how easily rumors could spread in Haiti, and he had felt the tension in the air as Haitians prepared to vote in less than two weeks. MINUSTAH was a campaign issue. Some Haitians rallied against the UN organization as occupiers. Others denounced MINUSTAH, and Piarroux believed the words of a foreign scientist should not add to that. Still, emotions continued to rise, stoked by an official in faraway Sweden.

Claes Hammar, Swedish ambassador to the Caribbean region, had visited Haiti in early November. Returning to Stockholm, he granted an interview to *Svenska Dagbladet,* one of Sweden's largest newspapers—and addressed the swirling rumors of cholera's origin among MINUSTAH troops: "I have had it confirmed by a diplomatic source that the cholera comes from Nepal."[6] Specifically, he meant the Nepalese peacekeepers.

Two days later, Hammar told a Finnish reporter, "I consider my source to be a reliable one. It is a United States official, but I cannot say who." He added that the tests taken by the official were at a camp of Nepalese UN workers.[7]

Mentioning a U.S. official raised eyebrows and some wonder, and within a few days Hammar's words went global. A dispatch titled "Swedish diplomat says Haiti cholera strain came from Nepal" showed up in newspapers and on news websites from Haiti to India and beyond.

During the same days, Piarroux was scheduled to give presentations at the Université Notre-Dame d'Haïti, the Haitian Medical Association, and the Institut Français d'Haiti. To prepare, he searched the Web for official cholera maps to augment those he had reviewed when he first arrived in Haiti. He had already discussed with Dr. Magloire that the online département-specific PAHO maps lacked crucial details necessary for local control programs. What he hadn't noticed earlier, though, was an accompanying table showing new cholera cases by epidemic week for each département.[8] The table showed no cholera cases in Centre département during the first week of the epidemic, from October 17 to 23, but more than 2,000 new cases in Artibonite *département.* Piarroux had just spoken with doctors in Mirebalais and knew the earliest cases during that week had come from the village of Mèyé in Centre département.

For the second week, October 24–30, the online PAHO maps showed about 350 new cases in Centre département and several thousand new cases in Artibonite département. Anyone studying these two Internet maps would have concluded—*erroneously*—that the epidemic started during the first week with thousands of cases in Artibonite département and then spread in the second week to Centre département. Piarroux knew this to be the opposite of what had occurred.

Were these clerical errors, perhaps the result of unfamiliarity with new surveillance programs? If so, they certainly focused attention away from the upriver Centre département, where the MINUSTAH camp was located, and toward the coastal areas. The same question nagged Piarroux: Were the mistakes part of a concerted effort to shift attention to the less controversial environmental view of cholera origin? Piarroux was finding it increasingly difficult to put these suspicions out of his mind.

There were so many other maps to review online. Even the series of cholera maps from OCHA, published between October 23 and November 10, were fraught with discrepancies and odd word choices from an epidemiological perspective. He was puzzled. Early cholera had been explosive in nature, appearing in many areas as an ever-expanding epidemic. Why did OCHA state that some areas experienced cholera "outbreaks" while others were merely "affected" by the disease? The October 28 OCHA map with the legend "zone where cholera began" (figure 6.3 in chapter 6) directly contradicted what Piarroux had found in Mirebalais.

Piarroux suspected that these choices reflected the growing suspicion—perhaps even proof—that Nepalese soldiers were involved. The Walker and Katz press dispatches surely caused alarm.[9] The UN must have calculated that deceptive maps—an altered reality—would go a long way to helping undo their damage. Unexpected were the revelations of the Swedish ambassador—continuing to fan the simmering flames.

Piarroux realized he was walking on eggshells. Surely President Préval and other high officials knew the truth about cholera's origin. He had, after all, made a trip with various officials to Mirebalais on October 23 shortly after the epidemic erupted. Yet he and his government were silent. The official UN OCHA maps were a blatant deception. Piarroux nearly uttered aloud the word he was thinking: *étouffer l'affaire*, to cover up the case. He could not fathom why, as a wave of death spread over Haiti, the main political leaders would say nothing publicly about its origin. All these elements—maps, official statements, silence—made him particularly uncomfortable and then anxious. He wondered whether continuing the investigation might expose him to danger.

Piarroux knew the expression in English, "Go along to get along." Instead, though, he was determined to get a full picture of cholera in Haiti—including how it really started. He also sensed that many of his Haitian colleagues did not accept the altered reality that was being presented publicly, and he imagined they faced far greater pressure. Having been commissioned by the Haitian government and French embassy to conduct an official investigation, not yet complete, he decided to avoid sensitive subjects in his public presentations and to mention the human-activity hypothesis only when asked. He would focus on several aspects of cholera in Africa and touch only briefly on the situation in Haiti. As for when he was back home and not in the immediate public eye—that would be another story.

Meanwhile, the embassy set up two important appointments for Piarroux. The first was the next day, Tuesday, November 16, with Edmond Mulet, special representative of the UN secretary-general in Haiti. On Wednesday, he would meet with President Préval and Minister Larsen. Undoubtedly, the French ambassador felt Piarroux's early discoveries should be discussed at the highest levels.

Edmond Mulet was among the most powerful people in Haiti. Many said he wielded even more power than President Préval. As the all-important head of mission for MINUSTAH, Mulet was responsible for managing the entire MINUSTAH annual budget of about $865 million[10]—a sum equal to $87 per year for every one of Haiti's ten million people, quite a sizable figure in the impoverished nation. Mulet was also accountable for a foreign force of nearly 9,000 UN troops and 1,500 police, along with some 3,000 trained Haitian police.

Piarroux had never met Mulet but knew of his impressive political résumé. A Guatemalan, Mulet was first elected to his nation's congress in 1982, ran for the 1984 National Constituent Assembly, and then served again in Congress from 1986 until 1996. He helped craft accords in the mid-1980s that brought peace to several war-torn Central American nations, served as a Guatemalan diplomat—including as ambassador to the United States—lectured extensively on politics and foreign affairs, and eventually became UN assistant secretary-general for peacekeeping operations. He was appointed to his Haitian post by the UN secretary-general just after the previous head of mission lost his life in the Haiti earthquake. Since Mulet had previously held the same position in Haiti during 2006–7, he was the logical replacement.

Ambassador Le Bret accompanied Piarroux to the meeting, where he was asked to assess the current cholera situation. Mulet—a man of medium build, elongated face, wire-rimmed glasses, and a prominent gray mustache—was fluent in French, which made discussion easier. Piarroux explained that all elements of his investigation pointed to the epidemic's having begun in mid-October in Mèyé just below the Nepalese MINUSTAH camp. Mulet did not seem surprised. Piarroux suspected he had heard this from others.

Piarroux went on to explain that the violent epidemic in the Artibonite delta a few days after the outbreak began was not typical of cholera epidemics in other poor countries. In fact, he had not seen a cholera epidemic spread so quickly, to so many people, since the Goma outbreak of 1994 in central Africa.

The discussion proceeded to the epidemiological mechanism that could account for the rapid spread of cholera in the first days and the role played by the river that flowed by Mèyé and the MINUSTAH camp and then on to the larger Artibonite River. Piarroux's field investigation had shown that the explosive outbreak in the Artibonite delta had begun sometime between the late afternoon of October 19 and the morning of October 20.

Typically, health-center doctors would be aware of severe diarrhea cases in their communities during the first days of a cholera epidemic. No such early warning signs or symptoms appeared in the lower Artibonite valley before October 19. This suggested that transmission was not primarily person to person but rather that a single source had spread to many people. While he admitted that some community cases might have gone unnoticed, Piarroux pointed out that hundreds of existing cases would be needed to trigger a near-simultaneous epidemic of the magnitude that had befallen central Haiti. The explosive outbreaks on October 19 and 20 had occurred almost all at once in many settlements irrigated by the Artibonite River—again, a situation far different from what epidemiologists would see in slower person-to-person transmission associated with road travel or movement.

Piarroux told Mulet that time constraints had made it impossible to do a rigorous statistical analysis. Instead, he used surveillance maps to show the day-by-day evolution of the epidemic. The maps left no doubt as to the role of the Artibonite River in the outbreak's early days.

The Artibonite is a large river, Piarroux emphasized, with flow exceeding 100 cubic meters per second (more than 3,500 cubic feet per second). To cause so many simultaneous cases and deaths, the concentration of cholera organisms in the contaminated river had to have been exceptionally high in the hours preceding the first cases.

A robust discussion of several explanations ensued. No other hypothesis, though, could account for what Piarroux had found. The only plausible explanation was that a massive fecal contamination of the river had caused the large wave of cases.

Mulet seemed to accept the river contamination point but wondered why some municipalities between Mirebalais and the Artibonite delta appeared to have been spared. Piarroux explained that he and his colleagues had visited those very communes, and that the main villages and towns were actually located away from the Artibonite River. People used water from hill and mountain streams. Further downriver, however, the villages and towns were located near rice fields of the delta, irrigated by canals that flowed from the Artibonite. Those communities experienced many cases from contaminated river and canal waters.

So, Mulet asked, where had this large concentration of cholera microbes come from? Piarroux surmised from Mulet's body language that he already knew the answer. From his investigation, Piarroux felt Annapurna Camp was the most likely source. To produce sufficient amounts of infectious feces to cause such a massive contamination of the river delta, many MINUSTAH soldiers must have suffered from pronounced diarrhea. Piarroux was very clear:

what happened could not have resulted from a handful of asymptomatic cholera carriers. There was no way just a few soldiers, unaware they were contagious and harboring the cholera microbes, could be responsible for such an extensive outbreak.

Mulet was clearly troubled. MINUSTAH's own physicians had assured him that no one had been ill and that there was no indication the Nepalese soldiers had brought cholera to Haiti. If he accepted Piarroux's hypothesis, wouldn't it be tantamount to admitting not only that MINUSTAH had made errors but also that some of his officers had concealed the truth?

Piarroux suggested the matter could be resolved by testing for cholera antibodies in the blood of soldiers, a method already used in several studies to measure recent cholera infection.[11] But this was not done.

The discussion shifted to current safety and security concerns. Both Mulet and Le Bret stressed the importance of maintaining the presence of MINUSTAH troops during what was a sensitive period for Haiti, especially with the looming November 28 election, and of the need to manage protests before and after the vote. It was clear to Piarroux that these two men had other serious issues to consider—again, security and stability. But they had brought him to Haiti to explain the nature of the spreading epidemic and propose management and control activities. His mission statement said nothing about finding a "political solution" if by chance the source of cholera was found to be a powerful organization.

Piarroux felt out of his element, but it wasn't the first time he had encountered politics while investigating cholera. In DR Congo and Comoros, he had been summoned repeatedly by the health ministers, sometimes for substantive issues but other times only to display the minister's concern for cholera victims to the public. Piarroux had learned to expect all types of inquiries from all sorts of political leaders. But he wasn't about to let politics interfere with science.

Late the next day, Piarroux was received cordially for a meeting with President René Préval and Haitian Minister of Health Alex Larsen. They sat in comfortable armchairs around a coffee table.

Piarroux opened his laptop computer and began to tell the president and minister what he had told Mulet the day before. Like Mulet, Préval did not appear fazed by what Piarroux said about the epidemic's starting in the immediate vicinity of the Nepalese camp. Obviously, thought Piarroux, this is not new information to these men. But he also knew that the president had made a public statement that he had no idea how the epidemic started. Was that his *official* position, a necessary façade to avoid trouble with the powerful United Nations?

The elections were only eleven days away. The president obviously needed MINUSTAH to maintain calm. Thus again, political considerations, expressed or not, were very present in the minds of Piarroux's interlocutors and changed substantially the way they perceived what he had hoped would be a straightforward scientific discussion.

Piarroux got more specific, going beyond where the first few cases had occurred. He spoke of the likely cause of the expanding epidemic only a few days after the initial outbreak started. When he mentioned a possible sewage spill or leaking septic pit, Piarroux again sensed they already knew, though they didn't let on. He showed them the epidemiological data that supported his hypothesis and called into question competing explanations. With a few clicks on his laptop, he generated maps that showed the day-by-day course of the epidemic. The two men followed closely.

When the question of what to do came up, Piarroux told Préval and Larsen that the cholera epidemic was still in its ascending phase and that government authorities still needed help monitoring its progress and targeting better intervention and prevention actions. Most important, he said, Haiti desperately needed a better sense for when and where new centers should be established to treat cholera. The good news was that Haiti would soon enter its dry season. With decreasing storm water, there should be less runoff from contaminated areas and less cholera pollution of rivers. Piarroux felt that in the months to come there would likely be a decrease in the transmission of cholera, providing more opportunities to reduce and even to eliminate it from some areas. Haiti, he said, must not miss these opportunities. In the Comoros islands, he had seen how a few months of a cholera epidemic can lead people to believe the disease is a permanent fixture—and they give up the fight prematurely. Unless the organisms were completely eliminated, the rainy seasons would cause iterative resumptions of cholera, with more outbreaks to follow.

Piarroux envisioned the cholera epidemic as a dragon's fiery breath scorching the land and leaving dying embers. The wind would surely begin to blow again, and the fires would flare up as before and even grow stronger. Haiti would need more help to make sure the dying embers actually died. At that moment, though, the epidemic was growing daily, and the most urgent task was to limit the damage.

Piarroux was scheduled to return to France the next day but felt his job was not yet finished. As the meeting came to a close, Préval and Larsen asked if he was willing to extend his visit another week. The president wanted Piarroux to work directly with the Unité de Crise—the crisis unit devoted to cholera that he had personally set up.

Piarroux said yes, assuming his employers back in France would approve. He would use the time to gain a better understanding of the evolution of the epidemic and continue training his Haitian colleagues. The extra time would also allow him to undertake a second field investigation.

The next morning, the French embassy sent a communiqué to the president of Piarroux's university and the general director of his hospital. "Professor Piarroux should have completed his mission today," it read, "but the President of the Republic, René Préval, and the Minister of Health and Population, Dr. Alex Larsen, have asked him to extend his stay until the system that he is responsible for developing has been established." Both employers granted permission.

Piarroux wondered where Le Bret stood on extending his stay. He wasn't sure the ambassador was as enthusiastic as Préval and Larsen, given broader political issues that had arisen back in France. Bernard Kouchner, a dynamic former student activist and physician, was outgoing as French minister of foreign and European affairs, to be replaced by Michèle Alliot-Marie, a politician with leadership experience in multiple ministries but not in the international arena. Following a doctrine that morality cannot stop at borders and that when confronted by extreme wickedness, politics and not just medicine should be *sans frontières* (without borders), Kouchner had cofounded both Médecins Sans Frontières in 1971 and Médecins du Monde in 1980.[12] Over the years, Piarroux had worked many times with Médecins du Monde. While Kouchner may well have understood the importance of seeking the truth about the Haitian cholera epidemic, Piarroux thought it just as likely that it was not even on Alliot-Marie's radar screen.

Once it was settled that Piarroux would stay, he was asked to meet again with Mulet. Ambassador Le Bret had been called back to Paris, and so Gérard Chevallier, a physician at the French embassy, accompanied him to the meeting.

This second meeting had a different feel than when Piarroux had met only with Mulet and Le Bret. This time the room was filled. Deputy Special Representative Nigel Fisher, many MINUSTAH staff members, and several other UN officials joined Mulet. It felt more like a formal hearing than a casual scientific discussion, a bit like appearing before a jury.

Piarroux was asked to bring the larger audience up to speed and repeat what he had told Mulet and Le Bret two days earlier. Again, he explained the preliminary results of his field investigation. He maintained that Nepalese soldiers as asymptomatic carriers could not explain the outbreak, since they would not have shed enough bacteria to contaminate even a small stream like the one that flowed by the camp, and certainly not the much larger Artibonite River.

The murmuring suggested his assessment was not well received. A lively discussion ensued, and Piarroux addressed many of the same questions and counterviews raised by Mulet in their first meeting.

After about an hour, Mulet asked Piarroux whether he would meet with the three MINUSTAH physicians who had gone to Annapurna Camp on October 21 to gather samples. Piarroux agreed and was surprised when they appeared immediately, as if by orchestration. Very strange indeed.

The three doctors, apparently from South American contingents of MINUSTAH, explained that they had seen nothing unusual during their visit to the Nepalese peacekeeping camp. Camp officers told them no soldiers were ill, so they collected no stool samples. They did collect samples in the latrines and river and sent them to a medical laboratory for analysis. All were reported to be negative—and relying on those results, the UN concluded that MINUSTAH had nothing to do with the introduction of cholera into Haiti.

Piarroux asked the doctors whether they had measured for the existence of chlorine in the latrines. After all, they could have been chlorinated just before their arrival, thereby killing the cholera organisms and testing negative. There was no response.

Piarroux described well-known tests for fecal coliforms that measure whether water has been contaminated by feces, separate from the presence of cholera that may have been missed. Had they tested water in the local river near where the contamination had taken place? Again, the physicians offered no answer.

Finally, Piarroux asked for details about how the "negative" tests had been conducted in the laboratory and requested the specific results. Again, nothing.

Piarroux wondered whether he was being too technical. Perhaps he was taxing their knowledge of cholera, which was a new disease in Haiti. Mulet's presence probably made it difficult for them; he was their boss and they weren't showing themselves in the best light. But Piarroux continued, reminding the audience that methodological issues are crucial, since searching for *Vibrio cholerae* in the environment is a complicated task mastered by only a few highly specialized laboratories.

He felt his every word being weighed carefully by this jury as it listened for flaws in his reasoning or misstated points—anything that might exonerate the UN. But Piarroux was confident his training had prepared him for such cross-examination. He believed the scientific quest to verify and validate, to find the facts, would prevail.

Through it all, everyone was polite and respectful to the distinguished professor and epidemiologist who had come to Haiti at the request of the Haitian authorities and under the auspices of the French embassy. But when the discussion came to a close, many issues were still unresolved, and the growing tension was palpable. In fact, that same day a riot broke out near the French embassy. Some 150 protesters threw stones and shouted that MINUSTAH had given them cholera and must go. Using tear gas and shooting into the crowd, soldiers finally dispersed the rioters.[13]

Piarroux would remain in Haiti for another nine days, continue his investigation, and share his thoughts on controlling the disease with local officials. He felt he had the implicit support of the nation's highest government officials to conduct an open inquiry. But he was becoming increasingly sensitive to the important relationship between Haiti and the UN and the politics that came with it.

Piarroux's plan: remain persistent in his investigation, be cautious in public, and add no fuel to the fire.

8

JOURNALISTS

Not everyone wanted the source of cholera to be found. Among those who did were three journalists who covered the initial outbreak of cholera.

Sebastian Walker of Al Jazeera had dispatched his first cholera report on October 22 from outside Saint Nicolas Hospital in Saint-Marc, where about 1,400 people were seeking treatment.[1] Less than a week later, Walker traveled to Mirebalais and the nearby MINUSTAH camp and made the first television broadcast suggesting possible cholera contamination of river water by UN peacekeeping troops from Nepal.[2] Three days after that, he expanded his initial observation and added the UN's perspective in an online Al Jazeera article.[3]

> Walker, reporting from Port-au-Prince, said there had been no confirmation of the accusations that excrement from the newly arrived unit of UN peacekeepers from Nepal caused the epidemic.
>
> "We certainly saw a lot of activity there when we visited the base recently, with UN soldiers digging around the latrines, trying to stop what looked like sewage from seeping down into the river," he said.
>
> "But we are not sure this could be a source of contamination. The UN has been very certain in denying that."

On November 3, 2010, Roberson Alphonse—a longtime member of the Haitian Association of Journalists—shared with readers of *Le Nouvelliste* details of early cases of cholera in Mirebalais near the MINUSTAH base.[4] Two videos, possibly broadcast that same day, were posted with the online version of Alphonse's article.[5] In Creole, he interviewed a government epidemiologist who had investigated the early cholera cases and, in the video, showed the septic pit where human waste from the MINUSTAH had been stored before it supposedly leaked into a neighboring stream that flowed north to the Artibonite River.

Then there was the reporting of Jonathan Katz, who had come to Haiti in 2007 on a three-year assignment for the Associated Press. He extended his stay for another year after the January 2010 earthquake and then covered the October cholera outbreak and its aftermath. His reports in late October (he was in Mirebalais the same day as Sebastian Walker) and throughout November provided important details on the source of cholera in Haiti.[6] Not only did his articles focus on the origins of the epidemic, but they also highlighted the political forces that would make any investigation difficult. As Katz wrote on November 4, 2010,

> The CDC, World Health Organization, and United Nations say it is not possible to pinpoint the source and investigating further would distract from efforts to fight the disease.
>
> But leading specialists on cholera and medicine consulted by the Associated Press challenged that position, saying it is both possible and necessary to track the source to prevent future deaths. . . .
>
> . . . Dr. Paul Farmer, a UN deputy special envoy to Haiti and a noted specialist on poverty and medicine, said . . . "Knowing where the point source is—or source, or sources—would seem to be a good enterprise in terms of public health."
>
> John Mekalanos, a cholera specialist and chairman of Harvard University's microbiology department, said it is important to know exactly where and how the disease emerged because it is a novel, virulent strain previously unknown in the Western Hemisphere.[7]

As the days went by, news of cholera in Haiti spread globally and other media outlets began to delve a bit deeper. The German newsmagazine *Der Spiegel*, in a November 2 article, included a figure with an early view of how cholera had spread from October 22 to 27, including a daily bar graph of those who became sick and those who died.[8] Its dark circles on an accompanying map showed death along the Artibonite River, with an increase in deaths in upriver Mirebalais and in the downriver communities of the Artibonite valley and beyond. It was a good illustration of how quickly cholera had made its way along the river.

That November, the situation in Haiti became tenser by the day. On Sunday, November 14, President Préval addressed the nation. He offered some advice regarding sanitation and hygiene and sought to dispel the swirling myths and rumors. Still, riots broke out the next day. Protesters who blamed the UN troops for the cholera epidemic attacked two MINUSTAH bases that housed Nepalese troops. One, in Cap-Haïtien in the Nord département, housed a Nepalese police unit, where—wrote Reuters reporter Joseph Guyler Delva—"hundreds of protesters yelling anti-UN slogans, hurled stones at UN peacekeepers, set up burning barricades and torched a police station." At the other in Hinche, in Centre département, "demonstrators threw stones" at the Nepalese infantry troops.[9]

The next day, Jonathan Katz added to his own dispatch what two local radio stations in Cap-Haïtien had reported. He explained that "UN soldiers and Haitian police had fired tear gas and projectiles to disperse at least 1,000 protesters at the Nepalese base" and that a national TV reporter had told him by phone that "at least three people were injured by Haitian police."[10] He also described the specific UN reaction to his own earlier report.

> After an Associated Press investigation, the UN acknowledged that there were sanitation problems at the [Mirebalais UN] base, but said its soldiers were not responsible for the outbreak. No formal or independent investigation has taken place despite calls from Haitian human rights groups and US health care specialists.
>
> Presidential candidates have seized on the suspicions to denounce the 12,000-strong UN peacekeeping force ahead of Nov. 28 elections.
>
> Nigel Fisher, the acting UN humanitarian chief in Haiti, said yesterday that the cholera had become a national security issue amid local protests. He said the UN is working with Haitian officials to ensure health precautions are taken so the elections can proceed as scheduled.

It did not take long for those involved in deflecting attention away from the origin of cholera to speak publicly. A November 17 *New York Times* article began, "Medical authorities in Haiti defended their decision Tuesday not to focus on finding the origins of a cholera outbreak that has killed more than 1,000 people and stoked violent demonstrations against United Nations peacekeepers, whom many people blame for introducing the disease."[11]

Notably, not a single one of the medical authorities quoted—all working in Haiti—was Haitian. Even if they had their own opinions, most Haitian medical authorities would not speak to reporters. They seemed to be taking very seriously the president's warning on October 23 that it would be "irresponsible and dangerous" to identify a country as the source of the epidemic.[12]

Daniel B. Epstein, Dr. Jordan Tappero, and Dr. David Sack, though, all offered their own views to *New York Times* reporter Randal C. Archibold to justify forgoing the search for cholera's origin. Epstein, a spokesperson for the Pan American Health Organization (the UN's regional health arm), said PAHO was focusing "on treating people, getting a handle on this and saving lives." Piarroux came to think of that as the "too busy" argument.

Tappero, a CDC epidemiologist, expressed the "too costly" argument when he told the *New York Times* that "it was unlikely that scientists would pinpoint where the outbreak began, and that he did not think mounting an all-out effort to find the answer 'is a good use of resources.'"

Sack, the cholera expert and epidemiologist from the Bloomberg School of Public Health at Johns Hopkins University, was more equivocal, acknowledging the need for origin studies but deferring to the "too busy" argument. While studying the genetics of the strain "would give a better idea where it came from," said Sack, he agreed that "it is more important to prevent the disease and control it. It should not be killing people."

These arguments all buttressed the remarks of the MINUSTAH spokesperson Vincenzo Pugliese, whose primary purpose seemed to be to disparage the motivations of Haitian protesters. "These are not genuine demonstrations," he told Archibold. "They are using spoilers paid to create chaos." Pugliese had nothing to say about whether UN peacekeepers might have brought cholera to Haiti.

Three days later, on November 20, the *New York Times* science and health reporter Donald G. McNeil Jr. elevated blame avoidance to an even higher level in an opinion piece. Its title—"Cholera's Second Fever: An Urge to Blame"—implied a feverish yearning among some investigators to assign blame. But, thought Piarroux, what McNeil called a "fever" is actually the scientific method.

McNeil did acknowledge that some "experts concede that the Nepalese soldiers are the most likely suspects," but even as officials in Haiti were tracing the origin of the epidemic, they were "dead set against announcing what they find, since scapegoating provokes violence."[13] "Scapegoating has a long and ignoble tradition in historic descriptions of pandemics," McNeil wrote, directly associating the investigation of possible UN culpability with some of the worst excesses in disease history. Blame avoidance would prevent violence, went McNeil's argument, which he seemed to suggest was more important than journalistic transparency.

McNeil's piece quoted two officials. Dr. Scott F. Dowell, chief of the response to the Haitian epidemic at the U.S. CDC, explained, "Naming individual countries is not productive. . . . We're focused on this really unacceptable number of deaths." The other official was Imogen Wall, identified as the United Nations spokeswoman in Haiti. "From our point of view," she said, "[the origin] really doesn't matter."

Infectious disease epidemiologists—including from CDC—typically have a much different view. While cholera was moving through Haiti, a giant outbreak of more than 1,900 cases involving the bacteria *Salmonella enteritidis*, occurred in multiple U.S. states.[14] A skillful investigation by CDC and the U.S. Food and

Drug Administration found the source: two huge egg farms in Iowa. The negligent owner was selling "old" eggs in filthy settings, and by mid-August more than half a billion tainted eggs had been recalled.[15]

No blame-avoidance campaign was mounted. No epidemiologist admonished reporters to leave the egg farm owner alone because he was "a community benefactor who shares his wealth and counsels prison inmates about Christianity"[16]—as some local community members said. Instead, the disease detectives executed a case study in how epidemiology should work hand in hand with government in a public health crisis, avoiding nothing in the quest for truth.

Just a day before McNeil's opinion piece came out, Katz had published another comprehensive piece on cholera in Haiti with many new details.[17] His was investigative journalism at its best—and the contrast with McNeil's piece could not have been starker. The article, headlined "U.N. Worries Its Troops Caused Cholera in Haiti," broke the story wide open.

"The mounting circumstantial evidence that U.N. peacekeepers from Nepal brought cholera to Haiti was largely dismissed by U.N. officials," Katz wrote. "Haitians who asked about it were called political or paranoid. Foreigners were accused of playing 'the blame game.' The World Health Organization said the question was simply 'not a priority.'"

Events on the ground, though, were forcing the UN to make a bit of an about-face—with the potential for some very significant consequences.

> But this week, after anti-U.N. riots and inquiries from health experts, the top U.N. representative in Haiti said he is taking the allegations very seriously.
>
> "It is very important to know if it came from [the Nepalese base] or not, and someday I hope we will find out," U.N. envoy Edmond Mulet told The Associated Press.
>
> The answer would have implications for U.N. peacekeeping missions around the world, he said.

Katz also addressed the "scapegoating provokes violence" theme.

> When riots broke out across northern Haiti this week, the U.N. blamed them on politicians trying to disrupt the upcoming vote. But observers say the U.N.'s early stance fanned the flames.
>
> "If the U.N. had said from the beginning, 'We're going to look into this' . . . I think that, in fact, would have been the best way in reducing public anger," said Brian Concannon, director of the Institute for Justice & Democracy in Haiti. "The way to contribute to public anger is to lie."

The AP reporter also provided further information about the Nepalese soldiers. "The latest Nepalese deployment came in October, after a summer of cholera outbreaks in Nepal," he wrote, referring to an article from the *Himalayan Times*.[18] He then connected the dots in what became a major international news story, explaining that 454 Nepalese troops were assigned to the UN camp in Mirebalais and that the changeover at the base there was done in three shifts on October 9, 12, and 16. "The U.N. says none of the peacekeepers showed symptoms of the disease. But 75% of people infected with cholera never show symptoms but can still pass on the disease for two weeks—especially in countries like Nepal where people have developed immunity."

Katz also revealed more details of what he had seen on October 27. An executive with Sanco, the sanitation company contracted by the UN, stated that her workers "emptied the septic tanks on October 11, after the first shift of Nepalese troops arrived, and did not return again until after the outbreak began. This was contradicted by local villagers. At some point in mid-October, neighbors said a new Sanco driver they did not recognize came one day and dumped outside of the usual pits." Sanco next returned on October 27, the same day Katz had been on site for several hours, and the executive told him there was more waste than usual.

Katz presented some intriguing news about testing. "The U.N. said none of the Nepalese soldiers had shown signs of cholera, which some news outlets misreported as saying the soldiers had specifically tested negative for it. [The UN spokesman] confirmed on Oct. 30 that they had not been tested for the disease." Then he revealed that what testing *was* done was far below any reasonable scientific standards.

> The U.N. also tested environmental samples the soldiers took from the base. It says they came out negative at an independent laboratory in Santo Domingo [the capital city of neighboring Dominican Republic].
>
> But the Santo Domingo lab, Cedimat, has been under contract to MINUSTAH since 2004, said Dr. Maximo Rodriguez, the doctor whose name appears on the tests. Rodriguez is a general medicine doctor whose specialty is treating obesity. Cedimat is a patient-treatment facility. In fact, the [environmental] test results were written on forms meant for people: The results provided to the AP by the U.N. had the "patient's" name listed as "Minustha Minustha (sic)"—age 40, male.
>
> Rodriguez said "any well-equipped laboratory" can do tests for cholera. But epidemiologists say examining environmental samples for cholera takes extra expertise, because the disease can be hard to isolate.

Katz's article pointed out the "unique implications" of UN troops' bringing cholera to Haiti. The country, ravaged by political instability since the early 1990s and by the earthquake, relied heavily on "foreign governments, aid groups and the U.N. for everything from rebuilding to basic services. . . . Some Haitians see the peacekeepers as the only hope for security in a nation where towns are ruled by drug lords and coups d'état are more common than elections. Others resent heavily armed foreign armies on their soil and see the soldiers as a threat to national sovereignty and pride."

In his reporting, Katz showed politics to be clearly at the epicenter of the unfolding investigation into cholera.

> Earlier this month, Dr. Paul Farmer, who founded the medical aid group Partners in Health and is U.N. deputy special envoy for Haiti, called for an aggressive investigation into the source of the cholera, saying the refusal to look into the matter publicly was "politics to me, not science."
>
> The CDC acknowledges politics played a role in how the investigation unfolded.
>
> "We're going to be really cautious about the Nepal thing because it's a politically sensitive issue for our partners in Haiti," said CDC commander Dr. Scott Dowell.

Politics, in fact, were trumping science—and scientists knew it. Katz addressed the apparent conflicts in CDC's actions and the head-in-the sand stance of the World Health Organization.

> The CDC agrees that the movement of pathogens from one part of the world to another is an important public health issue. Its scientists are working on samples of bacteria from 13 infected Haitians to sequence the cholera strain's genome, the results of which will be posted on a public database.
>
> But the U.S. government agency has several caveats. First, it has not taken environmental samples or tested the Nepalese soldiers. Second, it will not go public with its analysis until all its studies are complete. And third, it may not get enough information to say exactly how cholera got into the country.
>
> "The bottom line is we may never know," Dowell said.
>
> "At some time we will do further investigation, but it's not a priority right now," WHO spokeswoman Fadela Chaib said this week.

Noting at least one position shift, Katz ended his article with the MINUSTAH head Edmond Mulet, who acknowledged that Farmer had been right all along that "there has to be a thorough investigation of how it came, how it happened and how it spread." Mulet even mentioned "a French epidemiologist who met with him this week to discuss how to investigate the Nepalese base." That was Piarroux.

Said Mulet, "One thing I can assure you: There has been no cover-up—there has been no cover-up from our side—and we have done everything we can to investigate. . . . Eventually we will find out what happened and how it happened."

9

SECRECY

Piarroux did not see Jonathan Katz's November 19 article when it first appeared, and the next day he was already back in the countryside. Before leaving Port-au-Prince, though, he visited the Unité de Crise, devoted to cholera and personally set up by Préval. The use of the French word *unité*—which means both "unit" and "unity"—seemed a good sign.

The president had asked Piarroux to work directly with the unit, housed in a prefabricated building on the grounds of the collapsed Palais National. Several dozen people from national and international organizations occupied the offices. Some staff of LNSP, Haiti's national laboratory, had been relocated there, and WHO, UNICEF, the UN's OCHA, and even the Brigada Médica Cubana were all present. CDC scientists came by frequently for extensive discussions with Dr. Magloire, the epidemiologist and DELR head. Representatives of NGOs came for meetings.

Piarroux had been told the best time to find people was just before lunch. He found a relatively calm atmosphere. Small groups of people here and there spoke in whispered conversations. Others sat at their computers, one even playing a game. Telephones rang continually, but judging from what he could hear, Piarroux surmised some people were talking to friends or family. Everything seemed rather subdued.

The French epidemiologist had been wanting to meet Dr. Thimothé, director general of the Ministry of Public Health and Population, who came often to the crisis unit. One of the Haitians introduced the two men. Thimothé struck

Piarroux as very serious, even intimidating, with an imposing frame, skeptical eyes and full, dark mustache. He played an important role in the Haitian health system and was devoted to making sure the flow of epidemiological information was handled appropriately. Appointed personally by Préval, Thimothé had almost as much power as Health Minister Larsen.

President Préval had specifically asked Piarroux to give the crisis unit a presentation on his investigation and the surveillance map system he wanted to implement. Some forty people assembled, nearly all Haitians—many from the Haitian Civil Protection Agency responsible for the country's domestic disaster response. He spoke openly and comprehensively, having gotten a surprising "yes" when he asked Préval directly whether he was allowed to tell all he had found.

Préval himself refused to speak to the press about the origin of the cholera outbreak and had prohibited his ministers and their staff from talking about the issue publicly. But it was clear to Piarroux that Préval wanted the Haitian people to know the truth. He had asked Piarroux to extend his stay. He encouraged Piarroux to present his results, often in meetings with dozens of participants. He never once asked him to stop saying anything in particular.

On Saturday morning, November 20, Piarroux set out again with Robert Barrais for another field investigation with several objectives. One was to recover data missing from the Centre département epidemiology office in Hinche. The office had no Internet access; even telephone contact was difficult. They also wanted to understand what was happening in rural communities in the Chaîne des Chaos mountains near the town of Petite Rivières de l'Artibonite in the north plain of the Artibonite valley. The monitoring system indicated that mortality from cholera was much higher there than elsewhere. They wanted to get to the town of Saint-Michel-de-l'Attalaye in particular, where many more than expected had died of cholera since the epidemic had begun.

With no vehicle available from the French embassy, Dr. Gérard Chevallier—the physician who had accompanied Piarroux to his second meeting with Edmond Mulet—offered to join the disease detectives on the journey and provide transportation. At dawn, Piarroux came down from his hotel room to find Chevallier waiting in an extended-cab pickup truck with two rows of seats. Before picking up Barrais, Chevallier instructed the driver, Dominique, to get Stéphane Jourdain—a reporter with Agence France-Presse, one of the world's largest news organizations—and a Peruvian photographer. Piarroux knew Jourdain was coming along, but he was perplexed since he wasn't supposed to talk to the press. He assumed, though, that Chevallier must have cleared it with the embassy. In fact, the doctor had sent a note to the first secretary.

Piarroux worried that having a reporter and a photographer along might scare off people he hoped to speak with. Discretion is a valuable commodity in an epidemiological investigation, as is not making waves. But if it was okay with the embassy, who was he to question the presence of a reporter?

The journey to Hinche is 107 kilometers (66 miles). They traveled up Route Nationale 3 (RN3)—just as Piarroux had done the previous week—crossing the Cul-de-Sac plain, then the Chaîne des Matheux mountains, and on to Mirebalais. They passed by the small MINUSTAH camp at Terre Rouge and the much larger Annapurna Camp in Mèyé.

Jourdain wanted to interview Piarroux about the origins of the epidemic, especially since they were passing by the alleged source, but Piarroux had already told him the topic was off limits. He had no intention of feeding Haitian political instability during the election campaign. So Jourdain agreed to focus on how cholera was being managed in the remote areas far from the capital and on the humanitarian organizations involved.

The men drove on an unpaved but serviceable road through Mirebalais, continuing northeast on RN3. They stopped at Lac de Péligre, Haiti's second-largest lake, created in 1956 when the Péligre Hydroelectric Dam was constructed on the Artibonite River. Piarroux was particularly interested in doing a risk assessment of cholera transmission among residents there. Years before, in eastern DR Congo, he had found that lake water used for drinking, cooking, or laundry contributed to cholera transmission because it was so easily contaminated by sewage runoff from residential areas. He hoped to observe whether residents around Lac de Péligre consumed water directly from the lake or had other water resources less easy to contaminate.

In DR Congo, the main zones of cholera infection were in the densely populated areas around the lake, which served as starting points of outbreaks, following dry seasons when the disease was maintained at lower levels among fishing communities and merchant travelers. Then, with increased rainfall, contamination of the lake with cholera-ridden feces, and human movement, the disease was easily transmitted to persons living by the lake and then on to the major mining towns hundreds of miles away.

The epidemiology of cholera can vary considerably from one country to another. As it turns out, the lakes in Haiti generally are not critical to the spread of the disease, since they are much smaller than those in DR Congo and the local populations are more sparsely distributed. Many other characteristics of their country, however, make Haitians particularly vulnerable to cholera. Their rice fields, canals, and waterways create conditions for contamination that are especially favorable for disease transmission. DR Congo and Haiti share risk factors: overpopulation, poverty, poor access to drinking water, lack of latrines.

After passing the Lac de Péligre area, RN3 continues through Centre département, turning north toward Hinche, a small city of fifty thousand. In the late morning, they pulled up to L'Hopital Sainte-Thérèse, where a cholera treatment camp had been set up under tents outside the entrance to the main building. Activity was intense; apparent cholera cases had been pouring into the treatment center from the city and the surrounding villages. The medical staff seemed to be working as best they could with their limited resources.

Suddenly Chevallier's telephone rang. It was the first secretary of the French embassy calling, and he was furious. Outside the hospital entrance, the men stood and waited in the sweltering heat while Chevallier spoke on the phone. From his replies and body language they could tell the caller was yelling. The embarrassed doctor walked away so he could speak more freely.

The first secretary was fuming over a news article by Jourdain he had read that morning in *Le Nouvelliste*, Haiti's national newspaper.[1] Piarroux had skimmed it online before leaving the hotel. Jourdain had attributed to a UN spokesman a statement indicating that Piarroux was working with Dr. Chevallier of the French embassy and that Piarroux had met MINUSTAH staff members a few days earlier and told them he was "ready to participate in an investigation of the origin" of cholera in Haiti. The article also seemed to place Chevallier squarely in the camp of those who did not want that investigation. He was quoted: "It is useless to focus on this issue even if the epidemiological probability [of finding the source] is high."

Jourdain's article revealed little about Piarroux's work, but the damage was done, and the first secretary wanted no more—especially with the elections only a little more than a week away. Had he not seen Chevallier's note about Jourdain? Piarroux wondered.

The men were ordered to return to Port-au-Prince at once—something Chevallier did not tell the group immediately. He wanted to make sure the trip to Hinche was not a complete loss.

Piarroux and Barrais went into a small meeting room with the Centre département epidemiologists to analyze local data. Outside, Chevallier told Jourdain that an emergency had come up and the rest of the group would have to return to Port-au-Prince. He and his photographer decided to remain on their own.

When Piarroux and Barrais emerged from the hospital, they were quite upset to learn of the new plan to return to Port-au-Prince. Piarroux wanted to continue his fieldwork and was concerned about what was going on in the mountains of northern Haiti. Still, the men headed back down RN3 toward Port-au-Prince. As they came to Mirebalais, Chevallier—determined to save the investigation—phoned the French embassy and again spoke with the first secretary. He explained where they were and that they had left Jourdain behind. The secretary changed his mind.

The men stopped at the community hospital in Mirebalais, where they updated the data set on cholera in Centre département and spoke again with doctors from the Brigada Médica Cubana about the first cases. They then headed northwest to Gonaïves, the coastal city of about three hundred thousand and capital of Artibonite département.

Jourdain found plenty to write about in Hinche.[2] He interviewed the manager of the local cholera treatment center and learned that the dead were being laid out on the front lawn. The manager feared the outbreak was worsening. The article did not cite Piarroux but quoted Chevallier several times, including his warning that the "unusual" month-old epidemic could be far more severe than the figures suggested. Jourdain also wrote of the "disappointment" of UN Humanitarian Coordinator Nigel Fisher about receiving less than 10 percent of the amount requested in the international "appeal for 164 million dollars to help Haiti combat the epidemic." Fisher spoke with urgency: "We need doctors, nurses, water purification systems, chlorine tablets, soap, oral rehydration salts, tents for cholera treatment centers and a range of other supplies." He noted that the recent riots in Cap-Haïtien had slowed the response but didn't explain why that would have impeded international donations. It occurred to Piarroux that Fisher might have been implying that Haitians ought to ignore the rage-inducing rumors that the UN brought cholera to Haiti if they wanted international support to combat the epidemic.

Piarroux knew the next leg of his trip would be especially important. He was heading to remote inland communities, the kinds of places that all too often escape attention.

Once an epidemic that began outside the cities hits the urban areas, it can shift the focus dramatically. City-based leaders, even ones with national responsibilities, concentrate on their own backyards, giving less thought to faraway rural areas. It's the same as people in Europe or the United States learning of the death of one of its citizens, perhaps an aid worker or someone just traveling through an Ebola zone in Africa. Attention shifts to the publicized citizen away from the thousands of anonymous Africans who are victims of Ebola.

Something similar had happened when Piarroux was in DR Congo. When cholera hit the provincial capital of Lubumbashi, politicians and the press were very concerned. Decisions were taken to ramp up the fight against the disease. But earlier, when cholera had stricken the most remote areas of the province, few in the city had paid any mind.

Knowing the stakes, Piarroux began the next part of his fieldwork in Gonaïves, the "City of Independence," where Jean-Jacques Dessalines had declared that the former slave colony would become independent Haiti. The slaves had risen up in 1791, forced the French to abandon slavery two years later, and settled back into colonization until a new rebellion culminated in the Act of Independence, read by Dessalines in Gonaïves's central Place d'Armes on January 1, 1804.

Piarroux, Barrais, Chevallier, and Dominique arrived in Gonaïves after dark. They were greeted by a team from International Medical Corps (IMC), an NGO working in the area long before the cholera epidemic. The IMCers were quite familiar with the mountain villages north of Gonaïves. With the arrival of cholera, they had shifted their focus to managing patients in two treatment centers in the city and the inland town of Ennery. IMC also supported primary health care facilities in the surrounding villages, including mobile clinics that helped manage cholera patients in rural areas, providing care and medicines, chlorine for water and waste, and awareness sessions on the critical importance of good hygiene.

The cholera situation seemed under control in Gonaïves, but it remained a major problem in the rural hills. Many villages were largely inaccessible because of dirt roads that would wash out in the heavy rains. In theory, thought Piarroux, such isolation should have prevented cholera from appearing, but instead the disease had erupted, brought by workers returning home from the Artibonite valley. The consequences cascaded beyond sickness and death: for instance, local farmers were told to avoid coming into the major towns to sell their produce, which spared some from the disease but created greater economic hardship in an already impoverished country.

The local health workers made clear to the visitors that cholera was penetrating deeper and deeper into the Haitian countryside, a problem compounded by tremendously difficult access to health facilities for people there. Details were sparse. The IMC field coordinator said many cholera patients had died, but he had no numbers. Piarroux and the others wanted to see the situation for themselves, and IMC offered a driver and a four-wheel-drive vehicle to take the visitors to Saint-Michel-de-l'Attalaye and the surrounding villages the next day, along with two IMC nurses.

They spent the night in Gonaïves, fighting some very aggressive mosquitoes at what seemed to have once been a cottage resort. Damaged some years earlier during heavy flooding, it was now almost deserted but for a few houses occupied by volunteers working for NGOs.

Sunday began early for Piarroux, Barrais, and Chevallier. They rode with the IMC nurses, leaving Gonaïves and passing through Ennery—a city Piarroux and Barrais had visited the previous week on their way to Cap-Haïtien. They wanted to get in the most difficult part of the journey as early as possible—a habit Piarroux had developed over many years. Overcoming obstacles in the daylight hours, with the most time available, is always better than taking the risk of being trapped in the dark with a broken-down car or having to ford an unexpected stream with no bridge. It was the right choice. The road to Saint-Michel-de-l'Attalaye—actually more like a track—was fairly well maintained but was still a difficult drive. It rose in the hills along a valley and switched back and forth over the river, requiring ten crossings. Fortunately, the river was low. The ride was bumpy, but the IMC vehicle performed well.

Saint-Michel-de-l'Attalaye—or Saint-Michel by its French nickname—is a town of about thirty thousand inhabitants, part of a larger commune of the same name situated in the Marmelade arrondissement. Some distance to the north lies the village of Marmelade, where President René Préval had moved to his family farm in 2001 after his first five-year term in elected office.[3] He remained during the presidential term of his successor ,Jean-Bertrand Aristide, as Haiti gradually descended again into violence and political chaos. After Aristide's forced exile in early 2004 and then MINUSTAH's arrival, Préval began to consider reentering public life. Elected once more to the presidency, he began his second five-year term in May 2006, only to be confronted in 2010 by two devastating events—the January earthquake and the October cholera epidemic.

The town of Saint-Michel appears much smaller than its population would suggest. It is famous for *vodouisants*—believers in vodou—who make a June pilgrimage to the nearby grotto of Saint Francis of Assisi to pray and make offerings to *Iwa* (or spirits) and attend special religious ceremonies.[4] The town and surrounding villages of the commune suffer from lack of many services, including health care. The commune's 140,000 residents were served by only five basic health centers and two clinics—but no hospital, not even in Saint-Michel itself. Basic health centers in Haiti typically offer nursing care and the occasional services of a physician but no possibility of staying the night if needed. They stock few drugs. Clinics are much like basic health centers but are typically run by nurses from religious orders.

Two doctors and a few nurses serviced the town and surrounding villages, doing what they could to organize care with resources always in short supply. Anyone seriously ill or requiring surgery had no recourse but to make the trip to Ennery or Gonaïves—difficult travel given the bad road and paucity of available vehicles, including even bicycles.

Access to safe water and sanitation was equally problematic. Only Saint-Michel and two nearby villages had water systems, but even those were vulnerable to the frequent floods that interrupted the water supply and diminished the microbial quality of the water.

Referring cholera patients to faraway health facilities was not an option. The doctors and nurses established a makeshift cholera treatment unit. Yet it lacked chlorinated water at the entrance and exit, making hand washing impossible. Family members had to be pressed into duty to perform basic nursing tasks—which increased the likelihood of passing on the disease, especially absent any special precautions or training. Even with only a few dozen patients when Piarroux visited, moving around was impossible without stepping over people in the cramped space.

The doctor who welcomed them explained that some cholera patients needing immediate rehydration over a twenty-four-hour span would die because there was no one available to renew their infusion fluids overnight. But most deaths resulted because patients simply couldn't get to the facility. Many in the surrounding villages had to walk, and the nurses told story after story of cholera cases who died on the way. Others never tried and died at home.

The physician in charge of the Saint-Michel clinic had been carefully collecting epidemiological data since October 21 when the first cholera cases appeared among those who had come from the Artibonite plain. While hundreds of cases were seen, most patients were from the rural regions of the commune, not the town itself. By the time of Piarroux's visit on November 20, the local medical staff had treated more than nine hundred cases, hospitalized nearly four hundred, counted thirty-one deaths in the clinic, and knew of more than one hundred other deaths among those who had never reached a health facility. Of course, the doctors and scientists all understood that many other cholera cases and deaths were not listed—people who had been unable to get anywhere or be reached by health workers. So far, though, people living in the town were relatively unscathed, perhaps because of better water access.

Many cases that made it to a facility for care still died; the case-fatality rate exceeded 4 percent. The epidemic was only a month old.

The dramatic cholera outbreak in the lower Artibonite valley and the recent arrival of the epidemic in Port-au-Prince had diverted the attention of policymakers away from the crisis in the mountains of Haiti, just as Piarroux had suspected it would. Millions of people lived there without access to health care. What was happening in Saint-Michel was also occurring in many remote communes throughout the country.

Given the tremendous hardships, Piarroux could not help but wonder why people would stay in such remote places. The answer had much to do with Haiti's unique history. His companions told Piarroux of the slaves brought from Africa, the *Neg Mawon* ("black maroon" in Creole), who fought for independence. A famous Neg Mawon statue in Port-au-Prince, across from the President's Palace, stands as a symbol of the Haitian struggle for independence. The statue depicts an unknown slave holding a machete in one hand and a broken chain in the other and blowing into a conch shell.

When the French took over Haiti from the Spaniards in 1697, they focused on developing the agricultural sector, including sugar and coffee. Slave laborers were brought to do the harsh plantation work. By the end of the following century, more than four-fifths of the Haitian population were slaves. As they began to escape from the plantations, they established communities in remote mountainous regions. In the decades after independence, the land was parceled out in small sections, creating a large group of subsistence farmers.[5] Many of their descendants remained in the remote mountains in the heart of rural Haiti; these were the ones whom Piarroux and his companions were visiting.

The vast majority of patients arriving in Saint-Michel had come from only a few locations. One was Camathe, just a few miles back on the road to Ennery, where Piarroux and his colleagues now headed with the IMC nurses. Along the way, one of the nurses asked the driver to stop by a group at the side of the road. Two people were assisting an exhausted third person. The nurse spoke with them for less than a minute, offered some advice in Creole, and returned to the vehicle. The driver continued on.

The tired one was probably a cholera case, the nurse said, and was being brought to the treatment center—only a short distance farther. They had come from Camathe and had walked the entire way.

As they drove on, Piarroux felt a wave of guilt. Should we have left them? Driven them to the clinic? He said nothing, not entirely sure of what had transpired in Creole. Several months later, Chevallier recounted that he had felt the same regret.

The short trip to Camathe was only about five kilometers (a little over three miles). They came upon a hamlet of houses scattered on either side of Road 306, just south of the passing river. Supposedly, Camathe residents did not drink river water but rather drew their water from a rock wall outlet. Yet cholera had been raging there for more than a week, with new cases reported every day. Had it not been for the local radio, people would probably have had no idea what was afflicting their tiny community and how to provide basic care when cholera symptoms appeared.

The team made brief introductions to local officials and asked to be taken to where the villagers usually drew their water. Piarroux and Barrais felt that water from the rock wall was likely free of cholera and probably had not contaminated Camathe's inhabitants. So why so much cholera? The culprit, they hypothesized, could have been lack of chlorination to protect their stored household water.

Many villagers couldn't even afford soap. Without these resources, and without trusted community health workers to show them hygiene techniques, the mostly poor, set-in-their-ways inhabitants were on their own.

Piarroux wanted to stay in Camathe and figure out the exact cause of the village's cholera outbreak. Time would not allow him to. It was one of many instances when establishing the main mode of transmission proved impossible, but Piarroux was pleased that at least the team could highlight a major problem in how cholera was being fought. Clearly, there needed to be distribution of soap and chlorine, and immediately.

They left Camathe, fording the river again and again on the way back until they reached Ennery for a very short stay—just long enough to unload the medical supplies they had been carrying from IMC and tour the local cholera treatment center. Then it was back to Gonaïves, where Piarroux and his colleagues warmly thanked the IMC team for their invaluable assistance. The time had come to switch back to the pickup truck and return to Port-au-Prince. It was already getting dark.

The driver navigated the route quickly. He honked the horn freely and often, even at night as they drove through villages and towns. Piarroux was quite tired, but the jerky ride made dozing off difficult. Hours later, near Port-au-Prince, they found themselves caught in yet another of the city's incessant traffic jams. Creeping along, they heard music in the distance, interrupted by slogans and a responsive crowd chanting approval. It was a campaign rally for presidential candidate Michel Martelly, whom they could see on the platform in a white T-shirt, doing the occasional dance step. The former dancer—stage name "Sweet Micky"—knew how to captivate his audience.

Piarroux finally returned to his hotel around midnight. He slept like a log but had to rise early the next day to make the epidemiological surveillance meeting at DELR in the national public health laboratory—in the same room where, on October 18, members of the Brigada Médica Cubana had first sounded the alarm that there were suspected cholera cases in Mirebalais.

10

OBFUSCATION

It was Monday morning, November 22, 2010. A CDC team was presenting the results of an epidemiological case-control study. The researchers had set out to identify risk factors for contracting cholera in the town of Petite-Rivière-de-l'Artibonite, in the heart of the Artibonite valley. Did cholera come from food—perhaps brought from a coastal city? Did it come from kitchen practices or river water?

The findings were limited to people in that one community, although others in the valley region might well have responded in a similar manner. The investigators interviewed forty-nine people with cholera, asking about their diet and hygienic precautions taken in the three days before onset of their illness. They asked the same questions of ninety-eight healthy people from neighboring households—the "controls." By linking the responses of the cases and controls statistically, the CDC team could estimate the relative risk of cholera associated with the factors of interest.

The presentation offered two main—and rather puzzling—conclusions: drinking untreated water from the Artibonite River was not a risk factor; consuming meat and raw vegetables protected people from cholera. These unexpected results created quite a buzz in the room.

Piarroux sat quietly listening to the presentation, reflecting on what he had learned about the likely dynamics of Haiti's cholera epidemic from his field investigation. For a moment, his mind channeled Sherlock Holmes and his classic deduction about the dog that did not bark in the night.[1] Holmes and a detective colleague at Scotland Yard were addressing a mystery that involved the disappearance of a famous horse the night before an important race and the apparent murder of its trainer.

Regarding that night, the Scotland Yard detective asked Holmes, "Is there any other point to which you would wish to draw my attention?"

Holmes replied, "To the curious incident of the dog in the night-time."

The Scotland Yard detective thought for a moment. "The dog did nothing in the night-time."

"That," replied Holmes, "was the curious incident."

Holmes reasoned that the dog made no noise because no stranger had appeared. Instead, the late-night visitor was someone the dog knew well, and hence no barking was required.

"That you found no cholera risk from the Artibonite is, in fact, the curious cholera risk of the flowing river," thought Piarroux. He immediately recognized a timing problem with the CDC study. Since the new cholera cases were asked about their exposure to river water up to three days before they became ill, the first possible exposure time was October 31 minus three days—October 28. If his own preliminary investigation was correct, a large mass of cholera had likely entered the Artibonite River on October 17, then flowed past where the CDC study took place around October 18–19. In other words, by the time the CDC study began on October 31, the river was no longer the main transmission agent of cholera. Instead, new waves of cholera cases were probably infected mainly by previous human cases, household food or water, or contaminated well or storage water—like what happened in Saint-Marc. This explained—using the language of Sherlock Holmes—"the curious cholera risk of the flowing river."

Because of their timing, the CDC epidemiologists were correct—drinking river water was not a risk factor for *recent* cholera. However, they had failed to look for root causes, which led them to ignore the fact that drinking river water most certainly had been a risk factor when the local explosive outbreak began on October 19–20.

There was another timing problem. When the cholera epidemic was first discovered, MSPP had rapidly implemented a prevention campaign. It began on October 22, 2010. Surely, thought Piarroux, local people must have become aware that the water of the Artibonite River conveyed a deadly disease. If so, both the *current* cases and the controls would have drunk less river water than before, which would have given CDC investigators a false impression of the percentage of Petite Rivière de l'Artibonite residents who consumed river water when the initial outbreak began on October 19–20.

Yet CDC's water findings did add another piece to the puzzle. While Piarroux's own investigation was not yet complete, he had made some firm observations and had several important hunches about point source versus continuing source exposure.

He hypothesized that the Artibonite River transmitted cholera. Since exposure to the river was not a risk factor in the CDC study, he inferred that the risk had been transient with a contaminated plume serving as a passing *point source* of infection. Once the plume had flowed by and the initial wave of cholera cases had occurred, the risk of future cases was more associated with secondary human transmission or contaminated wells or stored water than with the drinking water from the river.

If CDC had reported that river drinking water was still a risk factor, this would have suggested continued soiling of the river by sewage from many cholera-ridden persons, with the river serving as a *continuing source* of infection. Each finding—whether *point source* or *continuing source*—would take the investigation in a different direction. Most important, the CDC team should have ended up at the Nepalese peacekeepers' doorstep had they only followed the clues. Piarroux was convinced that there were only two explanations for why they didn't: either they misunderstood the relevance of their study findings, or they didn't want to go anywhere near that MINUSTAH camp.

People in the room were eager for discussion. Dr. Donald Lafontant, deputy to Haiti's head epidemiologist, spoke first, followed by Barrais and then by Dr. Denis Coulombier, a French epidemiologist from the European Centre for Disease Prevention and Control who was visiting Port-au-Prince to assess several projects. The three men immediately recognized that when the study was conducted, the most likely route of contamination was contact with sick people and household transmission by soiled food and water, not river water. The percentage of people drinking Artibonite River water when the epidemic began had probably been underestimated because people avoided drinking that water after hearing the MSPP education message. And what about the observation that meat and raw vegetable consumption protected people from cholera? Wasn't it possible that the healthy controls were more prosperous than those who became cholera cases? Because of a higher standard of living indicated by eating meats and vegetables, they would have access to cleaner water and uncontaminated food. Finally, separate from risk factors, they asked why CDC had limited its study to one Artibonite département town and didn't study upriver communities in Centre département. Perhaps, thought Piarroux, they were looking under the proverbial lamppost because that was where there was light, not because it was the best place to find what they were looking for.

Piarroux got the distinct sense that CDC had seriously underestimated the knowledge and experience of the Haitians. But he saw another, more overarching problem in the agency's approach. Clearly, cholera—a disease absent from Haiti for a hundred years or more—had to have started somewhere. There had to be a point of origin in the country and an explanation for what triggered the massive outbreak. One would expect that conscientious epidemiologists would also focus on the many ways the disease was spreading in different regions of the country, noting the role of personal habits and the physical and social environment—information vital for formulating intervention and prevention programs. A single case-control study done in one geographic location is not enough to clarify complex geographic patterns. To Piarroux, when the disease was like a raging forest fire sweeping through community after community, their approach was like studying a single, smoldering tree.

It was true that the Haitians lacked specific training on the use of sophisticated statistical software and computer mapping. But aside from these practical limitations, Piarroux felt they at least had a clear sense of epidemiological fieldwork.

After the meeting, Piarroux and Barrais spoke with Dr. Lafontant, who hinted that some people in the LNSP had had accurate information on the early days of the epidemic that had never been made public—probably for political reasons, Piarroux assumed. Little by little, he was piecing together the puzzle of what had happened in Mèyé and Mirebalais. Apparently a fact-finding mission had been sent to the area soon after doctors from the Cuban brigade had reported the first cholera cases. Investigators had probably documented what had occurred, but so far there was no trace of a report.

So much remains to be discovered, thought Piarroux. But he would have to be patient. The wall of silence that had been erected was a difficult one for a foreigner to breach.

Piarroux returned to the Unité de Crise with an urgent message: the collection of epidemiological data from the communes must continue. It was the raw material crucial to analyzing the evolution of the epidemic. It would help guide decisions that could mean life or death for thousands of Haitians.

The cholera crisis was unrelenting. Since the beginning of the epidemic, the daily number of cases had risen steadily, reaching three thousand new cases per day. Only a fraction occurred in Port-au-Prince, perhaps one in five, but they had become the main concern of most Haitian leaders. Local and international health specialists had been stressing the risk of epidemic outbreaks in the slums and squalid tent camps of the city ever since the earthquake.[2] When the cholera epidemic appeared, however, public health officials quickly realized that people in the emergency tent camps were actually better protected than those in the slums—at least they had clean water.

Port-au-Prince and the immediate suburbs had thirty cholera treatment centers. The authorities wanted to double that number. They were being prudent, preparing for the worst. But the emphasis on protecting the capital city worried Piarroux. Wouldn't it hinder the ability to deploy resources to the outlying départements and more specifically to the rural communes within them?

If his weekend trip had taught Piarroux anything, it was the crucial need for a comprehensive response. He suggested setting up small, easy-to-implement treatment units in remote areas. To emphasize their importance, he pointed out that in absolute numbers there were three times more deaths so far in the rural town of Saint Michel de l'Attalaye than in Port-au-Prince.

It was with cholera maps, though, that Piarroux was most persuasive. He had developed maps showing cholera mortality for each of Haiti's 140 communes. He had used these maps in his earlier presentation to President Préval and Health Minister Larsen. Now he used them at Unité de Crise meetings with representatives from WHO, UNICEF, and the NGOs and to brief the Cuban ambassador—at Préval's request—and members of the Brigada Médica Cubana.

Piarroux was deeply impressed with the Brigada Médica Cubana, and meetings with BMC team members were especially rewarding. The Cuban government had a great reputation for helping out in crises around the world. After Hurricane Katrina devastated New Orleans, Cuba was one of the first foreign countries to step up, offering to send "some 1,600 medics, field hospitals and 83 tons of medical supplies to ease the humanitarian disaster."[3] The U.S. State Department said no—for political reasons.

In Haiti, the Cuban brigade had already deployed a large number of mobile teams in remote areas. Piarroux was able to provide the Cubans with maps of the evolving situation that complemented their own data provided from that extensive medical network.

He also wanted to engage the many humanitarian groups working in Haiti and with the UN and other international organizations. Préval, though, seemed to have a different opinion. He hadn't set up the Unité de Crise only to have to chase down the international community; he expected international organizations to recognize the problems and show up. Perhaps he felt, like many others, that the international community's long-standing use of Haiti as a laboratory for cashing in on disaster was wearing thin[4] and it was time for something different, on Haitian terms.

Piarroux never quite knew the true nature of the relations between Préval and the UN. But he sensed that the president harbored some deep-seated resentment toward many of the international organizations active in Haiti.

Most epidemiologists at the LNSP and the Unité de Crise had a pretty good idea of how the epidemic had started. The foreign humanitarian organizations in Port-au-Prince and outside Haiti largely ignored what the epidemiologists seemed to know. As time went by, it became apparent that there was an active effort to obfuscate the role of the Nepalese UN peacekeepers, aided by those who believed that cholera originates from climatic or environmental changes rather than human transmission—and theirs were strong voices.

During his final days in Haiti, Piarroux experienced again the pervasiveness of the environmental theory. The managing director of the Veolia Environment

Foundation forwarded him a message from a fund-raising specialist working with the Global Alliance Against Cholera (GAAC), started in DR Congo in early 2010 but since expanded to other cholera-affected countries. Months earlier, Piarroux and others had asked foundations and organizations to help DR Congo enhance access to safe water in its eastern cities where cholera was most prevalent. Veolia was heavily involved.

The fund-raiser had read an article about the origin of cholera in Haiti.[5] It quoted David Sack of the Johns Hopkins University School of Public Health: "Cholera is an environmental bacterium [that] can persist in the environment for many, many years without any human infections." Further, the fund-raiser explained that Sack thought the "most likely explanation [for the origin of cholera in Haiti] is a rise in temperature and salinity in the river estuaries around the Bay of Saint-Marc in the Artibonite Department of Haiti. That area, 70 miles or so northwest of Port-au-Prince, is the epicenter of the current cholera outbreak."

The same article quoted Professor Rita Colwell, one of the world's foremost experts on cholera and a member of GAAC's advisory council. She described *Vibrio cholera* as "an organism that can never be eradicated but only controlled"—a position she has espoused for many years.[6]

Never eradicated? Colwell may have been referring to eradication as a global process in the sense of eliminating cholera altogether from all populations worldwide (as with smallpox). The fund-raiser, who was not an epidemiologist, seemed to have confused global *eradication* with local *elimination*. To epidemiologists, these words have different meanings: elimination is about ridding a region or country of cholera, far different from global eradication.

The fund-raiser, though, worried that the goal of eliminating cholera in eastern DR Congo would be discredited by the scientific community. He wrote, "The article reminds us to be careful to avoid the words or implications that the GAAC Procedural Manual will lead to the 'eradication' of cholera as opposed to its 'control' as this is sure to bring the scientific community, led by Rita, down on our heads."

The foundation official tried in vain to explain that while cholera has not been globally eradicated, it had already been eliminated in some countries—England being the classic example—but to no avail. "While the context of the article [Colwell] was quoted in was clearly Haiti," the fund-raiser wrote, "the nature of the cholera bacillus is such that it will remain in the environment waiting for the right environmental conditions to allow it to become active."

Piarroux worried about the implications this exchange would have on the effort to reveal the true origin of cholera in Haiti. His investigation thus far had found no evidence of what Sack asserted. As for the claim that cholera would take root in Haiti and thereafter could never be eliminated, only controlled, Piarroux had heard that story everywhere. Comoros, Madagascar, Senegal, Ivory Coast, and Guinea had all suffered outbreaks of cholera followed by a period of total calm, and even when there were no cases for a very long time, there were always scientists who insisted they were endemic cholera areas. Scientists from the very countries with cholera would come to believe it was rooted in the environment—contradictory data be damned.

In the African countries Piarroux had visited, there was no evidence that the environment played the role of a cholera reservoir; rather, it served only as a transient site for the microorganism. Piarroux suspected that the situation in Haiti was similar. And yet the environmental theory is always center stage whenever an outbreak occurs, and officials end up believing that only economic development and massive water and sanitation programs will allow their countries to limit the resurgence of cholera epidemics.

Piarroux's experience as a scientist told him otherwise. In the early 2000s, several Latin American countries had each successfully eliminated cholera in ways that had little or nothing specifically to do with economic development. Colwell's and Sack's assertions about cholera in Haiti were only hypotheses, but he believed they were being used by others as part of something larger: the obfuscation campaign.

More immediate consequences also worried Piarroux. Predicting failure for a control program is a self-fulfilling prophecy. If the goal is elimination, public health officials need to remain aggressive even when cholera begins to weaken its grasp. Believing the scientific assertion that cholera would forever lurk in Haiti would only sap the energy of public health workers, slow or stop the funding of critical ongoing efforts, and undercut the very notion of elimination. It's folly to leave *Vibrio cholerae* alone when the microbes seem to be retreating. When transmission conditions are again favorable, such as the onset of the rainy season, the organism takes full advantage, creating epidemic havoc once again. The association with rainy weather reinforces the environmental hypothesis—even though it's wrong.

The French epidemiologist had seen a striking example in Comoros. The cholera epidemic there began in January 1998; its first peak was the following March, and then the number of cases began to decrease slowly. Piarroux and his team had set up a community-based strategy involving groups of people in what were called "hygiene committees" that went to every affected village to help people protect themselves against cholera. The strategy of hygiene and water chlorination seemed to be working. Then so-called experts insisted that cholera would be a permanent fixture of Comoros's mangrove areas and that any effort to halt transmission was useless. The money for the fight dried up, and there was an even more violent outbreak of cholera than the initial peak—precisely what Piarroux had warned would happen. Fortunately, the European Community funding agency reversed its decision and put money back into the fight until complete elimination of cholera was achieved.

Even high-profile individuals in the humanitarian sector, not wanting to criticize the UN peacekeeping mission or challenge famed researchers, embraced the environmental theory. Comments made by Dr. Rony Brauman, member and past president of Médecins Sans Frontières, in an article in the French daily newspaper *Le Monde* on November 23, 2010, were particularly disturbing.[7] Brauman was very concerned about the weakness of the international response to the cholera epidemic and the violence directed against UN peacekeepers. He drew a parallel between Haiti and the riots, fueled by social tensions, that had followed cholera outbreaks in nineteenth-century Europe. He also focused on the environmental theory. "*Vibrio cholera* thrives in stagnant and brackish waters where plankton can survive for years," wrote Brauman, "which suggests that outbreaks will persist permanently."

Piarroux knew Brauman and e-mailed him with his own findings:

> I'm still in Haiti, where I read your article as well as the interview with the American scientists who suggested climate as a cause of the current epidemic. I conducted a thorough investigation on the workings of this epidemic, which has very specific characteristics (it is particularly violent, and disseminated very rapidly compared to all other cholera epidemics I've studied).
>
> In this context, I am interested in what occurred in the early days of the epidemic. The facts I found are unfortunately very clear, showing that the epidemic began in the village below the MINUSTAH camp, and was then compounded by the release of a monstrous amount of *Vibrio cholerae* into the Artibonite River. The particularly violent character of the epidemic is the result of this phenomenal pollution of the Artibonite River, and of the flight of people frightened by the sudden deaths (140 in two days among those who drank water from the Artibonite).
>
> Climate anomalies played no role in triggering the epidemic.
>
> So far, refugee camps have been almost completely spared, while more than 60,000 cases are reported overall. Everything I state above has been covered up for various reasons, not always honorable, and appears only as an unfounded popular rumor.
>
> If I am silent about what I have found, it is because I do not want to trigger riots as the epidemic is in full swing and the election is in three days.
>
> I'll explain to you when I am back.

Brauman's response came a few hours later, startling Piarroux with its first words.

> I learned (through the back door and personally . . .) the main elements of your report on the day *Le Monde* published my article. I would have presented it differently had I read it in time! It's very compelling. You probably know that people from the *Quai* [French Foreign Affairs Ministry] are prohibited from acknowledging its existence!
>
> Anyway, as we reflect on our attitude toward this fact, the idea held by many of us here is that the price of lies (the *omertà* [code of silence] or active denial) is at least as high as that of truth. But there can be no question in this electric atmosphere that the information should be thrown to the wind, without warning. Of course, your name would not appear. We know nothing officially of your report, unless you say otherwise.

What report was he writing about? Piarroux was sure his opinions would have changed Brauman's mind, but he couldn't possibly have read a report that didn't exist. What Piarroux didn't realize was that his preliminary findings had already been shared with officials in France and elsewhere as part of the secret diplomatic communiqué sent on November 13 by the French ambassador. Although Brauman had probably seen it or heard about it, he seemed not to understand that Piarroux was not its author.

Piarroux was still unaware of the official position of the French embassy: "There is no evidence that [the cholera epidemic] was introduced by elements of the Nepalese battalion."

Piarroux had only a few more days before returning to France, and he wanted everyone battling cholera to have the most accurate information possible. He worked with Barrais to prepare monitoring maps of cholera by commune—a process slowed by many obstacles. All this disheartened Piarroux, although he retained hope.

Knowing his trip was coming to an end, he had pushed the French government to provide the services of another epidemiologist who could consolidate what had been achieved thus far and move the process forward. He proposed a military epidemiologist with infectious disease experience; the ones he had encountered had mastered the art and science of field investigations in difficult settings better than most of their civilian counterparts. The French embassy agreed to continue funding the mission and contacted CESPA, the French Armed Forces Epidemiological and Public Health Center, which in turn recommended the physician epidemiologist Rachel Haus-Cheymol. She left France immediately for Haiti and arrived on Thursday, November 25.

Meanwhile, Piarroux spent most of Thursday at the Unité de Crise. Everything was fairly routine. Then late in the afternoon a surprise envelope appeared that cast light on the rumor about an early investigation report. It was quietly handed to Piarroux by someone who wished to remain anonymous, fearing possible reprisal. Inside the envelope was the official Haitian government report that described the investigation of the initial cholera outbreak in the Mirebalais area by medical and hospital staff of both Centre département and the communes of Mirebalais and neighboring Lascahobas, including two epidemiologists.[8]

The contents were monumental. He had heard from Haitian colleagues that such a report might exist. That it had not come into his hands previously spoke volumes. He remained calm, not wanting to draw any undue attention, and scanned the document very quickly. A full and careful read would have to wait until later that evening, when he was alone at his hotel.

Piarroux spoke briefly with the anonymous envelope-deliverer about the report's timing and the need for anonymity. He stressed the importance of also getting access to any early laboratory results that might be available. The messenger promised them, matter-of-factly. Then the two parted company.

Back at the hotel, Piarroux pored over the well-written MSPP report. The narration began on Monday, October 18, when members of the Brigada Médica Cubana came to the LNSP situation room in Port-au-Prince and told of unusual cases of watery diarrhea seen over the weekend at the community hospital in Mirebalais. The DELR staff immediately telephoned Millande Tulmé, the nurse epidemiologist stationed in Hinche, who gathered her gear and headed to Mirebalais. The chief nurse at the community hospital told her the first five cases had all come from the small village of Mèyé, a few kilometers south. Tulmé was able to review the records of only three of the five cases, including a twenty-year-old man who died on October 17—but those three cases told her enough. Piarroux had met Tulmé in Hinche but had no idea she had participated in the initial investigation of the outbreak.

On Tuesday morning, October 19, Tulmé briefed her bosses in Hinche and Port-au-Prince and quickly assembled a team to investigate the situation in Mèyé. They searched households near the five cases that had come to the Mirebalais hospital and found another ten cases of diarrhea in sixteen homes. They took stool samples from six suspicious cases and sent them to LNSP for analysis.

Over the next few days, Tulmé's team disseminated information on diarrhea prevention through loudspeakers on vehicles and on the radio. They pressed local NGOs to provide sanitation and medical assistance and searched for additional cases in Mirebalais and environs.

On Thursday, October 21, another Haitian teamed arrived with senior officials from DELR. They learned that repair work on Mirebalais streets had created a water supply problem. Fewer than 10 percent of the city population was getting safe drinking water. That team met with local engineers, urging them to solve the problem quickly.

That same day both teams also went to Annapurna Camp. They were not allowed to enter but spoke with the camp doctor, who told them there had been no reported diarrhea cases over the previous two weeks. It was an incredible claim, thought Piarroux, since diarrhea is so common among travelers. Two community members then showed the teams the wastewater being discharged from the camp and an open septic pit local villagers said was used to hold the camp excreta. The report stated that the open pit by the UN camp was near the two streams by the camp, both flowing into the La Theme River, a tributary of the Artibonite River. The Haitian team collected water samples from the Artibonite and sent them as well to Port-au-Prince for analysis.

Tulmé's local team returned to Annapurna Camp the next day, accompanied by the regional health officer. They took samples of the wastewater in the open septic pit on the hilltop and from the river water that flowed near the discharge pipes coming from the camp and sent them to LNSP.

The report left no doubt as to the epidemic's starting point. The investigators did everything right.

Why had Piarroux not seen the report sooner? The information was critical to his field investigation. This early report by Haitian health officials was nothing short of a *bombshell.* Its contents would probably enrage the Haitian public and certainly could sway the upcoming elections. The UN's bringing a deadly disease to a country it was ostensibly helping had ramifications well beyond Haiti. It could alter the course of international relations and focus disturbing attention on UN peacekeeping. Piarroux speculated that the powerful international organizations that essentially "ran" Haiti would have worked overtime to make sure all copies of the report were destroyed had they known of its existence.

Why was he given the report at that particular moment? Did President Préval authorize it? Had he now shown himself worthy of the trust of the Haitians?

Piarroux was a knowledgeable and tenacious epidemiologist. He would be leaving Haiti very soon. He assumed that those who furnished him the report wanted it whisked out of the country so it could be widely circulated.

The day after the two MSPP public health teams had visited Annapurna Camp on Thursday, October 21, a new press posting appeared on the MINUSTAH website—perhaps reacting to the findings of the Haitian investigators. It seems either not to have been seen (until much later) or to have been largely ignored by everyone investigating cholera in Haiti, from scientists to journalists. Piarroux was unaware of it until long after he had left Haiti. (The press release remained on the MINUSTAH website for at least two years thereafter.)

The posting stated that the first case of cholera had occurred on September 24, 2010, in the lower Artibonite region, citing MSPP as the information source.[9] But this was not true. MSPP hadn't even known of suspicious cases of watery diarrhea until told of them by the Brigada Médica Cubana on October 18. Later, Haiti's national laboratory would report October 14 as the onset date of the first laboratory-confirmed case of cholera in Haiti. Figure 10.1 provides a timeline of the curious MINUSTAH reaction.

The start date for the cholera epidemic was clearly erroneous—weeks before the actual onset. What were the MINUSTAH officials up to? Trying to focus attention away from the Nepalese camp? To send anyone who might come sniffing around down a different path?

Piarroux didn't know it, but some Haitians had been given an inkling of the MSPP's initial investigation in Mèyé. Roberson Alphonse of the Haitian newspaper *Le Nouvelliste* had even interviewed Tulmé.[10] His article had appeared four days before Piarroux's arrival in Haiti. It focused on the cholera outbreak and the Nepalese peacekeepers and identified Rosemond Lorimé as the first "hospital death" in Mirebalais. He had lived in Mèyé, less than two hundred meters from Annapurna Camp.

Alphonse also mentioned that investigators had been to the camp. "Officially," he wrote, they "did not find any trace of the Asian cholera vibrio responsible for the deaths of thirty others and hospitalization of 1,672 others in the area." Using the word "officially" seemed to imply there was more to the story than met the eye, but it was unlikely Alphonse ever saw the actual MSPP report.

The *Le Nouvelliste* piece did not garner the international attention the articles by Walker and Katz received. Then the MSPP report itself was suppressed, resurfacing only when handed to Piarroux that fateful Thursday afternoon.

The next morning, the same person who had given Piarroux the suppressed report delivered the promised laboratory results of the six samples from Mèyé sent to LNSP on October 19. Five, from patients aged twelve to forty-three, were positive for cholera (figure 10.2). The twenty-year-old man's symptom onset date of October 14 appeared to be the first laboratory-confirmed case of cholera in a Haitian in Haiti.

Data on early cases from the report and laboratory results were especially important to Piarroux's investigation. There might have been earlier cases of cholera in Haiti, but these five were the first *laboratory-confirmed* cases. They provided clues to the origin of the outbreak based on true cholera cases, not a

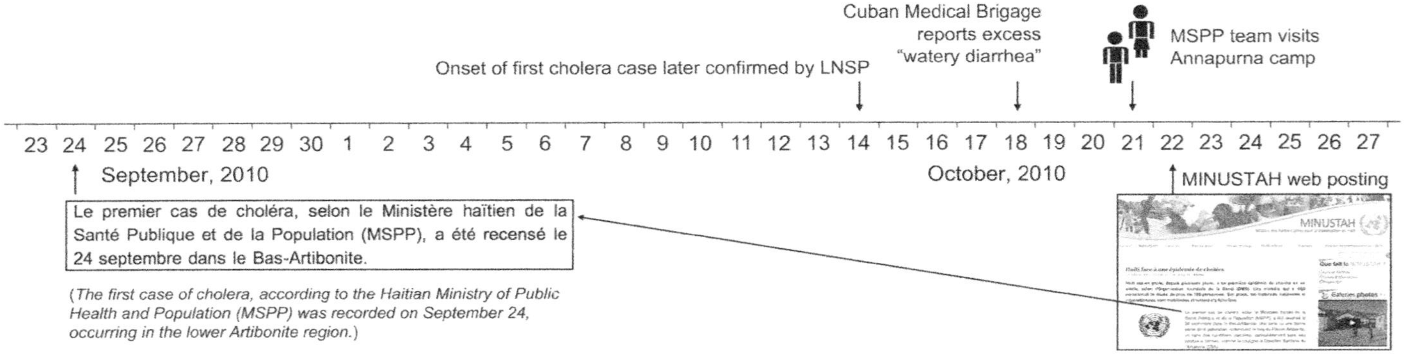

FIGURE 10.1. Events relating to MINUSTAH posting of September 24 cholera starting date. Website screenshot comes from MINUSTAH, "Haïti face à une épidémie de cholera" ["Haiti Faces a Cholera Epidemic"].

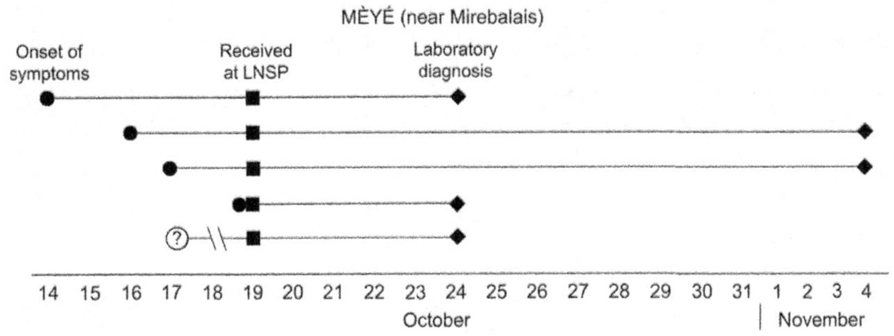

FIGURE 10.2. First five laboratory-confirmed cholera cases in Haiti. Based on data from Laboratoire National de Sante Publique, Port-au-Prince, Haiti.

mixture of true and false cases. The onset times of symptoms were gathered by the Haitian investigators for four of the five cases. Piarroux used his detective tool—knowledge of the incubation period—to count backwards from the onset times to assess when these cases had likely become infected.

But while the onset times gave Piarroux a general idea of when each case was infected, they did not allow him to distinguish between a point source of infection, a continuing source of infection, and person-to-person transmission of infection. Given the range of incubation periods, there was a small chance that all four cases had been infected by the same point source in Mèyé on the same day, perhaps October 12 or 13. Yet Piarroux couldn't rule out a continuing source of infection in Mèyé, with each case infected by the same source but on a different day. The data also supported the notion that the first case of October 14 had passed the microbe on to the remaining three cases. Still, while the incubation period was useful for guiding Piarroux's thinking, it was not biologically exact enough to indicate precisely what had happened. There was still an open question: *Where* and *when* did the epidemic actually start?

One nagging problem was that LNSP did not make the laboratory confirmation of *Vibrio cholerae* O1 Ogawa El Tor for the five cases from Centre département until five to sixteen days after receiving the specimens. In the ensuing months, that management delay for the early cases would become part of the campaign to shift the public perception of where the epidemic had actually originated.

Much of Piarroux's last full day in Port-au-Prince was spent with his replacement, Rachel Haus-Cheymol, discussing the ongoing mission. They visited the French embassy and went to the Unité de Crise for introductions—including to President Préval and Minister of Health Larsen, both of whom happened to be there.

It was Piarroux's last chance to speak with Larsen about the likely source of the cholera epidemic. Larsen already knew much of what Piarroux told him, and he didn't want any of it to come out publicly until after the elections. And he wanted someone other than the minister of health telling the true story. Piarroux understood: it was all about the dance of politics and power, a difficult dance for him. As a scientist, he knew that getting out the truth simply trumped all other considerations.

Piarroux's flight to France was scheduled for late Saturday morning. There was still time for a last visit to the French embassy with Chevallier and Haus-Cheymol. The French ambassador had returned the night before, and now he greeted them over coffee. The group took stock of Piarroux's three-week mission. The ambassador seemed pleased with how things had advanced. They discussed Haus-Cheymol's work, the prospect of Piarroux's returning in early 2011 when the dry season would contribute to cholera's decrease, and his plans to prepare a scientific publication. The ambassador had no objections—it was the role of an academic, after all, to write such articles.

First, though, Piarroux had to prepare a report on his visit. He wanted to describe the spread of the epidemic, especially in Haiti's remote rural areas. Ambassador Le Bret warned Piarroux to be cautious with journalists but suggested he speak with Deborah Pasmantier, a reporter for Agence France-Presse in Paris. She was someone in whom he had confidence, and he gave Piarroux her personal telephone number.

The entire visit was cordial. As they parted, the ambassador complemented Piarroux, saying he was "the right man at the right moment."

Piarroux's long flight home was an ordeal. He had planned to begin mentally organizing his trip report, but soon lack of sleep caught up with him. Before drifting off, he found himself contemplating fate and marveled at how its winds had brought him to Haiti during a tumultuous cholera epidemic. He had learned so much and had even more to share about the spread and impact of the deadly disease. But his thoughts kept returning to something very specific: the peculiar origin of Haitian cholera and his disturbing findings.

It was apparent that most Haitians wanted the truth. They wanted a full report of what had caused the dramatic early spread of the disease. More and more foreigners, though, and even some Haitians, wanted the opposite. Fate had dropped Piarroux right in the middle. He was an epidemiologist comfortable with investigations, with facts, and with truth. He had no interest in dealing with politics, but he felt he had no choice but to speak truth to power.

11

SPECULATION

Piarroux found sleep pointless. He kept thinking about the report and lab results he had received just before he left Haiti, wondering whether the person who had actually handed him the document was authorized to do so. Surely, given the report's importance, that person wouldn't have taken action unilaterally. No, Piarroux thought, only one explanation made sense: it had been leaked on the authority of President René Préval, acting through Minister of Health Alex Larsen.

The plane was largely silent as other passengers tried to sleep despite the discomfort of economy-class seats. Piarroux thought about still voices and then specifically about the deafening silence of the Haitian leaders regarding the epidemic's origin. Apart from statements on the day the epidemic was announced, not much had been said about the origin. Préval and Larsen in particular had seemed to avoid saying anything publicly—giving the impression that at the very moment a deadly epidemic was sweeping across their country, already devastated by an earthquake, it was not important to seek the cause. Now, though, Piarroux began to see that silence differently. Convinced that Préval and Larsen were behind his being given the report and lab results, he realized that they did want the truth to come out—a truth they knew. That they hadn't spoken said more about the stronger power at work that was capable of controlling a president and the ministers of a sovereign nation, and that could muzzle respectable institutions such as PAHO and CDC, than it did about the two Haitian leaders.

ırroux thought more about Préval and Larsen. Préval was sixty-seven years old, a distinguished national leader in the last year of his second five-year presidential term. The election for his successor was slated for the very day Piarroux would arrive home. Only much later did it become clear to Piarroux and the world just how tumultuous Préval's relationship had been with the MINUSTAH leader Edmond Mulet, who enjoyed tremendous power. Préval had little to no control over national security, neither police nor military. He had no say over MINUSTAH's activities or budget in his own country. Meanwhile, a Guatemalan acted as if he were the man in charge of Haiti because he led a gigantic outside force.

To add insult to injury, there were thousands of NGOs in Haiti that did not answer to Préval's government but were instead responsible only to their respective leaders and donors.[1] Many conducted their activities and moved throughout the country without consulting or even informing local or national officials. Thus, in a proud nation that had won its independence from colonial rule less than a half century after the United States defeated its own British colonizers, the country's president was subjected to challenges, orders, and other indignities from all sorts of foreigners. Everything was coming to a head as the election loomed at the end of November, including a slight by another international organization.

The Organization of American States (OAS) is a very influential group that brings together thirty-five countries, including Haiti, as a "political, juridical, and social governmental forum in the [Western] Hemisphere."[2] Over time, it became disenchanted with Préval and wanted him to stay out of the election for his successor. Ricardo Seitenfus, then the OAS special representative in Haiti, revealed later that "the international community had 'offered' President Préval a plane out of the country during Haiti's chaotic first-round election in November 2010."[3] Was his fate to be the same as that of former President Jean-Bertrand Aristide?

After the election, Préval's term was to continue until February 7, 2011, when the new president would be sworn in. But a runoff required because no candidate received 50 percent of the vote extended Préval's term to May 14.[4] Leaving early would have shortened his presidency by nearly six months and certainly affected his legacy.

Préval himself provided details of the November 28 "offer" in a 2013 documentary, *Assistance mortelle* (*Fatal Assistance*). "I got a phone call from [Mulet] . . . saying, 'Mr. President this is a political problem. We need to get you on a plane and evacuate you.'" "I said, 'Bring your plane, collect me from the palace, handcuff me, everyone will see that it's a kidnapping.'"[5]

Clearly, Préval had every intention of serving out the remainder of his term.

Asked about Préval's allegation, Mulet told a *Toronto Star* reporter, "I never said that, he never answered that" and claimed he "was worried if [Préval] didn't stop the fraud and rioting, a revolution would force him to leave. I didn't have the capability, the power or the interest of putting him on a plane."[6] By the time he spoke with the reporter, Mulet was gone from Haiti and back in his earlier post as the UN's head of peacekeeping operations.

The truth of this attempted "evacuation"—addressed by both Seitenfus and Préval—may never be known.

Then there was Alex Larsen, who had joined the Préval government in 2008 as minister of health. Like Préval, he was in his sixties. Trained as a cardiologist, in 2004 he became director of Office d'Assurance Accidents du Travail, Maladie et Maternité (OFATMA), a government medical care organization funded from workers' compensation insurance Haitian employers are required to pay.[7] Larsen and Préval got along very well, and Préval—not known for delegating—seemed to have no problem anointing Larsen as his administration's main spokesperson for health-related matters.

Piarroux was struck from the beginning by Larsen's friendly, open personality. With his well-groomed white mustache, glasses, and alert eyes, he had the appearance of a kindly country doctor who could relate to ordinary people. But he also had an international reputation and traveled outside Haiti to discuss public health and policy matters.[8]

In May 2010, Larsen attended a World Health Assembly meeting in Switzerland, where he met the then U.S. secretary of health and human services Kathleen Sebelius, his American counterpart in the agency that presides over CDC. They spoke of CDC's work "to help public health surveillance and improve laboratory capacity and epidemiological and laboratory training." It was four months after the earthquake and five months before the onset of cholera. Larsen expressed his appreciation for CDC and U.S. development assistance.[9]

When cholera first broke out, Larsen demonstrated real leadership. The Health Ministry was "the first to diagnose the outbreak" and took "the lead, telling non-governmental organizations that the Haitian government—not the international community—will confirm casualty numbers and dictate where treatment centers are set up."[10] Piarroux imagined how upset Larsen must have been that CDC was less than forthright in its initial assistance and then actively ignored how the devastating cholera epidemic had reached Haiti's shores.

Like Préval, Larsen was critical of the NGOs and their lack of coordination, permission, or guidance from the Haitian government. At the launch of the UN's annual "State of the World's Population 2010" report in Haiti he said, "There are good NGOs and bad ones. There are more bad ones than good ones here."[11]

Larsen then articulated the same feelings Piarroux had heard so many other Haitians express about MINUSTAH and the other foreigners in their country. "They go where they want and do what they want, and we do not accept that.... We are poor and we are in need, the clothes that I am wearing are not in good shape . . . but it is clean. I demand respect, and I demand respect for the people of the republic. Come and help me but respect me."

Piarroux never felt any of that wrath when speaking with Larsen, who always seemed to appreciate his presence and value his respectful nature and commitment to letting truth, not politics, be his guide. Now on his return flight to France, he imagined Larsen and Préval discussing whether or not to give him the secret MSPP October 21–24 report and early laboratory data.

Now Piarroux could better understand why authorities affiliated with or part of the United Nations would, at least officially, advocate not looking for the source of Haiti's epic cholera epidemic. It was political. But what nagged at him, what still kept him from sleeping, was fellow epidemiologists who were working for CDC. Already there was suspicion that the UN peacekeeping base near Mirebalais was involved. Yet in no uncertain terms, CDC's associate director for communication had told a reporter that CDC was not directly investigating the base. In the weeks that followed, three CDC epidemiologists—including two up-and-coming leaders of the organization—also chimed in, stating it was not the time to pursue cholera's origin.

How could any epidemiologist possibly think looking for the source was wrong or not timely? And yet not a single CDC epidemiologist had ever said, "We are going to get to the bottom of this origin issue."

CDC's politics wasn't the only thing disturbing Piarroux. There was also the matter of the report and laboratory results he had been given before leaving Haiti. He couldn't stop wondering why he had been entrusted with the Haitian report. His strong suspicion was that Préval and Larsen had wanted him to know the truth, even though, because of politics, they couldn't reveal it to others. And it was probably already clear to them that CDC wasn't interested in the truth.

When CDC first learned of the cholera outbreak, the organization, including its 119 employees deployed to Haiti, sprang into action.[12] The agency had been closely involved with the Haitian government for a long time prior to cholera. In 2002, two years before MINUSTAH arrived, CDC opened an office in Haiti to assist the government in dealing with HIV/AIDS, including support for a national laboratory.[13] In 2006, it joined others to establish LNSP,[14] later rebuilt after the earthquake with the assistance of U.S. charitable foundations. To this day, the building houses personnel in DELR, the epidemiological unit of the Haitian government, and CDC staff stationed in Haiti.[15] The collaborative partnership between the two countries, including joint authoring of many scientific publications, continues.

One would have thought, then, that CDC epidemiologists would put themselves at the forefront of the investigation of how cholera came to Haiti. To call CDC's lack of interest unusual is an understatement. CDC has a worldwide reputation for investigating outbreaks and for its extensive training activities and many helpful publications specific to such investigations.[16] In the United States, it is often the lead coordinator among investigators "to detect the outbreak, define its size and extent, and to identify the source." When food is involved, CDC offers clear guidance, stating that a source investigation "suggests ways to control the outbreak and prevent similar outbreaks from happening in the future."[17] That's basic infectious disease epidemiology.

Between 2001 and 2011, some 111 reported cholera cases appeared in the United States.[18] CDC epidemiologists showed their detective chops by tracing the origin of all but one. More than 80 percent were associated with international travel to named countries, while the others were domestically acquired, mainly from consuming infected seafood.

The bottom line: given the chance, CDC epidemiologists know how to investigate the source of a cholera outbreak. In Haiti, enterprising journalists pointed out the road to Mirebalais and the nearby Annapurna Camp, making the job even easier.

Something else baffled Piarroux. While some CDC epidemiologists were saying the agency had neither the time nor the interest in uncovering the source, CDC's own weekly report—*Morbidity and Mortality Weekly Reports*—was suggesting otherwise. The publication provided several interesting findings about the cholera microbe, including its potential arrival in Haiti. The *MMWR* authors stated that initial laboratory tests of fourteen isolates from persons in Artibonite département were caused by a single strain and wrote, "If these isolates are representative of those currently circulating in Haiti, the findings suggest that *Vibrio cholerae* was likely introduced into Haiti in one event."[19]

What that "one event" might have been, or where it might have taken place, was left to the reader's imagination. Piarroux had his theory; the *MMWR* authors allowed for a very wide scope of possibilities: "*Vibrio cholerae* strains that are indistinguishable from the outbreak strain by all methods used have previously been found in countries in South Asia and elsewhere."

In an accompanying comment, the *MMWR* editor wrote, "The initial cholera outbreak investigation suggested that exposure to contaminated water was the likely cause of the initial cases in Artibonite Department."

So, CDC investigators recognized that cholera was probably introduced to Haiti in one event. They acknowledged that contaminated water had caused the initial cholera cases in the downriver Artibonite département. They obviously knew the news reports that focused on Annapurna Camp but decided not to follow through with an investigation there. Even more certain was that they knew of the data at Haiti's national public health laboratory, with which CDC collaborated closely, that showed the first cases came from Centre département.

Two CDC epidemiologists spoke to the press when the cholera outbreak began: Dowell and Dr. Jordan Tappero. Both held prominent positions in the agency, had considerable international experience, were highly regarded, and had published extensively on a wide variety of public health and epidemiological topics. Tappero—a physician, epidemiologist, and administrator—had become director of a new unit in CDC's Center for Global Health just after Haiti's January 2010 earthquake. When cholera first appeared, he was among the leaders of CDC's response team in Haiti, along with Dowell.

Piarroux had connected with Dowell many years before in Africa. In 1994 Dowell—who had already built a body of international experience and spoke French—was deployed to Zaire (now DR Congo). A massive influx of about eight hundred thousand Rwandan refugees had crossed the border into Zaire, and epidemics of cholera and dysentery soon followed, with much loss of life and many abandoned children. In short order, about ten thousand unaccompanied children were being cared for in more than twenty centers in and around the town of Goma.

Piarroux, like Dowell a pediatrician by training, was also in Zaire with Médecins du Monde organizing public health assistance programs for children in a camp near Goma. The two men met. Each had respect for the other's work. A few weeks after he returned to France, Dowell invited Piarroux to coauthor an article about the children in the Goma camps. Piarroux agreed, and in 1995 their "Letter from Goma" was published.[20] Two years later, they met again when Rwandan refugees in Zaire were forced to flee from eastern Zaire and, in some cases, return to Rwanda.

Though Piarroux respected Dowell and his work, he was troubled by his and CDC's seeming lack of interest in finding the source of cholera in Haiti. Was this stellar scientific organization actually so subject to political influence?

As it turns out, Piarroux's question had been addressed a few years earlier. A "frighteningly virulent strain" of tuberculosis appeared in the United States in 2007 and questions were raised about how CDC was handling the crisis. An ABC News reporter wondered about "the extent to which [CDC] is an agency influenced by politics." He noted that it "enjoys a reputation for being independent" despite being part of the U.S. Department of Health and Human Services, and is "among the government's most trusted institutions." But he found several instances that caused him to wonder whether CDC was, in truth, "above the [political] fray." One was in 2006 and dealt with a highly charged U.S. political issue, when the agency "agreed to a politician's request that it insert two pro-abstinence speakers at a national sexually-transmitted-disease-prevention conference in Florida. It also removed panelists who would have discussed links between abstinence-only programs and rising STD rates."

Adding fuel to the fire was Dr. James Mason, who ran CDC from 1983 to 1989. He acknowledged that politics had always been a force to be reckoned with at the agency, then stated that it "should come as no surprise. . . . Of course you are going to have some political oversight and political influence. It's inherent and necessary."[21]

Given the long shared history of Haiti, the United Nations, and the United States, and the unusual statements of Dowell and Tappero, Piarroux was finding it easier and easier to understand that politics played a big role. Who would have enough power to constrain a nation's leaders and prevent every epidemiologist from PAHO and CDC from seeking the origin of the epidemic? Only highly influential U.S. officials, Piarroux suspected—and it was not an idea he liked.

Now another question occurred to him: Why was it so important for these unknown high-level U.S. officials to cover up what was probably the consequence of negligence on the part of foreign UN peacekeepers?

For more than a half century, the UN has been involved in peacekeeping efforts.[22] During much of that period, the United States has been a major supporter and financial contributor to these efforts, including the stationing of peacekeeping troops in Haiti.

Political turmoil has been a hallmark of Haitian history since U.S. troops left in 1934. The country experienced elections and then military coup d'états overturning the results in a seeming cycle. From 1957 to 1986, the Duvalier family dominated Haitian politics, with both father and son nominally presidents but actually dictators. They were brutal men who robbed the nation of its wealth and violently suppressed dissent with the Tonton Macoutes, a paramilitary force created in 1959. The death squad's name comes from a Haitian Creole mythological figure ("Uncle Gunnysack" in English) who kidnaps and punishes unruly children, taking them away in a macoute to be eaten for breakfast. Even after the Duvalier era, the Tonton Macoutes remained in one form or another, and Haiti continued to be ruled by presidents or the military, often in rapid succession.

The second major military occupation of Haiti during the twentieth century had its genesis in 1990, when the popular Roman Catholic priest Jean-Bertrand

Aristide was elected president, followed less than a year later by a military coup and ferocious suppression of human rights. In 1994, the UN Security Council adopted a resolution encouraging the removal of the military leadership and new democratic elections. The United States was prepared to send troops into Haiti, but held off when President Bill Clinton convinced the military leaders to step down and restore Aristide to power until 1996, when the constitution barred his reelection to a consecutive term.

In 1996, Haiti experienced a historic first: the transition from one democratically elected president to another, when René Préval—an Aristide ally—won a five-year term as president with a resounding vote total. But unrest continued. In 1999 Préval, frustrated by political gridlock, dismissed the elected parliament and assumed total rule.

Aristide accused Préval and his party of "distance from the people." He formed a new party and ran for election again, winning with more than 90 percent of the vote and returning to the presidency in 2001. Even before he was inaugurated, Haiti verged on bankruptcy and social programs were in disarray. While many viewed Aristide as close to the people, especially in poor neighborhoods, others considered him a self-serving demagogue. His time in office was again turbulent, with gangs, political rivals, and wayward police adding to the mix, eventually leading to open rebellion. "Aristide was a virtual prisoner in the midst of his own security apparatus," wrote Peter Hallward about those days.[23]

In early 2004, open rebellion was common in the countryside. In Port-au-Prince, Aristide supporters "dragged out large objects—containers, rusted-out trucks, boulders, discarded refrigerators, rubber tires—and mounted them into a protective corridor around the National Palace." Once the government talked them into removing the barriers, the turmoil continued with the opposition calling for "the president's unconditional departure from Haiti," although as noted by Randall Robinson, "none of Aristide's foes argued that he had committed an impeachable offense."[24] Aristide was forced from power in the early hours of Sunday, February 29, and taken to the Central African Republic—not unlike what nearly happened to Préval years later, in November 2010. Aristide "claimed he'd been kidnapped and didn't know where he was being taken until, at the end of a 20-hour flight, he was told that he and his wife would be landing 'in a French military base in the middle of Africa,'" wrote the same Paul Farmer who later called CDC's inaction on cholera's origin "political." Meanwhile, back in Haiti, Boniface Alexandre, chief justice of the supreme court—having just been sworn in as interim president—petitioned the UN to send international peacekeepers. That same day, the UN Security Council authorized the "immediate deployment of a Multinational Interim Force for a period of not more than three months" that was extended for over a decade and became known by the French acronym

MINUSTAH, a multinational force eventually composed of more than eight thousand troops and police.[25]

Among other concerns, the Security Council worried about the safety of NGOs and demanded that "all parties in Haiti provide safe and unimpeded access to humanitarian agencies to allow them to carry out their work."[26] While human rights and many other issues were raised, the main concern of MINUSTAH was always security, the rule of law, crime, and political violence. The UN recognized that charitable work and lawlessness do not fit well together.

It didn't take long for UN peacekeepers to become Haiti's most dominant military, economic, and political force. By November 2004, about 4,500 foreign troops and nearly 1,000 police from more than thirty different countries had descended on the country. Some 60 percent came from four South American countries: Argentina, Brazil, Chile, and Uruguay. But other countries also sent troops, including Nepal, with 137 troops to begin with.[27] Soon, though, Nepal's troop contribution grew significantly larger. By August 2010, Nepal—the poorest country to contribute to the force—provided about 1,200 soldiers and police, second only to Brazil.[28]

For Nepal, participating in UN peacekeeping is a moneymaker. In 2013, the flat-rate annual compensation by the UN for all countries that contribute personnel to MINUSTAH was about $12,000 per person, independent of actual incurred expenses.[29] That's far below typical salaries in some contributing countries, but for the Nepalese it is five or more times the average annual salary back home. On top of that, the UN salaries benefit the entire Nepalese military, since some money goes into a welfare fund that provides medical and educational support for military families.[30] The financial appeal of UN peacekeeping helps explain why Nepal is the fourth-largest troop-contributing country to UN peacekeeping missions globally,[31] and perhaps why the troops would be so keen to make sure their reputations were not tarnished by something as sordid as bringing a deadly disease to Haiti. The country wanted to make sure opportunities to participate in peacekeeping continued.

The United States also benefits from troop arrangements with the UN, especially by comparison with the troubles it once endured in occupying Haiti directly. Having troops from multiple countries makes it hard to pin the "U.S. imperialism" tag on the mission—a particularly sensitive issue given U.S.-Haitian history.[32] "Increasing the effectiveness of UN peacekeeping is one of the highest priorities for the United States at the United Nations," declared a U.S. State Department Fact Sheet posted barely a month before the Haiti cholera outbreak.[33] "Multilateral peacekeeping shares the risks and responsibilities of maintaining international peace and security, and is a cost-effective way to help achieve U.S. strategic and humanitarian interests."

MINUSTAH takes pains to state publicly and frequently that it is deployed with the consent of the Haitian government, expected to use only very limited force beyond self-defense, and that it always remains impartial among contending parties in the country. In short, MINUSTAH gives the United States the stability it desired in the Caribbean region, without encouraging direct anti-U.S. resentment among the Haitian people. It saves a lot of money too. The annual cost of the Haiti operation from 2008 to 2012 ranged from about $550 million to nearly $795 million dollars. The U.S. contribution was about 29 percent of the required budget.[34] Such a hefty contribution makes the United States a very influential partner of MINUSTAH, but its contribution is only a fraction of what would be necessary if the United States were fulfilling the role of peacekeeper by itself with U.S. soldiers, police, and higher-standard facilities.

The U.S. military stayed out of Haiti until January 14, not entering until two days after the 2010 earthquake. "This is a time when we are reminded of the common humanity that we all share," said President Barack Obama, characterizing it as a humanitarian intervention and encouraging donations from the public.[35] By month's end, the U.S. military had seventeen thousand personnel in and around Haiti.[36] They remained until late March, when UN peacekeeping troops again took the dominant role.

Piarroux wondered about all this on his flight back to France. He could not help but think that word had come down from the U.S. government to CDC to downplay the possible role of the UN in the cholera disaster. So much was at stake for the United States and the United Nations, including potentially long-term negative effects on peacekeeping efforts around the world.

Piarroux's mind continued to race as he flew home. He imagined how a U.S. government scientist might find it difficult to ignore political pressure from senior officials. A scientist with especially strong personal ties to Haiti might find it even more difficult. Scott Dowell had spent part of his youth in Deschapelles, where his father was a pediatrician, and he had served from 1999 for five years as medical director at Albert Schweitzer Hospital—the institution inundated with cholera cases in the 2010 outbreak. Years later, after becoming a high CDC official with considerable global health experience, he joined the board of that hospital, helping secure funds for many health and humanitarian projects. It didn't surprise Piarroux to learn that Dowell was among the first to hear from Dr. Ian Rawson, the hospital's managing director, when cholera first appeared.

The French epidemiologist tried to put himself in the shoes of a scientist like Dowell or anyone else working for an agency of a powerful government with interests that go well beyond science. How would he deal with a request from that government to abandon a critical aspect of an epidemiological investigation?

What if his government insisted that safety and security were more important than scientific integrity at a given moment? What if he were told flat out that the political consequences of revealing the truth could be devastating, perhaps sparking rage and mayhem?

Piarroux wanted to believe he would always uphold scientific truth, but he had never confronted such a situation in his own work. He understood the notion of cover-ups and that they can be a double-edged sword. He imagined what would happen anywhere if multiple witnesses saw a policeman shoot a teenager in cold blood, and there was no follow-up investigation. A riot would no doubt ensue. What if investigators found that an accidental wildfire was caused by a careless off-duty fireman and then covered it up? Big or small, cover-ups usually provoke anger, rage, cynicism, and distrust—especially when authorities publicly refuse to investigate.

The Swedish ambassador, Claes Hammar, told a Swedish journalist he "had it confirmed by a diplomatic source that the cholera comes from Nepal" and then revealed to a Finnish journalist that his source was "a United States official, but I cannot say who." Piarroux wondered whether that source was a CDC employee so unhappy with the political pressure that he had taken that huge risk. Was the whisper to the Swedish ambassador an effort to get the cholera investigation back on track, and was the whisperer torn between internal forces?

12

PANDEMICS AND SOUTH ASIA

South Asia—identified as the original home of Haiti's cholera, first by CDC and then by scientists in the *New England Journal of Medicine*[1]—is loosely defined as the southern region of the Asian continent, typically including seven countries. They are nations that touch or cross the Himalayan mountains—Pakistan, India, Nepal and Bhutan—as well as the sub-Himalayan countries of Bangladesh, Sri Lanka, and Maldives. Some definitions include Afghanistan to the west and Myanmar to the east.

The seven core countries account for well more than 20 percent of the world's population and together comprise the most densely populated region on earth. South Asia is also the world's second-poorest region, after sub-Saharan Africa. While there are areas of considerable wealth, many feature a toxic mix of crowded cities with people almost piled on top of each other, crushing poverty, miserable water problems, and deplorable sanitary conditions. Water and sanitation issues are pervasive in rural areas too. Such poverty creates breeding grounds for diseases and their transmission.

Cholera is an ancient infirmity. Evidence suggests it was present nearly ten thousand years ago when changes in agricultural practices led to more sedentary communities, creating new niches for the disease.[2]

Seven cholera pandemics have been described since the early nineteenth century, when global reporting got under way. "Pandemic" is a word epidemiologists use to describe a disease that has actively spread to many countries, often worldwide. Pandemics, which can last for years or even decades, typically begin as outbreaks or new cases in a local setting and then expand to an epidemic as cases spread to multiple regions or even an entire nation. When cases occur in many countries, the pattern becomes a pandemic. By its nature, a pandemic is defined well after it has begun since the earlier stages of outbreak and epidemic take time to unfold. Because of inexact beginning and ending dates, historical researchers differ in their dating of pandemics, sometimes by years. This has been the problem with cholera, which has been particularly hard to quantify because the causative agent was not clearly identified until 1884.

The first six pandemics (the first beginning in 1816–17)—all caused by the classic biotype of *Vibrio cholera*, serogroup O1—began in or near the Ganges Delta of South Asia, the largest of the world's deltas. It flows into the Bay of Bengal and is considered the "homeland of cholera."[3] This gave rise to the notion of an aquatic coastal environment as a reservoir of *Vibrio cholerae*, sheltering the organism between pandemics.

The seventh and current pandemic began in 1961 and is perhaps the easiest to describe. It started in Indonesia and then appeared in the Bay of Bengal. From there, "at least three independent but overlapping waves with common ancestor in the 1950s" ultimately described as one pandemic emerged and flowed to other regions of the world.[4] This seventh pandemic eventually found its way to Haiti in October 2010.

The seventh pandemic is different from its predecessors in three ways. It is the largest, with more than seven million cases in over fifty countries since 1961.[5] The disease first became evident nearly 2,700 miles southeast of the Ganges Delta in the main islands of Indonesia, starting in Java and Borneo in March–July 1961, then on to Sumatra and Sulawesi.[6] And the agent itself is different, although still *Vibrio cholerae* O1. Rather than the classic biotype of earlier pandemics, the seventh features the biotype El Tor of *Vibrio cholerae* O1.

After beginning in the Indonesian islands, *Vibrio cholerae* O1 El Tor spread through much of the Malay Archipelago, on to Southeast Asia and South Asia, and then to the Soviet Union. Eventually, it reached the Middle East, Africa, and Latin America. In early 1991, cholera appeared in Peru, then Ecuador and Colombia followed by other South and Central American countries. Despite its relative proximity, though, Haiti was spared until 2010, years after the regional pandemic ended in 2002.

Piarroux confronted the seventh pandemic in Africa, witnessing the devastation during the 1994 Goma outbreak in what is now DR Congo. The disease among the many refugees pouring in from Rwanda was believed to have caused twelve thousand deaths in a few short weeks.[7]

An odd thing happened in 1992, three decades into the seventh pandemic. Throughout the previous six, damage from *Vibrio cholerae* was caused by the O1 serogroup. But then in South Asia's Ganges Delta, a new serogroup emerged—O139. The "new" cholera caused explosive outbreaks in Bangladesh and India and spread to neighboring countries. Some suggested this was the beginning of an eighth pandemic. But then *Vibrio cholerae* O1 El Tor reappeared on the Indian continent and temporarily displaced the O139 serogroup. In 1996, *Vibrio cholerae* O139 reemerged, and both O1 and O139 remained in cholera endemic areas of India and elsewhere. All strains are considered part of the seventh pandemic.[8]

Cholera pandemics are created by the interplay between microbe and people—crowding, poor sanitation, dirty water, and stress—and are intensified by religious pilgrimages, political havoc, wars and troop movements, and mass transportation such as boats, trains, or planes. Susceptible persons are brought into close contact with infectious cases or contaminated food and water, which results in more new cases.

When the first cholera pandemic began in India in 1816–17, the disease was known as "Asiatic Cholera." Since accurate records were not kept, deaths were poorly tallied.

Troops fighting in two wars were pivotal in spreading the disease. The Arab state of Oman experienced cholera following a war in which infected soldiers brought the disease from India. Thereafter, it spread to Turkey and then was brought home to Persia (now Iran) by soldiers waging war.[9] It continued to spread to the Near East, southern Asia, and Japan, partly as a result of increased shipping from infected to susceptible ports.[10] The first pandemic finally ended in 1823.

The second pandemic occurred in 1829–51, although historians differ on its start and end. The *Vibrio cholerae* agent was still unknown, as were appropriate methods to treat patients and prevent epidemic spread. From its source in India, the pandemic expanded to Russia, on to continental Europe, and to the port of Sunderland, England, likely coming with ships from Germany. London and Paris both experienced outbreaks, as did the United States and Canada, with cholera accompanying ships carrying Irish immigrants. Cholera also traveled home with pilgrims returning from Mecca, Saudi Arabia, who spread the disease throughout the Middle East and Eastern Europe.

John Snow, the famed father of epidemiology, was involved with the second pandemic, which made its way twice to England. He confronted the national epidemic of 1831–32 while still learning his craft and again in December 1850 when he and others founded the Epidemiological Society of London to advise the government on ways to combat the disease.[11]

Although the Italian microscopist Filippo Pacini had written of the causative organism in 1854, few outside Italy were aware of his work. Hence, the agent remained unknown to most of the world. During the third pandemic of 1852–60, when cholera again found its way to London in 1853–55, Snow conducted the epidemiological research on the Broad Street Pump Outbreak and the Grand Experiment that made him famous—comparing London households that received polluted river water with those that received unpolluted water. The third pandemic was considered the most deadly up until then; cholera devastated large swaths of Asia, North America, Africa, and Europe, including England.[12]

The fourth pandemic of 1863–79 included a major epidemic during an 1865 Mecca pilgrimage and the 1866 epidemic associated with two wars—between Austria and Italy and between Germany and Austria. There were many deaths in Russia, some countries of Europe, and much of northern Africa. When cholera arrived in the United States in 1865–66, the disease spread from New York City's docks to much of the eastern half of the country, including New Orleans to the south. Several countries in Central America that traded through the port of New Orleans also had cholera outbreaks, and other countries in South America were affected.

Although John Snow had written much about cholera transmission on the basis of clinical and epidemiological observations, and Filippo Pacini had actually seen *Vibrio cholerae* with his microcope, skepticism during the fourth pandemic was widespread, which led many public health officials to continue the errors of the past.

It was during the fifth pandemic, 1881–96, that *Vibrio cholerae* became widely known. Cholera was epidemic in Egypt in 1883, when Robert Koch, a German physician and microbiologist, traveled in August with a group of colleagues to Alexandria.[13] Conducting autopsies of cholera victims, they found a bacillus in the intestinal mucosa. Koch reasoned it was related to the cholera process but was unsure whether it was causal or consequential. He postulated that the time sequence could be resolved only by isolating the organism, growing it in pure culture, and reproducing a similar disease in animals. He was unable to obtain such a pure culture but did try unsuccessfully to infect animals with choleraic material. His ideas and early findings were sent in a dispatch to the German government and shared with the German press.

Late in 1883, Koch and his fellow investigators set sail to Calcutta to continue their work. The epidemic had subsided in Egypt but was still very active in India. On January 7, 1884, Koch announced he had successfully isolated the bacillus in pure culture. One month later, he wrote that the bacillus was not straight like other bacilli but "a little bent, like a comma," was able to proliferate in moist, soiled linen or damp earth, and was susceptible to drying and weak acid solutions. Finally, he pointed out that the specific organisms were always found in patients with cholera but never in those with diarrhea from other causes, were relatively rare in early infection, but were extensively present in the characteristic rice-water stools of advanced cholera patients. He was, however, still unable to reproduce the disease in animals, reasoning correctly that they are not susceptible. In May 1884, Koch and his colleagues returned to Germany, where they had become national heroes.

After originating in the Ganges Delta, the fifth pandemic swept through Asia, Africa, South America, and parts of France and Germany. In 1893–94, cholera deaths in Russia reached two hundred thousand. Japan saw ninety thousand deaths in 1887–89. While the new knowledge explained how the disease was transmitted, it did little to slow the worldwide pandemic other than lead to quarantine measures that kept the disease out of Britain and the United States.

The sixth pandemic occurred in 1899–1923, again associated with pilgrimages to Mecca, notably in 1902 and again in 1907. Precursors of the organism that would dominate the next (or seventh) pandemic—*Vibrio cholerae* O1 El Tor—were discovered in 1905, recovered from the intestines of persons who had died of diseases other than cholera in the El Tor quarantine camp in Egypt's Sinai Peninsula. The sixth pandemic affected mainly Asia. Western Europe escaped the disease, as did the Americas.

Now we are in the seventh pandemic, also associated with the Ganges Delta of South Asia. Just how prevalent is cholera in South Asia? During 2010 alone, three of the seven South Asian countries reported cholera cases to the World Health Organization, although the cases were probably greatly underestimated.[14] For example, even though cholera is considered endemic in Bangladesh, the government there typically reports zero cholera cases to WHO.[15] Danger arises if infected persons (such as military troops), water, or food products from these countries—indeed, from any country where cholera has been detected—move to other regions of the world.

As noted in earlier pandemics, cholera often accompanies troop movements. In 2010, the UN prided itself on being the "largest multilateral contributor to post-conflict stabilization worldwide" and noted, "Only the United States deploys more military personnel to the field than the United Nations."[16] In South Asia, Pakistan—with 164 reported cholera cases in 2010—had sent 304 UN-sponsored troops or police to Haiti, and 310 had come from India,[17] which had reported 5,155 cholera cases that same year. Neither of these countries, however, had troops stationed by the village of Mèyé, where Piarroux reported that cholera had first appeared in October 2010. No, the MINUSTAH camp near Mirebalais was the Haitian "home" only for UN peacekeeping troops from Nepal, which reported 1,790 cholera cases to WHO in 2010 and which had 1,280 troops assigned by the UN to Haiti.

13

REPORT

Piarroux gave up on trying to sleep. As the plane soared through the night sky over the Atlantic Ocean, he remembered a fable from his childhood, "Le Loup et l'Agneau" ("The Wolf and the Lamb"), by the seventeenth-century French author Jean de La Fontaine.

> That innocence is not a shield,
> A story teaches, not the longest.
> The strongest reasons always yield
> To reasons of the strongest.
> A lamb her thirst was slaking
> Once at a mountain rill.
> A hungry wolf was taking
> His hunt for sheep to kill,
> When, spying on the streamlet's brink
> This sheep of tender age,
> He howl'd in tones of rage,
> How dare you roil my drink?
> Your impudence I shall chastise!
> Let not your majesty, the lamb replies,
> Decide in haste or passion!
> For sure 'tis difficult to think
> In what respect or fashion

My drinking here could roil your drink,
Since on the stream your majesty now faces
I'm lower down full twenty paces.
You roil it, said the wolf; and, more, I know
You cursed and slander'd me a year ago.
O no! how could I such a thing have done!
A lamb that has not seen a year,
A suckling of its mother dear?
Your brother then. But brother I have none.
Well, well, what's all the same,
'Twas some one of your name.
Sheep, men, and dogs of every nation,
Are wont to stab my reputation,
As I have truly heard.
Without another word,
He made his vengeance good—
Bore off the lambkin to the wood,
And there, without a jury,
Judged, slew, and ate her in his fury.[1]

Were the Haitian people the lamb? Was the UN, or at least its representatives in Haiti, the wolf? Were UN peacekeeping forces the teeth of the wolf? Could the streamlet be the Artibonite River? Piarroux understood the meaning behind La Fontaine's fable: it was first and foremost about the wolf's justification for eating the lamb. And so, Piarroux's mind returned to the UN's and CDC's justifications for not looking for cholera's origin. And the more he thought about what he witnessed in Haiti, the stronger his conviction grew.

By the time his plane landed in Paris, Piarroux knew he had no choice but to tell Haiti's true cholera story, with a clear, comprehensive, logical, and truthful argument. He had witnessed an avoidable health disaster. He had been entrusted to tell what he found. He had a moral obligation to the truth and a professional responsibility to uphold the integrity of his epidemiological investigation.

Piarroux thought back to his maternal grandfather, who had written a small family history and had adopted as a family motto *Fais ce que dois*—"Do what you must." He had long considered that his code of conduct. He had no illusions, though, regarding how his report might be received by the powerful devouring wolf. *Sans autre forme de procès* (without any form of judgment, without any due process, without a jury): the words that began the last line of La Fontaine's fable churned in Piarroux's mind as the flight neared its end. Could his report alone hold those responsible accountable?

Piarroux landed in Marseille on Sunday, November 28. Back in Haiti, it was Election Day. He wondered whether things were peaceful.

Later he learned of reports of violence at voting centers.[2] At midday, twelve of the nineteen presidential candidates held a joint press conference to demand a suspension of voting, citing voter irregularities and fraud that favored Jude Célestin, candidate of President Préval's party. Some voters were outraged; supporters of the opposing candidate, Michel Martelly, took to the streets. One reporter observed that "as they roamed, they tore down posters of Célestin." Another wrote, "Many polling centers opened late, producing queues of angry, suspicious would-be voters. In others, voting seemed slow, with police and observers outnumbering those who had come to cast a ballot."[3]

Piarroux also learned later that Election Day turmoil had mixed with ongoing rage and fear over cholera. The worst report came from Grand'Anse département in southwest Haiti, where a dozen or more people, most of them vodou priests, were accused of importing cholera and were killed with machetes and rocks before their bodies were burned in the street. Still others accused of cholera-related witchcraft were lynched.[4] It smacked of the darkest days of the Middle Ages. An epidemic is not always measured exclusively by the increase in cases. Sometimes it provokes the irrational and transforms a crowd into a thousand-headed monster. Piarroux was convinced that the more the origin of the raging epidemic was presented as an unsolvable "mystery," the more people would embrace illogical explanations and look for scapegoats.

Despite his exhaustion he set to work soon after arriving home. First he phoned Deborah Pasmantier of Agence France-Presse. He introduced himself, said the French ambassador in Haiti suggested he call, and gave an interview. She asked him directly about the Nepalese peacekeepers. He simply acknowledged that cholera in Haiti was imported and said he preferred that his forthcoming report—and a subsequent scientific study he hoped to publish—answer her questions more specifically. He was not going to make any potentially inflammatory statements.

After the interview, he shifted his attention to his mission report—a detailed account of his activities and conclusions that he would submit to the Ministry of Foreign and European Affairs in Paris and the French embassy in Port-au-Prince. He began by writing a summary of his findings. First and foremost, he wrote, foreigners had introduced cholera into Haiti. There was not a single piece of evidence to support the environmental hypothesis that *Vibrio cholerae* had been lying dormant and then came up like a monster from water because it was hungry or had been upset by the January 2010 earthquake. The outbreak had occurred nine months after the earthquake! No, human activity was the cause, and the starting point seemed to be a cholera outbreak in Kathmandu, Nepal. Piarroux had verified the outbreak with two sources—the U.S. embassy there and a Nepalese newspaper—and had confirmed that it occurred shortly before the Nepalese soldiers flew to Haiti.[5]

The suppressed October 21–24 MSPP report he had been given just before leaving Port-au-Prince left no doubt that the entry point of the epidemic in Haiti was the hamlet of Mèyé adjacent to Annapurna Camp. This was corroborated by the testimony of Brigada Médica Cubana members and Haitian medical staff at the Mirebalais hospital and during his first field investigation.

Notably, the tiny hamlet of Mèyé was not even in a part of Haiti affected by the earthquake, which made dismissing the environmental theory much easier. If cholera was "aroused" by the earthquake, why didn't it strike in the earthquake zone? As for the idea that cholera just came up out of the nearby Artibonite River or streams to slake its thirst, Piarroux asked whether it was just a coincidence that potentially infected Nepalese troops from Kathmandu were in the immediate vicinity. That was ludicrous and downright unscientific.

Piarroux knew human activity was the culprit and that someone from outside had transported cholera into the area. Mèyé was far from the capital and from the camps of persons displaced by the earthquake. It was even farther from the Caribbean Sea and brackish coastal estuaries. There were no NGOs in the area and no expatriates from cholera-infected countries living nearby. There was not a single foreigner living in the hamlet of Mèyé.

Epidemiologists use the vital clues of space and time (explained in chapter 4), and the only foreigners to have settled near Mèyé were the Nepalese soldiers (*space*). Piarroux also knew that the first cholera cases identified in Mèyé became ill on and after October 14, a few days after their arrival (*time*). The poor sanitary conditions in and around Annapurna Camp had been well documented. There were many opportunities for fecal debris to flow from the camp's toilets to the nearby stream and from leaks in a waste-receiving septic pit on a hill overlooking the stream. More *space* to be linked with *time*.

But what of the second mystery—the origin of the massive cholera contamination in the lower Artibonite valley, followed by the extensive epidemic throughout Haiti? How did that happen? The explosive phase in the Artibonite delta was too sudden to have been caused by human-to-human spread, and polluting a major river and subsequently launching a massive epidemic at a great distance downstream could not be explained by a contaminated waste pipe dripping into a stream, minor leaks of a hilltop septic pit, or even open defecation into the river by a few infected soldiers. It would require cubic meters of infected feces.

That was the science, but Piarroux had other questions. Who decided to discharge such a large volume of highly contagious feces into the stream? Did they have any idea the feces were infected? Were the military authorities aware? How could the United Nations tolerate establishing a camp of peacekeeping soldiers without basic sanitation services? He imagined what other diseases could have appeared easily and been transmitted in such an unsanitary setting—notably viral and bacterial diarrhea, viral hepatitis, and typhoid fever. Given its enormous peacekeeping task and its large presence in Haiti, how could the UN risk the respect it needed to do its work through such neglect—allowing septic waste from its troops to pass into local drinking water? Without an official inquiry, he doubted the answers would ever be known.

As Piarroux summarized his findings and drew his conclusions, he took note of the torrent of official denials, lies, and attempts at deception as the involvement of UN peacekeepers in bringing cholera to Haiti became more apparent. The UN spokesperson, Vincenzo Pugliese, assured everyone that the Nepalese soldiers were all asymptomatic. But the Annapurna Camp latrines had certainly contained enough fecal matter to contaminate an entire river. There were foul odors emanating from the camp. Reporters had seen the leaky sewage pipes being removed and the ditches being filled. The stealth and intrigue he had experienced in Haiti came into sharper focus.

Then there were what seemed like institutional errors but really looked more like deliberate deception: CDC "investigation," the PAHO maps, and so on.

By the end of the day, Piarroux's report was largely complete. It had four sections—mission activities, circumstances of onset of the epidemic, evolution of the epidemic, and conclusion and recommendations—and was dated November 29, 2010. He decided to sleep on it and review what he had written the next morning before sending it off.

The following morning, Piarroux searched the Internet for news on Haiti and saw a bold headline over Deborah Pasmantier's byline: *Choléra en Haïti: Une épidémie importée* ("Cholera in Haiti: An Imported Epidemic").[6] The article had been dispatched to hundreds of newspapers and websites around the world.

It began with a dramatic summary. "The cholera epidemic in Haiti is imported, and the strain could not have come from either the environment or camps housing victims of the January 12 earthquake, French Professor Renaud Piarroux, an epidemiologist just back from a mission for the Haitian government, told AFP."

Piarroux had deliberately avoided discussing MINUSTAH or troops from Nepal but Pasmantier had drawn the broader implications of what he had said and material from other sources. "According to Haitian officials, the first cases appeared in mid-October on the banks of a tributary of the Artibonite River, near the Mirebalais base of Nepalese peacekeepers of the UN Mission in Haiti (MINUSTAH), located in the center of the island nation. They have been accused by some of the population of importing the disease that, according to the latest report, has killed 1,721." The article included MINUSTAH's denial and its assertion that the water and latrine sample tests from the Nepalese camp were "negative" for cholera.

Piarroux realized he needed to get his report to the ministry quickly. He reviewed his draft and e-mailed it to the French embassy in Haiti.

Pasmantier's article began what became weeks of intensified interest in "French epidemiologist Renaud Piarroux," even though he had spent only a few minutes talking with the journalist. Piarroux's findings soon made their way around the globe, placing him on the world stage in a role he had never sought but ultimately, and reluctantly, accepted.

His report identified the Nepalese troops as the likely source: "No other hypothesis could be found to explain the start of a cholera epidemic in the village of Meille" (using the hamlet's French name). The massive contamination of the Artibonite River, which Piarroux called "unique in the recent history of cholera," could be explained only by "a spill all at once into the river by a tremendous amount of feces from a large number of patients"—that is, Nepalese soldiers.

The report ended with four recommendations. Two focused on disease management issues for health personnel in Haiti. The others addressed the legal and policy implications of his origin findings. Piarroux recommended creating "a judicial inquiry into the origins and development of the epidemic, because even if the epidemiological investigation leaves no doubt about what happened, it is not the correct means for establishing the responsibilities of the various parties." Further, he urged a review of "procedures at the earliest that might have prevented this biological catastrophe, particularly those relating to medical surveillance of troops involved in UN missions and those relating to sanitation (latrines, excreta) in camps housing those troops."

Although blame for the epidemic, after a truthful scientific investigation of the origin of cholera in Haiti, was not Piarroux's point, it was laid clearly at the UN's doorstep.

The trip from Marseille to Paris, just shy of five hundred miles, takes about three hours on the train. On Tuesday morning Piarroux headed to a midafternoon meeting in Paris at the Ministry of Foreign and European Affairs, preceded by lunch with several leaders of the French wing of Médecins Sans Frontières interested in his views on the cholera situation in Haiti.

Piarroux welcomed the discussion. MSF, the main NGO in Haiti involved with cholera, had already responded to more than 41,000 suspected cholera cases in thirty Cholera Treatment Centers located throughout the country. At a bistro near the organization's headquarters, Piarroux sat down for lunch with Rony

Brauman and Jean-Hervé Bradol, both former presidents of MSF-France; Marie-Pierre Allie, the current president; and Thierry Durand, the director of MSF-France operations. He expressed great concern that the catastrophic nature of the epidemic in the rural areas of Haiti was being overlooked as the disease entered the capital city. And he recounted what he had written in his report.

Brauman and Piarroux had corresponded by e-mail only a few days earlier, when Piarroux learned the report he hadn't yet written was already being read. After lunch, the group retired to the nearby MSF offices, where Piarroux's colleagues made a shocking revelation that explained Brauman's e-mail. He was handed a copy of the confidential diplomatic communiqué sent on November 13 by Didier Le Bret, the French ambassador in Port-au-Prince.

Piarroux was greatly disturbed. The ambassador had undermined his preliminary findings by boldly stating something he could not possibly know: that the "cholera is of the Asian strain, but there is no evidence that it was introduced by elements of the Nepalese battalion." It seemed the French embassy, at least officially, had turned its back on the scientific integrity of his work before it was even completed, calling into question the very premise of his investigation. Reading Le Bret's words, Piarroux realized what was coming: his results would be actively challenged.

How odd that the ambassador had never spoken to him about that communiqué, thought Piarroux. And how odd that Le Bret had put Piarroux in touch with Pasmantier, the AFP reporter. Piarroux weighed these two things carefully. Could it be, he wondered, another case of an official taking one position for public consumption while privately taking steps to buttress a different position? He remembered his musings on the plane about the ambiguous attitude of Haiti's president and health minister, who remained silent on the origin of the cholera epidemic while pushing him to conduct a scientific investigation that would lead conclusively to the truth. The Swedish ambassador also came to mind, as Piarroux pondered whether the source of Hammar's revelation about cholera's origin might have been a CDC official. If nothing else, Piarroux was getting an education in how politics and diplomacy worked.

Piarroux gave his MSF colleagues a copy of his mission report. Politics or no politics, they all agreed that covering up the origin of the epidemic, which meant deceiving the Haitian people and disrespecting cholera's victims, was unacceptable. Sooner or later, the truth would come out, and Piarroux thought that having MSF's company in *connaître la vérité* (knowing the truth) was a very good thing.

The French Ministry of Foreign and European Affairs is located some distance west of the MSF headquarters, on the left bank of the River Seine at 37 Quai d'Orsay, and it is that street name by which it is commonly known. Piarroux had high expectations for his meeting with officials in the Quai d'Orsay's Directorate for the Americas and the Caribbean. Perhaps too high.

He debriefed the officials and asked whether they would alert the UN's Department of Peacekeeping Operations of his findings. They said any further action would have to await the official position of France. Piarroux could not help but wonder whether his mission report would even be circulated in the ministry, let alone whether there might be any follow-up to his recommendations. Michèle Alliot-Marie, the new minister, had already shifted France's attention away from cholera and toward Haitian children orphaned by the earthquake and awaiting adoption in France. She wanted that settled by Christmas, less than a month away.

Piarroux went next to the Crisis Centre, a unit in the ministry that deals with humanitarian crises and supports the overseas activities of French NGOs. People there, including the director, were attentive and seemed to appreciate the importance of his investigation but were quite coy about what would be done about his conclusions.

If he hadn't realized it before, the day's events convinced Piarroux that his official mission was over. He would return to Marseille and catch up on the considerable backlog of work that had accumulated at the university and hospital. He would leave it to Bernard Valero, the ministry's chief spokesperson, to handle future discussion of his report. And he would begin the work of publishing his findings in a scientific journal. Ministry officials seemed fine with that, understanding it was expected of an academic scientist.

Piarroux, though, could not escape the ramifications of his mission report—not that he really wanted to.

The surprise phone call came on Wednesday, after he was back in Marseille. On the line was Eric Laroche, a French physician who was then the World Health Organization's assistant director-general of Health Action in Crises (since retired). WHO is a UN agency. Laroche had learned of his report—news travels fast, thought Piarroux—and asked for a copy. He and his colleagues wanted to review the epidemiological situation and get a better understanding of how cholera arrived in Haiti.

WHO had shown no interest in the cholera origin investigation while Piarroux was in Haiti. In fact, Claire-Lise Chaignat, head of the agency's global task force on cholera control, had done a lot to deflect attention away from what Piarroux was learning while he was there. So he was skeptical, but he agreed to send a copy to Laroche. After all, he had nothing to hide, and maybe his report would stimulate some discussion and debate among WHO's cholera specialists.

Laroche also told Piarroux he would be hearing soon from Chaignat. Piarroux knew her well; she had his contact information. He waited some days for her to finish reading his mission report but heard nothing. Laroche again assured him he would be contacted shortly by someone at WHO. He never was. During the year that followed, Piarroux learned that both Laroche and Chaignat had retired from the organization.

Although Piarroux did not know whether anyone at WHO had read his report, he soon became well aware that it had been read elsewhere within the far-reaching UN and its affiliates. On Friday, after weeks of accusations in the press that UN peacekeepers from Nepal were the likely source of Haiti's cholera epidemic, an informal meeting of the UN General Assembly took place at UN headquarters in New York City. Secretary-General Ban Ki-moon addressed the diplomats.

Ban spoke first about the many problems that had beset Haiti and praised the Haitian people for their "resilience in the face of the earthquake and the cholera outbreak."[7] He discussed UN activities aimed at shoring up Haitian democratic institutions and detailed some of the steps being taken to address the public health crisis caused by the outbreak. He ended by addressing some of Piarroux's findings without explicitly mentioning the report.

> Let me say directly to you that I am determined to understand and address the manner in which the cholera outbreak occurred and was spread. The people of Haiti are suffering. They are suffering enormously, and they are asking legitimate questions. Where did this come from? How did this happen?
>
> We may never be able to fully answer these complex, difficult questions, but they deserve our best efforts. MINUSTAH and the Government of Haiti have carried out a number of tests of water samples from the Nepalese military camp in Mirebalais and waters adjacent to the base. All have so far proved negative.
>
> We are continuing to take action on three critical fronts: first, MINUSTAH is monitoring the situation closely, drawing water samples from various sources and ensuring that waste waters do not flow into the rivers. Second, we are deploying a team of water, sanitation and hygiene experts to review all sanitation systems at MINUSTAH military, police and civilian installations. Third, I have instructed the Mission to actively follow up on any additional information it may receive on the origins of the current outbreak. This includes cooperating fully with

> national or competent authorities in any further effort to shed light on the source of the epidemic, to improve treatment for victims and to prevent further spread.
>
> The people of Haiti deserve nothing less.

Well, thought Piarroux, perhaps my report has done some good already. It was true that the secretary-general had repeated the same language MINUSTAH used in Haiti to deflect attention away from the Nepalese camp. But at the same time, he had ordered an expert review of sanitary conditions at all MINUSTAH installations. Clearly, the source of cholera in Haiti was on Ban Ki-moon's mind.

14

VODOU AND CHOLERA

From the mid-1340s until 1351, the Black Death—caused by another bacterium, *Yersinia pestis*—spread from the plains of Central Asia, traveling along the Silk Road, and reaching Crimea. From there, merchant ships full of black rats with Oriental rat fleas probably carried it to Europe. Upwards of 30 to 50 percent of Europe's population is estimated to have lost their lives in the pandemic, one of human history's most devastating.[1]

As the plague ravaged Europe, the confused populace looked first for explanations and then a scapegoat, someone "different" or "other." Often they targeted Jewish communities, where better hygiene and relative isolation from the population at large kept the disease from wreaking the same havoc. Responding to widespread antisemitic feelings, Jews were rumored to have deliberately poisoned wells to kill Christians.[2] Later, scapegoating over cholera would find other victims in Russia and then much later in Haiti.

Cholera first reached Russia in September 1823, then was absent for six years, reappearing in 1829 in the southern regions of the country. In the fall of 1830, it continued to spread, reaching St. Petersburg, the capital of Russia. The rumor that doctors had poisoned the wells sparked a wave of bloody riots throughout Russia, with large crowds sacking affluent households and killing medical personnel. In St. Petersburg the rioting came to a head in June 1831 when demonstrators gathered at the main cholera hospital, ransacked the building, and murdered several doctors. The riot ended when Emperor Nicholas I appeared, accompanied by two regiments with cannons, and convinced the insurgents to cease the destruction.[3]

Cholera in Haiti, like great epidemics before, put everyone on edge. There were occasional outbursts of violence, most notably aimed at vodou believers and priests. Why vodou?

During Piarroux's last week in Haiti, rumors of sorcery and cholera began to spread in a remote southwestern region.[4] Some people accused of witchcraft were lynched, while others narrowly escaped. The lynchings had continued, day after day—six hanged in one village and five in two others. A dozen other accused were killed with machetes and stones, their bodies then burned in the streets. The murderous anger could be traced, in part, to a report that local vodou practitioners "had fashioned a magic powder to spread the [cholera] infection."[5]

CNN reported that a senior *houngan*—a male Haitian vodou priest—had insisted "people who practice voodoo have nothing to do with the cholera epidemic."[6] Yet, by late December, at least forty-five suspected vodou priests were lynched because of suspected connections to the outbreak of the disease.

The rumors also involved Piarroux. Weeks after returning to France, he heard reports that his investigation had led to lynchings and street deaths, including an earlier attack on MINUSTAH camps in which dozens of protesters were killed. He understood the outrage of the Haitian people and their desire to blame someone for cholera, but when these lynchings and supposed attacks happened, he hadn't even written the first line of his report—not that he mentioned vodou when he did.

The actual lynchings, though, ended almost as quickly as they began.

Vodou, also known as voodoo, has played an important role in Haitian community life and death since before nationhood. When slaves were shipped from Africa in the eighteenth century to the island, they brought beliefs about the "spirit world" that were later formalized as Haitian vodou. Followers believe in spirits in both the seen and unseen worlds. They consider humans to be spirits (*Iwa*) in the visible world and to be the spirits of others—including ancestors and the recently deceased—in the invisible world.[7] Haitians pray to spirits in the invisible world for health, protection, and favors. They serve these spirits with rituals of devotion sometimes led by family members or village elders and, more formally, by *houngan* or *manbo*—male or female priests.

In the long 1791–1804 battle for independence from France, vodou bolstered the resistance of rebellious slaves. Its ceremonies were a time to gather and organize, important for bonding since the slaves had come from different parts of Africa.[8] But in the first four decades after independence, Haiti's political leaders actively suppressed it, fearing it might stimulate further revolt and that its followers might cast spells on them. This led to frequent anti-vodou purges throughout the nineteenth and twentieth centuries.

When U.S. Marines invaded Haiti in 1915, and during their nineteen-year occupation, a succession of local political leaders extolled vodou—and ever-popular vodou-inspired dance and music—as a defense against foreign cultures. The arts played an important role in bringing together social classes to appreciate their African heritage and to scorn outside domination.

During the nearly thirty-year reign over Haiti by the Duvalier family—first President François "Papa Doc" Duvalier from 1957 to 1971 and then his son Jean-Claude "Baby Doc" Duvalier, who served as president until 1986—things changed. Papa Doc was a physician, active in Haitian public health programs and politics. He won the presidential election in September 1957 with a "program of popular reform and black nationalism."[9] As president, he began to shift the country to a dictatorship, captivating and manipulating the Haitian people with his artful use of vodou.[10] He "affected the staring gaze, whispered speech and hyper-slow movements recognized by Haitians as signs that a person is close to the voodoo spirits." He swayed presidential audiences with vodou priests brought from the countryside and encouraged rumors of his supernatural powers—which helped forge a personal connection with vodou believers.

"My enemies cannot get me!" Duvalier told his followers. "I am already an immaterial being."

This close identification with the common people was part of Duvalier's demagogic effort to capture greater power, first with the backing of the Haitian army and then through his creation of the Tonton Macoute, a paramilitary organization that functioned largely as a death squad and brutalized Haitian society.[11] Through its leaders, the group was also closely associated with vodou. It developed an "unearthly authority in the eyes of the public" and linked the spiritual forces of vodou and nationalism with loyalty to the Duvaliers. Throughout the Duvalier dictatorships, the Tonton Macoute "murdered over 60,000 Haitians and many more were forced to flee their homes." The ongoing violence spurred a brain drain of Haiti's most educated citizens, who left in droves—further crippling the country.

When Baby Doc was exiled to France in 1986, Haitian villagers "attacked vodou temples and threatened and killed their occupants." Over the next three months, nearly one hundred priests and priestesses were "hacked, burned or otherwise put to death by mobs."[12]

It seems doubtful that past thoughts of the Duvaliers were the main motivation for the killings in late 2010. Nearly half of the Haitian population had not yet been born when Baby Doc was driven from office in 1986. Furthermore, the

Haitian parliament had legally recognized vodou as a formal religion in 2003, giving its ceremonies, such as marriage, equal legal status with other established religions.[13] Besides, vodou in Haiti does not really stand alone. "The mixture of gods and goddesses and Catholic saints is an integral part of Haitian life," the BBC noted. "One common saying is that Haitians are 70% Catholic, 30% Protestant, and 100% voodoo."

So when general hostility toward vodou is ruled out, what provoked the lynchings in 2010?

It is serendipity that mental health researchers in November–December 2010 were studying the lingering effects of emotional distress associated with the earthquake and cholera at roughly the same time as the lynchings.[14] Their study sites were two poor suburbs of Port-au-Prince and two rural areas (Petit-Goâve and Léogâne) in Ouest département, not that far from where the murders of vodou practitioners occurred.

They found beginning in December that Haitians they surveyed increasingly suspected cholera could be spread by *hougan* or *Vaudouizan* (vodou believers) using *pout kolera*—magic powder with cholera—to infect water. The researchers noted further that the uncertainty about cholera's origin "feeds feelings of insecurity and fear, which in turn, fuels stigmatization and potentially violent reactions towards individuals and institutions."[15]

Older Haitians already viewed Vaudouizan with suspicion for their past associations with the Tonton Macoute and what other religious groups said. For them and some of their younger followers, cholera may have been the last straw. In Russia in 1830–31, perhaps the marauding, murdering gangs of rioters—desperate victims of the czar's policies of deprivation and political repression—saw cholera the same way.

Haitians also told the researchers that cholera was a poison brought by foreigners "to divide us" and "to exterminate us and take our land."[16] When the rumor about the Nepalese peacekeepers became more widespread in early 2011, the lynchings stopped and the emotional rage shifted from vodou to a genuinely blameful target—MINUSTAH.

Unlike vodou priests, peacekeeping troops could easily protect themselves. Not a single MINUSTAH peacekeeper was killed or even seriously injured during the angry demonstrations. Piarroux thought back to La Fontaine's fable. *La raison du plus fort est toujours la meilleure.* The strongest reasons always yield / to reasons of the strongest.

In other words, might makes right.

15

INQUIRY

It didn't take long for Piarroux's report to attract the attention of other French journalists. Somehow, it and Le Bret's confidential diplomatic communiqué found their way into the hands of Béatrice Gurrey, a well-known writer for the French daily newspaper *Le Monde*. She never revealed her source, even to Piarroux.

On Sunday, December 5, 2010, *Le Monde* ran Gurrey's article, "Choléra en Haïti: L'hypothèse népalaise confirmée" ("Cholera in Haiti: The Nepalese case confirmed").[1] It began very directly, using the nickname often given to UN peacekeepers (for the color of their headwear).

> According to the confidential report of a French expert, the source of the epidemic is a UN Blue Helmets camp.
>
> The confidential report of a French physician, Dr. Renaud Piarroux, leaves no doubt about the origin of the cholera epidemic that has killed more than 1,800 people in Haiti since mid-October. This document, obtained by *Le Monde*, says the deadly bacteria comes from the camp of Nepalese soldiers of the UN Mission for Stabilization in Haiti (MINUSTAH), located in Mirebalais in the Central Region [, a] hypothesis UN officials have denied.

Gurrey concluded with a swipe at the French ambassador in Haiti. Piarroux's "investigation was not to the liking of its sponsor, the French Ministry of Foreign Affairs. In a confidential diplomatic cable prior to 28 November, Didier Le Bret, the French ambassador to Haiti, indicated he would ask Professor Piarroux 'to refrain from any public comment' because 'the government—Haiti—does not wish to embarrass MINUSTAH before the elections.'"

Gurrey's article even included a photo of Le Bret's document.

Deborah Pasmantier of AFP had also been busy, digging deeper after her article earlier in the week. She published a second article, this time delving into Piarroux's report.[2] Quoting her anonymous source regarding cholera's origin, likely someone in the Quai d'Orsay, she wrote, "The source of the infection came from the Nepalese camp." Bernard Valero, the Foreign Ministry spokesman, refused to reveal the conclusions of Piarroux's report but confirmed its receipt "and said it had been passed on to the United Nations for investigation."

Two days later, at his December 7 press briefing in New York, Martin Nesirky—spokesperson for UN Secretary-General Ban Ki-moon—said MINUSTAH was aware of Piarroux's findings, while not mentioning the French epidemiologist by name.[3] "MINUSTAH has neither accepted nor dismissed his findings," he said. "It's just one report among many, which the Mission has taken seriously." Nesirky also reiterated what Ban Ki-moon had promised the previous week: that the UN has "deployed a team of water, sanitation and hygiene experts to review all sanitation systems at MINUSTAH's military, police and civilian installations."

Meanwhile, as political rage gripped Haiti, conflict was brewing at Médecins Sans Frontières between staff in France and some colleagues in the field. Piarroux's report was sent to MSF teams in Haiti and other countries, and two MSF epidemiologists wrote to Rony Brauman about "major inaccuracies." Brauman e-mailed Piarroux with some of their critique:

> They found the report to be unscientific and noted it had not been subject to a critical review. . . . For example, the central hypothesis of the report does not provide a very powerful explanation as to how the Artibonite River could cause the epidemic explosion that took place in both Saint-Marc and Grand Salines since they are part of a different hydrological basin. . . . For the record, Saint-Marc is a major harbor, receiving cargo ships, including from Asia.

Piarroux saw the e-mail as a harbinger of things to come: a combined political and epidemiological assault on his conclusions, perhaps to serve the same purpose. He responded to Brauman, pointing out that cholera had occurred in the part of Saint-Marc located in the Artibonite River delta and reminded him that the epidemic did not begin in Saint-Marc on October 19 but rather in Mèyé on October 14—confirmed by the Brigada Médica Cubana and the official Haitian investigation. "How," he asked rhetorically and not without a hint of sarcasm, "could an epidemic that began in Saint-Marc on October 20 or 19 have resulted in deaths in the village of [Mèyé] on October 17 and 18?"

The response in France to Piarroux's report played out as cholera continued to spread throughout much of the country, with about 3,000 new cases per day into the first week of December. The epidemic then peaked in mid-December at about 4,000–4,500 cases per day, hitting a significant percentage of the population.

Increased rains contributed to the early-December rise in cases, but human activity again proved more decisive than the environment. Violent protests in Haitian cities continued for weeks following the election,[4] halting the distribution of clean water and chlorine and resulting in many new cases. With streets blocked, those seeking medical care couldn't get to health clinics, including cholera treatment units reported to have exhausted their supplies of clean water, body bags, and other supplies.[5]

Only when the riots ended, coincidentally as the rains subsided, were clean water and medical care again provided. From its peak, the number of cases fell dramatically to about 2,500 per day by the end of December.[6]

The riots made it impossible for the work Piarroux had begun to continue. His replacement, Rachel Haus-Cheymol, couldn't leave her hotel because of the danger in the streets. On Thursday, December 8, the U.S. State Department even issued a warning to American citizens considering trips to Haiti, urging them to avoid nonessential travel to the country. The U.S. embassy imposed a curfew on its personnel.[7]

More journalists began to write about Piarroux's report—including Jonathan Katz of the Associated Press, who had been one of the first on the scene at Annapurna Camp. He contacted Piarroux by e-mail, but Piarroux remained true to his word to Quai d'Orsay, having told Bernard Valero, the ministry's chief spokesperson, to handle future discussion of his report. In a widely circulated December 7 article titled "Haiti Cholera Likely from UN Troops, Expert Says," Katz wrote, "The AP obtained a copy of the report from an official who released it on condition of anonymity. Piarroux confirmed he had authored the report but declined in an e-mail interview to discuss his findings."[8]

In an opinion piece that appeared days before in the influential *New Scientist* magazine, the journalist Debora Mackenzie criticized WHO's unwillingness to investigate the origins of the cholera epidemic. Titled "Haiti: Epidemics of Denial Must End," Mackenzie's piece said WHO's argument that the question was unimportant "could not be further from the truth." After all, "Haitians themselves care deeply about how their country got cholera."[9]

The remainder of her piece focused on the growing cover-up:

> The UN insists it is in the clear because the tests on water on or near the base did not find cholera, and none of the peacekeepers had symptoms.
>
> A single positive swab from a soldier early in the outbreak would have strongly suggested they were the source. A negative result would not have entirely cleared them—tests can produce false negatives—but it may well have calmed public suspicion.
>
> But no such tests were done. The Nepalese government claims the water samples alone prove that its troops are not the source. The UN Mission in Haiti even phoned me out of the blue to claim that tests cannot detect cholera in symptom-free people.
>
> Why would the UN go to such trouble? I can only conclude that they are trying to protect themselves and their people. Many Haitians dislike the UN force; dozens of peacekeepers have been killed in violent clashes since the mission arrived in 2004 to stabilise the country in the face of political upheaval. . . .
>
> The big lesson from Haiti is the same as with every new disease outbreak: do the tests, find out as much as possible, and tell the truth. What part of this is so hard to learn? Denial may seem safer, but with scientists increasingly able to track pathogens, and bystanders increasingly armed with cellphones and the internet, it isn't.
>
> Accountability matters, vitally so in a networked world. It is too late now to do those tests in Haiti. It is not too late to learn why they should have been done.

CDC could still have tested those troops, looking for serological evidence of the disease. Piarroux knew it was *not* too late for that.

At least in the press, the tide seemed to be turning. The very next day, at his daily press briefing at the French Ministry of Foreign and European Affairs, spokesman Bernard Valero was asked directly, "Do you have any comment regarding the publication in *Le Monde* of Mr. Piarroux's report on the cholera epidemic?"[10] His answer was circumspect.

> France deplores the very heavy toll exacted by the cholera epidemic in Haiti: since October 19 when the epidemic broke out, more than 2,000 people have died and almost 92,000 people are estimated to be contaminated throughout the country. As soon as the epidemic broke out, France sent, at the request of Haitian Health Ministry, one of its leading cholera specialists to Haiti: Professor Piarroux, a head of department in the Public Hospital System of Marseilles. Professor Piarroux was personally responsible for a report that was submitted to the Haitian authorities.

The ministry forwarded Piarroux's report to the UN, "which opened an inquiry," Valero added. "We should wait for the results."

Politics makes strange bedfellows. The expression from American writer Charles Dudley Warren had made its way into many languages since he penned it in 1870. And indeed, on the same Wednesday that Valero was briefing the press in the Quai d'Orsay, Piarroux learned that politics had given him his own strange bedfellow: Fidel Castro, the ailing Cuban leader whose public pronouncements had become increasingly rare. The *Havana Times* ran a statement Castro had released titled "MINUSTAH and the Epidemic."[11]

Castro reflected on the weeks gone by during which "news and photos were published showing Haitian citizens throwing stones and protesting in indignation against the forces of MINUSTAH, accusing it of having transmitted cholera to that country by way of a Nepalese soldier. The first impression, if one doesn't get any additional information, is that this deals with a rumor born out of the hatred caused by any occupying army."

Castro, though, was up on the latest news. He commented on Pasmantier's AFP article of December 5 and a similar article the following day from EFE, the leading Spanish-language news agency. He had asked the doctors from Brigada Médica Cubana about the situation; they confirmed press reports with "remarkable precision." He then offered some details about the earliest days of the outbreak and explained that the cholera strain matched an Asian one. Castro's commentary, citing information provided by BMC, was an independent confirmation of what Piarroux had written in his mission report.

Reflecting further, Castro wrote, "Why did the UN insist on denying that MINUSTAH brought the epidemic to the Haitian people? We are not blaming Nepal which in the past was a British colony, and whose men were used in their colonial wars and today seek employment as soldiers."

This, Piarroux realized, was a political statement in the form of a question.

The flurry of press reports about cholera in Haiti and Piarroux's findings did not take long to reach Nepal and provoke a reaction in the capital, Kathmandu. Also on Wednesday, the Nepalese army reacted angrily "to a study linking its UN peacekeepers to a cholera outbreak that has killed more than 2,000 people in Haiti."[12] An army spokesman told an AFP reporter, "We strongly condemn the making of such allegations with no firm evidence or facts," and characterized the report's conclusions as "hypothetical." He added that there was "no evidence to support the conclusions" of Piarroux.

That indignation was challenged later the same day, when BBC News South Asia reported that the Nepalese Army's chief medical officer told its reporter, "None of Nepal's soldiers serving with UN peacekeepers in Haiti was tested for cholera before they went"—a statement that "contradicted previous statements by the Nepalese army which has maintained that all its troops were given a thorough medical test—including being tested for cholera—before being deployed to Haiti in October."[13]

Brigadier General Kishore Rana said that the UN did not require such a test unless a soldier had cholera symptoms and insisted, "UN protocol had been followed during the pre-deployment medical, but that none of the troops exhibited symptoms of cholera—so no follow-up tests were done."

What news would be next? wondered Piarroux.

Most publicly available findings about cholera in Haiti had come out in news reports. Scientific journals had largely not addressed the situation. On November 19, while Piarroux was still in Haiti, a CDC publication had reiterated that the cholera-causing organism was *Vibrio cholerae* serogroup O1, serotype Ogawa, biotype El Tor.[14] CDC had conducted a detailed analysis of fourteen isolates gathered in Artibonite département and concluded that "if these isolates are representative of those currently circulating in Haiti, the findings suggest that *V. cholerae* was likely introduced into Haiti in one event." The agency stopped short of investigating what that "one event" might have been.

The day after the Castro and Nepal stories came out, however, the advance publication of an article in the highly influential *New England Journal of Medicine* added scientific fuel to the fire.[15] It reported on a second laboratory investigation of the organism that had caused cholera in Haiti. The authors used an advanced method to determine the genome sequences of two clinical *Vibrio cholerae* isolates from the current outbreak in Haiti. They then compared the Haiti isolates with a diverse set of twenty-eight other strains, including one from Latin America in 1991 and two from South Asia, in 2002 and 2008.

The authors made three important observations. First, comparing their two strains from Haiti with three others collected previously by CDC in Haiti, they noted the "Haitian cholera epidemic is clonal"—meaning all five isolates shared the same ancestor or common human host. "Collectively," they wrote, "our data strongly suggest that the Haitian epidemic began with introduction of a *V. cholerae* strain into Haiti by human activity from a distant geographic source."[16]

Second, they wrote, "Our data distinguish the Haitian strains from those circulating in Latin America and the U.S. Gulf Coast and thus do not support the hypothesis that the Haitian strain arose from the local aquatic environment." To bolster the point, they added, "It is therefore unlikely that climatic events led to the Haitian epidemic, as has been suggested in the case of other cholera epidemics."[17]

Third, they wrote that their result "supports the conclusion that Haitian *V. cholerae* is more closely related to contemporary South Asian strains of *V. cholerae* than to Latin American strains."[18] Some scientists had suggested the outbreak in Haiti might be associated with the 1991 outbreak in Peru, previously spread throughout South America (but not Haiti)—so this focus on South Asia was a very important comment. This was the first laboratory-based epidemiological evidence to support Piarroux's own conclusions.

"Understanding exactly how this South Asian variant strain of *V. cholerae* was introduced to Haiti will require further epidemiologic investigation," the authors added.[19] Piarroux agreed. His report was insufficient; it was time to prepare a peer-reviewed scientific article—and he wanted to move quickly.

Peer-reviewed journals are not known for moving at a fast pace. So Piarroux asked a colleague to contact an editor he knew at the *Lancet*, one of the world's leading medical journals. "I am involved in a very hot manuscript on cholera in Haiti, reporting the spread from a unique source, investigated by R. Piarroux," he wrote. "Can this be fast-tracked?" The editor indicated he would be happy to consider it.

Then, though, the *Lancet Infectious Diseases*—a sister publication of the *Lancet*—entered the fray and published an unusual editorial commentary titled, "As Cholera Returns to Haiti, Blame Is Unhelpful."[20] Curiously, a few months earlier its editors had chided WHO for its lack of transparency in assigning pandemic status to influenza A H1N1.[21] Now came a justification for obfuscation in Haiti. In five paragraphs, the unnamed authors briefly reviewed the cholera situation in Haiti and then launched a direct assault on the quest for scientific truth. "Although interest in how the outbreak originated may be a matter of scientific curiosity for the future, apportioning blame for the outbreak now is neither fair to people working to improve a dire situation nor helpful in combating the disease."

"Scientific curiosity"?! Piarroux could barely believe his eyes. What if there had been a major foodborne outbreak in Europe, or a hospital-acquired outbreak in a large London medical facility? Would they have characterized searching for the origin of those as scientific curiosity? Why should Haiti deserve anything less than what other countries would expect—a genuine epidemiological investigation, especially when this disease had never appeared there in recorded history?

Piarroux could only conclude that the authors believed epidemiologists should investigate sources only under certain circumstances—and that smelled of politics. Was protecting the UN's reputation worth diminishing and discrediting science?

He also wondered what this might mean for publishing his findings in the *Lancet*. Still, he moved forward. And he decided to go on television.

From the moment Deborah Pasmantier's AFP dispatch reached readers, Piarroux was barraged with interview requests from newspapers and broadcast media outlets around the world. At first, he said no, but as things intensified he changed his mind. Reporters were implying that the French ambassador had tried to prevent him from investigating the epidemic or that he had traveled to Haiti as some sort of rogue epidemiologist working on his own. He wanted to set the record straight, especially after being hung out to dry by the Quai d'Orsay spokesman at a December 8 press conference: "Professor Piarroux was personally responsible for a report that was submitted to the Haitian authorities."

"Personally responsible"?! That unsettling remark had to be countered. Piarroux had collaborated extensively with his Haitian counterparts and met many times with Haitian officials and French diplomats to explain his findings in detail. That was *professional responsibility*—an attribute he held in high regard. Being professional, he informed the Quai d'Orsay and the French embassy in Haiti that he intended to accept an interview request from France 24, the international news and current affairs television channel. He offered to reverse his decision if they formally forbade him. No such message was forthcoming.

The following Tuesday, December 14, Piarroux again traveled to Paris. Sylvain Attal, host of *L'Entretien* on France 24, broadcast a thirteen-minute interview in which Piarroux summarized his findings, clarified how he had come to be in Haiti, and explained the full support for his investigation given by Haitian and French officials.[22]

The United Nations was taking a beating in the print press and online. The first step in the UN counteroffensive was announced on Wednesday, December 15, 2010. "The United Nations is exploring the establishment of an international scientific panel to look into the source of the cholera epidemic in Haiti," said Alain Le Roy, the under-secretary-general for peacekeeping operations, at a press conference.[23]

Le Roy announced that the UN would entertain all the possible theories about cholera. "Experts who have studied the epidemic have so far come up with different theories on the origin of the infection," he stated. "There is no consensus among scientists on this issue."

The UN hoped to find "the best experts to be in a panel, completely independent, and conduct the best investigation on the source of the outbreak," said Le Roy, and it would ask its health arm, the World Health Organization, to help find them. The UN report reiterated the complete independence theme, adding that the panel would have "full access to all UN premises and personnel."

To review evidence of its own culpability, the UN would appoint a panel of scientists in collaboration with its sister organization, WHO. Yet Claire-Lise Chaignat, who headed WHO Global Task Force on Cholera Control, had in the first month of the epidemic told a reporter that "speculation about the UN troops from Nepal having brought the disease to Haiti seems very unlikely."[24] And she was a wholehearted supporter of the climate-environmental theory of cholera, having coauthored an article in the *New England Journal of Medicine* on that very subject.[25]

It made perfect sense that Piarroux should be asked to serve on or consult to the panel, although he didn't expect a formal invitation. But he had hoped that a UN-sponsored inquiry would at least include scientists with open minds, ones not harboring loyalty to a particular theory or the political interests of the UN.

Meanwhile, as the UN put together its panel, any physical evidence of contamination at the Mirebalais UN base was eroding. It had been months since the initial cholera event. If the UN's panel made a visit, it would find an environment far different from that described in Piarroux's mission report. Further, the current UN review of MINUSTAH water, sanitation, and hygiene systems the secretary-general had promised would surely result in many changes—months before the panel could visit the alleged scene of the crime.

Jonathan Katz had written that the UN was unwilling to discuss details of that review of MINUSTAH camps.[26] The more Piarroux thought about that, the less he was surprised. The UN had something to hide.

Two days later, Ban Ki-moon announced the "creation of an independent scientific panel to investigate the source of the outbreak amid widespread media reports that Nepalese peacekeepers from the United Nations Stabilization Mission in Haiti (MINUSTAH) are the likely source, with infected water spreading from their base into a nearby tributary of the Artibonite River."[27]

The secretary-general said he had consulted closely with the WHO director, Dr. Margaret Chan. "There remain fair questions and legitimate concerns" regarding the source of the cholera epidemic, he noted, "that demand the best answer that science can provide."

A little over three weeks after returning to Marseille from Haiti, Piarroux and his colleagues sent an article to the *Lancet*, where it was assigned an editor. The "fast-track" designation was used mainly for presentations of randomized controlled trials of important new therapies. But Piarroux and his coauthors were still hoping that the unusual and massive cholera epidemic in Haiti would warrant an exception for their article, titled "Understanding the Cholera Epidemic in Haiti." The authors, from both France and Haiti, were Renaud Piarroux, Robert Barrais, Benoît Faucher, Rachel Haus, Gérard Chevallier, Martine Piarroux, Roc

Magloire, and Didier Raoult. An accompanying map clearly identified where the epidemic began.

Meanwhile, as the authors waited for the editorial process to unfold, the UN issued its final news release of the year, stating that the cholera epidemic in Haiti had already killed more than 2,760 people and infected another 130,000-plus, nearly 71,000 of whom had been hospitalized.[28] "There is an urgent need for massive mobilization activities to promote prevention and early treatment of a disease that is spread by contaminated water and food," the release said. "In addition, controlling the epidemic will depend on the level of access to safe water and basic sanitation and implementation of hygiene measures."

The release ended with a reminder about the "independent scientific panel" created two weeks earlier. As far as Piarroux knew, the panel members had not yet been announced. As 2010 came to a close, only two things were certain about the situation in Haiti: intrigue had become the order of the day, and many more Haitians would suffer from cholera.

16

POLITICS BEFORE SCIENCE

It was January 4, 2011, and Piarroux's article for the *Lancet* was in trouble. The editor said the manuscript did not meet the journal's criteria for fast-track review and that it was being passed on to other editors for regular consideration. Three days later, the editor delivered the fatal blow: "Our decision is that your manuscript is better placed elsewhere."

A dejected Piarroux couldn't fathom how an investigation of the largest cholera epidemic in the Americas didn't even merit outside review before being rejected for publication altogether. Did the editors believe they had already covered the topic sufficiently? A review of the journal's contents certainly suggested otherwise.

The *Lancet* had run an article in its late-November 2010 edition on the Haiti outbreak, the possible source, and violent protests against UN peacekeeping forces—but that was a news article.[1] Two issues later, there was a brief piece focused primarily on how the Haitian epidemic had changed the "public health landscape of the Western hemisphere . . . suddenly and dramatically"[2]—but not a single word regarding how cholera might have come to Haiti. Finally, there was a commentary in mid-December that focused on global steps required to address cholera. It did ask why the first cases had appeared in Haiti—the authors mentioned "speculations" about UN peacekeepers—but then shrugged off the question, suggesting "cycles of accusation will continue for years without helping to slow the cholera epidemic."[3] It fit hand in glove with the *Lancet Infectious Diseases* editorial about "unhelpful" blame.[4]

As Piarroux and his coauthors considered their options, Piarroux received some unwanted news from the French ambassador in Port-au-Prince: he couldn't return to Haiti to continue his investigation and help set up a cholera tracking system until after the final round of the presidential election, scheduled for March 20, 2011. The ambassador feared Piarroux's presence would make too many waves before the next vote.

Piarroux certainly didn't want to cause any trouble. Perhaps the ambassador was right, although others differed. The Catholic News Service had interviewed Archbishop Louis Kebreau, president of the Haitian bishops' conference, while he visited the Washington headquarters of the U.S. Conference of Catholic Bishops.[5] He spoke of the hope Haitians had felt after the earthquake, when so many throughout the world had responded with care and compassion, and how ten months later that hope had given way to a feeling of abandonment in the face of the cholera epidemic.

"The problem is that the government knows [the cholera epidemic] comes from Nepal," the archbishop said. "But the government doesn't have the guts to say it openly. . . . People are reacting . . . because the government hasn't acted."

"Truth and openness would resolve a lot of trouble," Kebreau concluded.

On January 6, the members of the "independent" UN panel were announced.[6] They had been selected on the basis of their "global stature, expertise and extensive experience working with cholera in all its aspects," said the UN, emphasizing that "the panel will operate completely independent of the UN" with "access to all UN records, reports and facilities."

Dr. Alejandro Cravioto was named as chair. A prominent pediatrician from Mexico with a PhD from the London School of Hygiene and Tropical Medicine, he was the director of the International Center for Diarrheal Research in Bangladesh (ICDDR,B)—a post he had taken over from Professor David A. Sack, the prominent proponent of the environmental-climatic theory of cholera who had already weighed in on cholera in Haiti. Cravioto had ten publications on cholera cited in PubMed, a premier online source for citations in the biomedical literature—including one written with Rita Colwell, the world's leading proponent of the environmental theory.

Dr. Claudio F. Lanata, a Peruvian physician and infectious diseases expert and a senior researcher at the Nutritional Research Institute in Lima, was also named to the panel. He too had connections to the environmental theory's best-known proponents. He had been a board member of ICDDR,B when Sack was director and had an appointment at Sack's Johns Hopkins University. He also had published on the previous cholera epidemic that began in Peru in January 1991, the origin of which remained shrouded in mystery. At the time, WHO officials had stated that the origin couldn't be determined while acknowledging that the microorganism might have been introduced by maritime traffic from the Pacific"[7]—much like what Piarroux was hearing from WHO about Haiti. One of Lanata's articles stated that "coastal sea water and zooplankton were a reservoir for *V. cholerae* in Peru"[8] and another concluded that "ocean and climate patterns are useful predictors of cholera epidemics, with the dynamics of endemic cholera being related to climate and/or changes in the aquatic ecosystem."[9] His coauthors were Sack and Colwell.

Dr. G. Balakrish Nair was by far the most prominent researcher named to the panel. Among the world's most cited investigators in the cholera field, he had already coauthored some 250 publications on the disease—including 19 with Colwell and 33 with Sack. Since 2007, he had been director of the National Institute of Cholera and Enteric Diseases (NICED) in Kolkata (formerly Calcutta), India. Before that, he had worked with Colwell at the University of Maryland and with Sack at Johns Hopkins and had spent seven years at the ICDDR,B while Sack was director, first as microbiologist and associate director and later as director of the laboratory sciences division.

A pattern was coming into sharper focus for Piarroux. The panel members were linked together and firmly tied to the environmental theory.

The final member, Daniele S. Lantagne, was the youngest and least experienced with cholera but brought particular expertise in sanitation and water systems to the panel. She had a master's degree in environmental engineering from the Massachusetts Institute of Technology, and was enrolled in the PhD program in infectious tropical diseases at the London School of Hygiene and Tropical Medicine. An American advanced doctoral fellow in sustainable science at Harvard University's Kennedy School of Government, she had worked in several less developed countries, including Haiti.

The UN panel's mandate was to "investigate and seek to determine the source of the 2010 cholera outbreak in Haiti." The four experts were expected to present their findings in writing to both the UN secretary-general and the government of Haiti. But the UN didn't seem to feel the panel members constituted enough of a united front, and it hired Sack as a consultant to them. Yes, thought Piarroux, the same David Sack who in late November, without having spent a single moment on site investigating cholera in Haiti, had stated, "*Vibrio cholerae*, the bacterium responsible for cholera, may have been dormant in water until weather-related conditions caused it to multiply enough to constitute an infective dose if ingested by humans."[10]

Dr. Marie-Pierre Allié, president of Médecins Sans Frontières in France, had written her opinion piece two days before the UN cholera panel was named, but it wasn't published until a week later.[11] The headline made abundantly clear where she stood: "Why It's Important to Know How the Cholera Epidemic in Haiti Began."

Notably, Allié focused her attention on CDC, calling out the organization for what appeared to her as hypocrisy. "For its part, [CDC] officially refuses to investigate the origin of the disease. Contrary to the principles on which it was founded, the U.S. government's epidemiological investigative and monitoring agency asserts that 'the answer to that question makes no difference in efforts to prevent the disease from spreading.'"

Allié was well aware, as a scientist and physician, of what was at stake. "In fact, the lack of investigations and documentation leaves the field open to several theories," she wrote. Allié explained the "two competing hypotheses" for the epidemic's source, one relying on "global warming" and the other "on an imported Asian *Vibrio*." She identified Sack as the champion of the "green" environmental hypothesis and discussed the Harvard University microbiologist John Mekalanos, a leading proponent of what she called "the 'Nepal' hypothesis."

Piarroux was mentioned, too, as supporting the Mekalanos hypothesis and placing in his report "the first cases near the MINUSTAH camp in Mirebalais, in the center of the country and far from water that might carry zooplankton. This theory may also explain the suddenness with which cholera began in Haiti."

The "two explanatory models" had many different implications, Allié explained, insisting that priority be given to "the confirmation or rejection of one or the other by an independent, multidisciplinary team." She demanded transparency, too. Noting the repeated claim by the UN's Office for the Coordination of Humanitarian Affairs that "the issue of the origin of the epidemic is actually not important," she wrote that MSF could not support such statements. "It is counterproductive to hide epidemiological data and keep investigative reports confidential. It prevents us from establishing an accurate diagnosis and can result in misdirected relief efforts."

But it was too late: the UN panel was set.

The panel commenced its work in mid-January 2011, meeting first in Delhi, India, and then communicating through e-mail and conference calls. Panel members began by gathering information and discussing with experts outside Haiti who had voiced perspectives on the source of the disease. Piarroux was not contacted.

Early on, the UN panel began with three hypotheses considered credible.[12] First was that an environmental strain of *Vibrio cholera*, normally inhabiting the Gulf of Mexico, had traveled to Haiti via ocean currents as a consequence of the January 2010 earthquake and caused the October cholera epidemic. Second, a local, nontoxigenic *Vibrio cholerae* strain endemic to the Haitian environment naturally mutated into a virulent pathogenic strain, then quickly spread throughout the human population. To Piarroux, these were the monster-waiting-to-strike hypotheses. Third, an infected human carried a pathogenic strain of *Vibrio cholerae* into Haiti from a cholera-endemic region outside the country. The panel also mentioned a variation of the third hypothesis—that soldiers at Annapurna Camp were the direct source.

In late January and early February, the UN panel invited presentations from cholera experts, including Sack and Colwell. In his role as consultant, Sack shared with the panel his report to the UN and a related slide presentation.[13] His material addressed many issues. One section in particular caught Piarroux's attention when he finally saw the documents. Sack posed two questions: "Did the Nepal peacekeepers bring cholera into Haiti as proposed by Professor Renaud Piarroux?" and "Are there simple ways to insure that UN personnel do not introduce cholera into an area?" The first question was the one most germane to the UN panel's mandate.

In his slide, Sack informed the panel that he had reviewed Piarroux's mission report and carefully considered the evidence for and against Piarroux's conclusion. What he had not done was contact Piarroux.

Sack acknowledged that the arrival of the Nepalese troops and the onset of cholera were associated in both time and place and that Annapurna Camp had sanitation problems. He cited the *New England Journal of Medicine*'s statement that *V. cholerae* found in Haiti was closely related to South Asian strains of the microbe.[14] And he observed that the antibiotic sensitivity profile done by others for the cholera organism found in Haiti was similar to the pattern seen in Nepal. He offered no references for the latter, but likely was thinking of two articles that described the organism and antibiotic sensitivity patterns and showed that both the Haitian and Nepalese strains were susceptible to tetracycline and ciprofloxacin and resistant to furazolidone and nalidixic acid.[15] He used the antibiotic issue to dispute Piarroux, writing that "strains with this sensitivity pattern are found widely throughout South Asia. The sensitivity pattern changes from time to time, so the antibiotic sensitivity pattern does not provide useful information to answer the question of the strain's true origin."[16]

In his "evidence against," Sack seemed to ignore press reports about the obvious clear path from the MINUSTAH camp to the river. He stated that there had been only minor contamination that could not possibly have caused an explosive outbreak. He then posited that there was no way Nepalese troops could have started the widespread epidemic, writing, "None of the Nepalese soldiers had any diarrheal illness, and fecal samples from a sample of them were tested for *V. cholerae*. These were negative." Again no source was given. Sack had essentially repeated what MINUSTAH spokesman Vincenzo Pugliese had told reporters the previous October.[17] Finally, Sack made a serious charge that Piarroux had failed to consider the role of environmental conditions, ignoring a hypothesis he surely knew existed. Piarroux noted that Sack presented not a shred of scientific evidence to back up his claim of cholera's coastal presence in Haiti.

Sack's overall conclusion was also only an opinion: "I do not believe that the personnel from Nepal brought cholera to Haiti."[18] He had taken on Piarroux's report without addressing what the French epidemiologist had actually observed and written. The two men did agree on one thing, however: "Cholera appeared very quickly over a wide area of the Artibonite Valley within a matter of days." From there, though, Sack did not present epidemiological evidence from Haiti to support his views.

Sack's argument, on its face, seemed to Piarroux to boil down to this: I am an expert and I can make my chosen hypothesis fit the situation. My years of experience tell me the Haiti epidemic was "consistent with other epidemics" and that coastal cases of cholera were "mild or unrecognized infections, that later became explosive epidemics." Sack also directly attacked Piarroux's epidemiological method in his consultant report:

> If the first case in Haiti truly was this patient [October 14, 2010] in the village of Meille, near Mirebalais, [Piarroux's] conclusion would be logical. However, in an epidemic such as this one in Haiti, it is extremely difficult to identify the true "index" case, and much of my efforts were focused on attempting to find where these very early cases were occurring. Did the epidemic start in the area adjacent to the Nepal camp, or were there other cases occurring simultaneously suggesting that the case identified by Professor Piarroux was simply one of many such cases occurring at about the same time?[19]

Ironically, the only cholera case data Sack had were in Piarroux's report. On January 5, he had e-mailed colleagues familiar with Haiti and asked for "dates and places of the earliest cases of cholera, between October 10 and 22 . . . especially . . . cases along the coast near Saint Marc," as well as "information on ships which came to the port in Saint Marc following the earthquake."[20] Sack seemed to be looking for information to buttress the conclusion he had already drawn. His colleagues sent none.

Piarroux had written nothing about asymptomatic carriers, but he agreed with Sack that "such a massive contamination from an asymptomatic person is virtually impossible." What Piarroux *had* stated was that a tremendous amount of feces from a large number of *symptomatic* cholera patients would have been needed to create such outbreaks. His conclusion: a lot of soldiers in the camp must have been symptomatic. The Haitian public health team that conducted the October 21–24 field study had wanted to verify this, but they were turned away at Annapurna Camp.

Sack's slide presentation and report likely put the UN panel in a quandary. It was clear that his sponsor, the UN itself, wanted a particular outcome from what was supposed to be an independent and transparent investigation. Should the Sack material be released? It would be subjected to intense criticism. Sack was certainly a leading scientist in the cholera field but also was personally connected to three of the four panel members.

They kept the documents secret. A year later, I asked Sack directly to confirm their existence, which he did.[21]

The e-mail on Sunday, January 23, came as a surprise. Piarroux did not expect a request for assistance from Dr. Alejandro Cravioto, chair of the UN panel—even if such a request made perfect sense.

Of course, Piarroux responded immediately that he would do his best to provide all relevant information—cautioning, however, that much was in the manuscript he and his colleagues had recently submitted to the journal *Emerging Infectious Diseases*. This had been the group's second choice after rejection by the *Lancet*, and the article had been accepted subject to peer review. Piarroux said he would ask the *EID* editor for permission to share the manuscript, but when he did so, he was told that sharing it would violate the journal's guidelines and disqualify it for publication. So Piarroux offered to discuss his findings with Cravioto by telephone. During the call, Piarroux agreed to submit in writing some information about the initial spread of cases.

Piarroux next heard from Cravioto by e-mail the following Thursday. The panel chair wrote that he would be sharing Piarroux's information with Colwell and Sack and suggested "an open scientific discussion about the start and spread of the problem in Haiti based on the information you have all gathered and made available to the panel." The e-mail also included a curious attachment—an unsigned "consensus paper on the future management of the cholera situation in Haiti" Cravioto thought would interest Piarroux. It included the following paragraph.

> Some have suggested that the culprit strain of the outbreak is endemic to a region of South Asia, home to a group of UN peacekeepers stationed in central Haiti. The resulting conflict between UN peacekeepers and the public has further interfered with efforts to respond to the outbreak. If AIDS and previous pandemics offer any lessons, cycles of accusation will continue for years without helping to slow the cholera epidemic.

Unwilling to endorse what seemed to him to make a sham of investigating the source of the cholera outbreak, Piarroux didn't even mention it when he wrote back to Cravioto. He did, though, share his thoughts about asymptomatic cases, mentioning a review article on cholera transmission from a few years earlier that included a table describing the number of *Vibrio cholerae* organisms discharged from an infected case, typically measured as vibrios per gram of stool

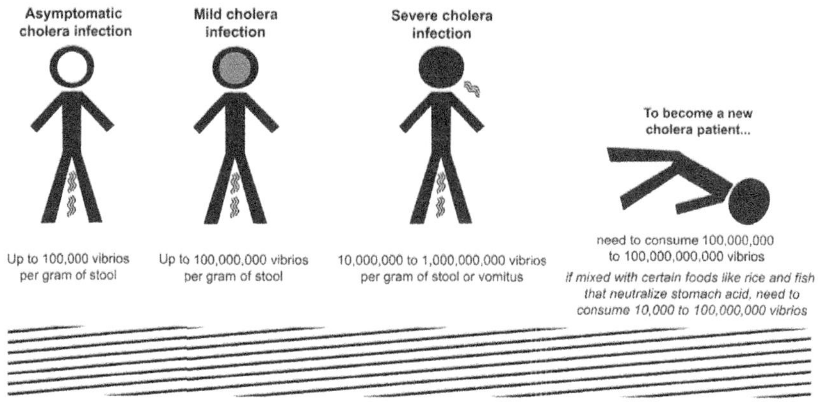

FIGURE 16.1. Transmission of cholera from infected person to susceptible person. Based on Nelson et al., "Cholera Transmission," 695 (table 1), 697.

or vomitus.[22] The numbers in that table lent themselves to the graphic depiction in figure 16.1.

Piarroux reasoned in his e-mail to Cravioto that the paucity of vibrios meant that the epidemic in Mèyé and Mirebalais could not be due to an asymptomatic cholera carrier who remained unnoticed in the Nepalese UN camp. Asymptomatic cases do not discharge very many vibrios, at least not enough to infect a typical susceptible person drinking water obtained from a stream. Instead, he concluded that one or more soldiers incubating the disease must have arrived with the replacement Nepalese battalion and soon became ill. Then, in the close contact of the camp, they infected others and generated new cholera cases among the troops. If mild or severe and sufficiently plentiful, the new cases would have discharged a much larger number of vibrios into the leaky toilets or nearby stream—enough contamination to create new cholera cases in the hamlet of Mèyé across the road from the camp.

Also, Piarroux shared a slide presentation showing the location of the MINUSTAH camp in relation to Mèyé, along with the important October 21–24 MSPP report and initial LNSP lab results.

"I will share them with the panel and get back to you with our questions and comments," Cravioto wrote back later that day.

A week and a half went by before Cravioto wrote to acknowledge receiving the materials—and asked for more. He mentioned that the panel had asked the UN to comment specifically on Piarroux's report, a request "essential to have a more clear perspective of the events around the beginning of the epidemic." He also noted that the panel had reviewed a large number of documents and opinions from other people working in Haiti that would be used when it wrote its final report.

Piarroux responded with a much longer description of his investigation. He provided important information about the people and communities in the Artibonite River basin and the expanding valley and wrote, "I could not find one suspected case that occurred before October 19 in the six communes of the lower Artibonite basin. The epidemiologist of the Artibonite department told me the health department received its first alert from the town of Bocozel in Saint Marc commune on October 19. This alert involved three children who died from acute watery diarrhea while they were at school. None of the three children had any health problems before October 19."

The French epidemiologist explained the cluster of cases in the area, the rise and fall in the number of cases, and how the disease spread or did not spread to upriver communes. Focusing on the facts, he then took on issues mentioned in Sack's report—even though Piarroux did not yet know of its existence.

> Our investigation showed that the contamination occurred simultaneously in the six communes of the lower reaches of the Artibonite River. Moreover, the epidemic curve peaked very rapidly and started to decrease on the third day. I have investigated numerous cholera epidemics in the Congo and the Comoros islands and have epidemiological data from various other countries in Western Africa. This, however, was the first time that I have seen an epidemiological curve like the one in Artibonite department.
>
> If you scan the data for other departments of Haiti, you will notice that none exhibited a similar unusual epidemic curve. Even in 1994 in the camps around Goma, Zaïre [later DR Congo], the peak of the epidemic was not reached so abruptly (the epidemic started in mid-July with the arrival of the refugees and peaked on July 26th, at least ten days later).
>
> Taking into account the incubation period of cholera that usually ranges from a few hours to five days, the epidemic curve in the lower six communes is what you might expect in a common source outbreak, provoked by a single contaminating event that persisted in each commune for at least one to two hours while people are drawing water from the river and canals, but likely no more than one day.
>
> . . . The only plausible hypothesis is a massive but transient contamination of the Artibonite River with a large cholera plume flowing downriver toward the ocean. During October, the river flows at a rate of 150,000 liters per second, or one billion liters during a two-hour span.

> If we assume that the population is highly susceptible to cholera, perhaps an inoculum as low as 100,000 vibrios per liter of water would have caused disease, but likely would have needed many more. The only way to reach transient concentrations of 100,000 or more vibrios per liter of Artibonite River water for at least two hours is to discharge a huge amount of *Vibrio cholerae*-contaminated stools into the river or into one of its feeding streams.
>
> The smaller outbreak that started in [Mèyé] and Mirebalais could not have stimulated such a massive and short-duration contamination of the Artibonite River. Indeed, after October 22, the epidemic was still increasing in Mirebalais whereas it exhibited a marked remission in the communes of the lower Artibonite River, suggesting that the infecting cholera plume had flowed past the communes.
>
> As I had previously explained to Edmond Mulet and the MINUSTAH staff in Haiti, only the dumping of a septic tank containing a large number of cholera vibrios from many infected persons could have led to such a huge contamination of the Artibonite River. I really want to discuss this point with the UN panel, as it is very important to find if a credible alternative explanation is forthcoming.

Cravioto's response was quicker. The next day, he wrote that Piarroux's information was "very impressive," but he would "need time to digest [it] all." He promised to forward it all to his panel colleagues and assured Piarroux that any questions they might have would be sent back.

Piarroux wrote again to Cravioto on Saturday, February 12. He knew the UN panel would soon travel to Haiti, and he wanted the chair to have the names of his colleagues there who had participated in his investigation. He asked Cravioto for feedback on the documents and lengthy e-mail he had sent five days earlier, wondering whether there were any questions.

Cravioto responded immediately. The information had been shared, he wrote, but the panel had been working either alone or in small groups gathering information. He planned to discuss more with them while in Haiti and thereafter, once they had a better picture of "what happened in the days just before and after the start of the epidemic."

There was no further communication for more than a month. Finally, Piarroux grew weary of waiting, so on March 17—several weeks after the panel had concluded its trip to Haiti—he prompted Cravioto with a brief note of inquiry. The response was terse.

> The Panel is working hard to finish the report, which of course will take into account your findings, as well as those of many others who have

> also shared their work and findings with us. The members of the Panel have no further questions about your work and thank you for sharing it with us.
>
> We will be finishing our report soon to hand it in to the Secretary General. Once this is done we will be doing a dissemination of the results.

The panel issued its report in early May. Piarroux was surprised when he read the introduction.

> Two previous investigations that commented on the source of the outbreak came to opposing conclusions: Sack (personal communication) concluded that the outbreak was caused by a local event; whereas Piarroux (2010) concluded that the outbreak was caused by cholera being imported to Haiti by an infected MINUSTAH soldier. Neither report presents sufficient evidence to support its conclusions with reasonable certainty.[23]

Piarroux was incensed but not beaten. He knew facts have a very nasty habit of persisting even when deliberately ignored.

Even before the panel's report was released, Piarroux had suspected what the outcome would be. So he and Benoît Faucher, a colleague from his university and hospital, decided to go on the offensive while they awaited a decision from *Emerging Infectious Diseases* regarding publication of their scientific paper.

The two men wanted to address the reluctance of officials and scientists to conduct field investigations on the exact origin of the Haitian cholera epidemic. In an editorial in *Clinical Microbiology and Infection* posted online in late January (prior to hard-copy publication), they presented four reasons for their disagreement: the importance of getting information on the spark that starts an outbreak; the importance of gathering data on causative factors that explain the full dimension of an ensuing epidemic; the need to understand whether the organism was in the environment or was brought by human activity so as to forecast the future course of the disease; and the consequences of failing to maintain the public's trust.[24]

They saved their most powerful admonition for the end. "Nobody would dare to claim the uselessness of the determination of the source of the outbreak if its location was Europe or the United States. Haitians deserve as well to know why, and how, thousands of them died."

17

NEPAL

Nepal experienced much cholera over the course of the seven great pandemics, but beginning in the latter half of the twentieth century it was political turmoil that posed the nation's greatest challenge. Years of power struggles between the monarchy and elected government came to a head in 1959 when thirty-nine-year-old King Mahendra—the ninth king in the 191-year rule of Nepal's Shah dynasty—shut down the democracy "experiment" and established a "partyless" system. That lasted until 1989, when a popular movement forced King Birendra—Mahendra's eldest son and successor—to accept constitutional reforms. A multiparty parliament was elected and seated in 1991. Five years later, civil war broke out as the Communist Party of Nepal (Maoist) launched an assault. Eventually, the ongoing guerilla war claimed more than 160,000 lives.[1]

A peace process began to unfold in 2006. In 2007, the United Nations Mission in Nepal (UNMIN) was established, and UN peacekeeping forces arrived to help stabilize the country—an ironic turn of events for a country that had been, since the late 1950s, a supplier of more than one hundred thousand troops and police to UN peacekeeping efforts elsewhere in the world.[2]

The Nepalese Army ("Royal" was dropped from its name in 2006) had taken its first UN peacekeeping assignment in Lebanon in 1958 and in the intervening years had served as part of UN contingents in more than three dozen missions.[3] The accusation that its troops had brought cholera to Haiti was a terrible stain on its reputation and threatened a longtime source of considerable financial revenue to the army and its welfare fund in a very poor country. The welfare fund takes about a fifth of the peacekeeping soldier's monthly income while abroad and provides medical and educational assistance for soldiers' families, including those not serving as peacekeepers. Reduce or eliminate the welfare fund, and Nepal would be unable to provide that support. Simply put, bringing a deadly disease to Haiti could deliver a devastating blow to Nepal's "peacekeeping industry."

The accusation came amid preparations for departure from Nepal by UNMIN troops, which happened on January 15, 2011. Self-described communists of various stripes had expanded their influence throughout the country, and the Maoist hold on the Ministry of Health and Population was growing stronger.[4] Tensions between former combatants persisted, especially since part of the country's stabilization plan was to merge former Maoist troops into the regular army. Unlike her predecessors, the new Maoist minister of health and population had no loyalties to the army and no concerns about safeguarding the reputation of the Maoists' former military nemesis.

The change in leadership sent political ripples down to the National Public Health Laboratory, directed by Dr. Geeta Shakya, a highly regarded scientist and administrator. Over the years, she had helped establish the Antimicrobial Resistance Surveillance (ARS) system that guided medical care in Nepal and was funded first in part by the U.S. government and after 2006 largely by WHO. A surveillance system, with eleven laboratories, monitored *Vibrio cholera* and other microbial agents in the country.[5] Yet "political instability and insurgency" had made maintaining the ARS difficult.[6]

Meanwhile, Shakya was feeling pressure from international groups to help determine the possible role of the Nepalese in bringing cholera to Haiti. The Nepalese Army, with its weakened influence, had no choice but to go along with the comparative analysis of cholera specimens.

Details of the intricate scientific analyses were left to Shakya. To avoid potential charges of bias, she decided to seek an outside, objective assessment of whether there was a Nepal-Haiti cholera link and engaged three world-class international organizations. The International Vaccine Institute (IVI) in Seoul, Korea, had successfully addressed cholera outbreaks in northern Vietnam[7] and had been collaborating on an anti-typhoid fever vaccine for use in Nepal. IVI received cholera specimens from various years and areas of Nepal. The Technical University of Denmark (TUD) housed a respected WHO collaborating center focused on antimicrobial resistance in foodborne pathogens and had led a training course in Thailand attended by one of Shakya's staff. TUD scientists received Nepalese cholera samples and planned to employ state-of-the-art high-resolution genotyping analysis, previously used with anthrax and plague. Finally, there was the Wellcome Trust Sanger Institute in Cambridge, England, famous for sequencing approximately one-third of the human genome as well as genomes of more than ninety pathogens, including cholera. Wellcome received about eighty cholera strains from various regions of Nepal collected between 2007 and 2010.

As Shakya and the world awaited the results of these independent analyses, political events continued to unfold. The peacekeeping mission in Nepal had finally ended in mid-January 2011, about a month before the samples were sent out. Then Nepal again began a plummet into turmoil and disarray. In February, Jhala Nath Khanal—chairman of the more moderate Communist Party of Nepal (Unified Marxist-Leninist)—became the country's thirty-fifth prime minister. During the preceding seven months, no candidate had been able to win enough votes to take that office, but Khanal had finally won the weighty backing of the Maoists. The promise of stability was soon shattered, though: Khanal was unable to form a unity government, and the Constituent Assembly—in which the Maoist party made up the largest voting bloc—failed to meet its May deadline for drawing up a new constitution. In August, Khanal resigned after his government failed to reach a compromise on a new constitution and on how the former Maoist fighters—many of whom had been languishing in camps since 2006—would be integrated into the Nepalese Army.

Parliament elected a new prime minister from the Maoist party itself. Baburam Bhattarai vowed to address the constitutional crisis and resolve the army integration challenge. He, too, failed, and in May 2012 he dissolved parliament and called elections for the following November. Bhattarai remained in charge of what could only be called a "caretaker" government.

Political turmoil shared the spotlight with explosive scientific information on August 23, 2011, when TUD scientists—who had joined forces with colleagues at the Translational Genomics Research in Flagstaff, Arizona—published the results of their analysis in *Mbio*, a peer-reviewed online journal published by the American Society for Microbiology.[8]

An internationally known molecular geneticist in Arizona, Paul Keim, had heard about the Danes' getting samples and became very interested in the potential link between Nepal and Haiti. He had demonstrated his own considerable detective skills in 2001 when he helped the Federal Bureau of Investigation solve an anthrax outbreak in the United States.[9] Since then, he and colleagues at Northern Arizona University had created a state-of-the-art forensic laboratory for doing sophisticated molecular genetic analyses.

The *Mbio* publication, with coauthors from Denmark, Arizona, and Nepal, presented the analyses of twenty-four isolates gathered between July 30 and November 1, 2010, from five different Nepalese districts. They had been compared with ten *Vibrio cholerae* isolates—including three from the 2010 Haitian outbreak—that had previously undergone whole-genome sequence typing (WGST), a powerful new tool for describing the complete hereditary information of an organism. WGST showed that all twenty-four isolates from Nepal belonged to a single group, but that group also contained isolates from nearby Bangladesh and faraway Haiti.

The single group was then further divided into four closely related clusters, one of which contained three Nepalese isolates collected on August 1 and 30, 2010, in the Banke and Rupandehi districts of south-central Nepal. Those three were then compared with the three Haitian isolates from 2010 previously collected and characterized by CDC. All six were virtually identical, with only very small differences of one- or two-base pairs (i.e., the building blocks of the microbe's DNA double helix) out of more than four million base pairs reported in the *Vibrio cholerae* genome.[10]

"Results in this study are consistent with Nepal as the origin of the Haitian outbreak," wrote the authors—an explosive statement. They acknowledged the possibility that "this genetic group [of isolates] will be discovered in countries other than Nepal and Haiti" and added "the current conclusion that Nepal is the source of the Haitian cholera outbreak can be reached only if both classical epidemiology and highly suggestive WGST are used together." Piarroux's investigation, employing "classical epidemiology," was the only one mentioned in the *Mbio* article.

Denying Nepalese involvement had become more difficult.

18

CONCEALED IN THE FIELD

Epidemiologists may not all work exactly alike, but they do have some standard operating procedures for outbreak investigations. For instance, they typically list disease cases by the date symptoms first appear—the "onset date"—not when they are confirmed in a laboratory. The onset date provides the most accurate picture of an outbreak's beginning; laboratory analyses may be held up because of workload and other priorities.

CDC epidemiologists in Haiti knew these standard operating procedures, outlined in CDC's own manual—*How to Investigate an Outbreak*—used to teach the approach.[1] The manual explains the importance of correctly identifying infectious disease cases and then using a frequency distribution of the onset dates to estimate the outbreak's start time.

CDC had ignored its own standard procedure by using the "first confirmed case" in its Haiti Cholera Outbreak map of mid-February 2011.[2] It based the onset on laboratory confirmation time, which falsely implied that cholera had first appeared on October 21 in downriver Artibonite dépkartement, then two days later in Ouest dépkartement, and finally a day after that, October 24, in upriver Centre dépkartement—findings entirely different from Piarroux's and the Haitian public health team's.

Charitably, Piarroux gave CDC some benefit of the doubt. Perhaps its epidemiologists were troubled by the absence of onset information for many of the early laboratory-confirmed cases, especially those from the explosive outbreak phase in Artibonite dépkartement. Persons with cholera appeared at medical facilities but either were not asked for or did not know the onset date. Because much of the onset data were missing, CDC may have decided that the date of symptom onset was simply not reliable enough to include in the map.

Piarroux, though, knew CDC could have done something different. Its epidemiologists could have used the date when the soon-to-be confirmed stool specimens arrived at LNSP rather than the sometimes-delayed date when the specimens were finally confirmed and reported as cholera. With that, they could have correctly reported that the epidemic began in Centre département and then appeared in Artibonite département.

Piarroux suspected that CDC had released the map in anticipation of the UN panel's arrival in Haiti and was helping the UN shift attention away from the Nepalese peacekeeping base in Centre département. Implying that cholera had started elsewhere served that purpose.

It was the first in a series of online maps from CDC that used the poorest available measure to show when cholera had first appeared in Haiti's ten départements. The CDC information remained widely circulated through updates in September 2011.[3]

To its credit, CDC was becoming convinced that cholera had arrived in Haiti via a single source, discounting the environmental theory. In spite of this, the organization still seemed determined to help focus attention away from the UN peacekeepers.

So, if not from coastal estuaries, how might cholera have first come to Artibonite département? The editors of CDC's *Morbidity and Mortality Weekly Report* planted an alternative seed in December 2010, writing that "transnational spread of cholera is caused most commonly by importation by travelers."[4] But rather than tourists, they had maritime travelers in mind: "Toxigenic *V. cholerae* also can be transported by ships' ballast water." Earlier researchers had suggested that Indonesian cargo ships, for instance, brought cholera to Peru in 1991.[5]

Cargo ships need weighted bottoms for stability and maneuverability in turbulent ocean waters. Typically, the cargo itself serves this function, but if there is insufficient cargo the crew typically pumps water into ballast tanks in the boat's hull. The water may become contaminated with microbial agents such as *Vibrio cholerae* from soiled cargo or from feces or vomitus of infected crew or passengers.[6] A partially loaded ship entering Saint-Marc harbor in coastal Artibonite département could have discharged excess cholera-ridden ballast water to accommodate the weight of new cargo, launching an outbreak among consumers of harbor water or shellfish.

Well, thought Piarroux, that's an interesting theory. But his findings of inland origin near Mirebalais had made clear that it did not apply to the Haiti outbreak of 2010. Still, CDC persisted with its misdirection. In January 2011, the ballast notion was raised again but this time in a CDC map titled "Map—Ship Ballast Discharge Evaluation" that highlighted Haiti within the Caribbean region.[7]

CDC's unusual onset map and ballast theory may even have confounded some of its own scientists. In a November 2011 article, a CDC laboratory group wrote that cholera "quickly spread from its origin along a main river in the Artibonite Department north of Port-au-Prince to all 10 departments in Haiti and to the Dominican Republic."[8] Yes, as Piarroux had confirmed, cholera in Haiti had spread rapidly. But CDC's map of first cases, coupled with its ballast theory, led the authors down the wrong path. They simply repeated CDC's incorrect assertion of where cholera originated.

Whether the UN panel was influenced by the CDC map or the ballast theory was never clear to Piarroux. There were so many other problems with the panel's work in Haiti.

The flight that brought the four panel members to Haiti landed at the Port-au-Prince airport on Sunday, February 13, 2011. The plan was to remain for one week and gather input for the final report. But the panel's field investigation faced several challenges. From press reports, Haitians knew they were coming, and there was widespread skepticism that any panel appointed by the UN to investigate the epidemic's origin would actually be seeking the truth, especially when most Haitians by then believed cholera had been brought by UN peacekeepers.

Another challenge was the panel's timing: put bluntly, they were late to the investigation. The first cases of cholera had occurred four months earlier. Then there was the team of water, sanitation, and hygiene experts the UN had sent in early December to "review all sanitation systems at MINUSTAH military, police and civilian installations."[9] Surely their findings, which hadn't been released publicly, would have helped MINUSTAH clean things up and thus alter the evidentiary landscape.

Right from the beginning of the panel's visit, there was trouble. In his January 27 e-mail to Cravioto, Piarroux had shared a photocopy of part of the spreadsheet LNSP used to tally results for cholera testing. It made clear that LNSP had received stool specimens from the field, tallied important dates, and conducted laboratory diagnoses of cholera. It showed onset times for the first cases. The panel knew LNSP had a larger database with a completed roster of submitted specimens for suspected cholera since the beginning of the epidemic, but it never obtained those data. Piarroux wondered why. Later, Daniele Lantagne, the panel member designated as spokesperson to the press, offered specific information on the panel's activities and intentions beyond what was cited in its ultimate report.[10] Still later, Piarroux also learned of some local Haitian views of what had taken place.[11]

Before their trip, panel members said they wanted to see the LNSP data, and CDC staff arranged for a meeting in Haiti. Once in Haiti, they met with local Haitian government officials, including three Haitian epidemiologists, and toured the LNSP site where cholera specimens were being confirmed. When the panel members requested the raw cholera data, the Haitians referred them to CDC in Atlanta to process their request—but no one on the panel ever followed up. Perhaps panel members felt that less valid clinical information gathered in the field would still be sufficient for their report.

The Haitians, though, told a different story. Dr. Gabriel Thimothé, director general of the MSPP, was at the meeting with the panel members and sent them to the Department of Epidemiology, Laboratory and Research to meet Director Roc Magloire, Deputy Director Donald Lafontant, and epidemiologist Robert Barrais. The meeting did not go well: there was an argument regarding the origin of the cholera epidemic and the planned starting point for the panel's investigation. The Haitians insisted on Mirebalais; panel members were determined to visit the Artibonite delta first.

To the Haitian scientists—well aware of the epidemic's true origin—this only confirmed their suspicions about the UN panel's bias.

Also in that meeting, panel members never said a word about the findings of the October 21–24, 2010, MSPP investigation. The Haitian scientists knew Piarroux had shared those seminal findings with the members and were disturbed by their silence. This only intensified their distrust, and the three men made no further effort to assist the panel members.

One member, the prominent microbiologist G. Balakrish Nair, did meet later with LNSP director Jacques Boncy to discuss the laboratory findings. The early cases from Mèyé were not yet recorded in the laboratory database, since they had come from the team of public health investigators rather than through the official route from local hospitals. Nair never asked Boncy about those specimens, even though Piarroux had shared the spreadsheet output with early laboratory-confirmed cases with the panel.

The bottom line: UN panel members never reviewed the laboratory-confirmed cholera data from LNSP that Piarroux had used. Instead, they relied first on interviews with unnamed persons who supposedly had knowledge of early cholera cases but who could provide no data to support whatever they told the panel. Then, citing a lack of "physical evidence to confirm this anecdotal data," the panel decided to search for "clinical information in the form of medical records of MINUSTAH personnel and admission records at Centre and Artibonite Department regional hospitals."

While the UN panel was in Haiti, Piarroux received word from *Emerging Infectious Diseases* that the peer review of his coauthored article was complete and that some changes were necessary before a second round of reviews. One reviewer suggested the authors consult a "spatial epidemiologist" who might help with a better presentation of the geographic spread of cholera and help "assess the relative risk associated with exposure to key rivers, water sources," and the like. So Piarroux enlisted the assistance of Dr. Jean Gaudart, a fellow faculty member at Aix-Marseille Université in Marseilles. Gaudart, a physician with a PhD in mathematics who had published space-time analyses of malaria risk, had developed new statistical approaches for viewing spatial clusters that Piarroux felt would strengthen the analysis of the cholera investigation. Gaudart joined the coauthor list.

The same reviewer had also written that the authors should "avoid drawing too many conclusions about what is a highly charged political issue"—a comment that troubled Piarroux, who wondered whether it was part of a general campaign to deflect attention away from the UN's culpability. He agreed to make some wording changes but pointed out that discussing plausible explanations for a first-time epidemic in a scientific report was hardly "political." Did the reviewer really believe the authors should not fully discuss their own findings?

After some of the typical back and forth, the editor emailed Piarroux on April 27, 2011, that the article was accepted for publication in the July issue. It would appear online as an "Epub ahead of print" on May 6,[12] which turned out to be two days after the official release of the UN panel's report.[13]

As previously stated, the panel had omitted mention of the Haitians' October 21–24 field investigation report, which clearly indicated when and where the outbreak of cholera had truly begun. By contrast, Piarroux and his coauthors' *EID* article did not shy away from the early LNSP data and certainly didn't ignore the MSPP's own investigation of October 21–24, writing, "On October 18, the Cuban medical brigades reported an increase of acute watery diarrhea (61 cases treated in Mirebalais during the preceding week) to MSPP. On October 18, the situation worsened, with 28 new admissions and 2 deaths. MSPP immediately sent a Haitian investigation team, which found that the epidemic began October 14."

The UN panel members did visit the Annapurna camp by Mèyé in the first days of their investigation. They wanted to review the medical log book maintained at the small clinic that served the Nepalese troops stationed there—as well as at the Terre Rouge camp to the south and possibly at the Hinche camp to the north. The worn log showed the date a patient was first and last seen and the patient's medical condition and had years of data entered in various hands. The panel members looked for tampering but found no evidence. Convinced the entries were valid, the members focused on September–October 2010.

Piarroux thought about the word "tamper." It means to interfere with something, and in French it has many synonyms, not all involving direct physical action. Making alterations is a form of tampering, but you could just as easily tamper by omission. Had the panel considered that the log might have been used selectively—that once Nepalese troop commanders realized there was an explosive diarrhea outbreak among soldiers, they might have ordered that no patient entries be made? Nothing in the panel's report indicated that members had given this a moment's thought. Instead, the log was deemed a valid, inclusive, and truthful source from which the panel drew a very strong conclusion: "No cases of severe diarrhea and dehydration occurred among MINUSTAH personnel during this period" and, even more emphatically, "no clinical cases of cholera occurred among MINUSTAH personnel before or during the start of the cholera outbreak in Haiti."

According to WHO, the field definition the panel seemed to use—severe diarrhea with dehydration—accounted for only about 10–20 percent of all cholera cases. The remaining symptomatic cases—considered mild or moderate in severity—accounted for 80 percent.[14] Were moderate and mild cases omitted? Piarroux wondered, acknowledging that the two clinical members of the panel undoubtedly knew cholera's clinical features.

Later, panel member Lantagne revealed that even diarrhea cases of the mild and moderate form were not reported in the medical log. No surprise, thought Piarroux, considering that on December 15, Alain Le Roy, the UN under-secretary general for peacekeeping operations, had insisted that during the two weeks between their arrival and the confirmation of Haiti's cholera outbreak "none of the Nepalese soldiers have been sick or have been shown any sign of diarrhea."[15]

Piarroux had read about Le Roy's statement when he was back in France and wasn't the only one to wonder how so many troops recently arrived from Nepal could have avoided experiencing *some* level of diarrhea. Later, Dr. Jody Lanard used published data on the incidence of diarrhea in travelers to analyze the expected pattern of diarrhea among the newly arrived Nepalese troops. She and her husband are risk assessment pioneers called on time and again by WHO to analyze risk in disease outbreaks. She estimated that the 454 Nepalese troops identified by journalist Jonathan Katz as in the camp[16] should have had between 13.5 and 65 episodes of diarrhea in the two-week period. Writing on the *Peter Sandman and Jody Lanard Risk Communication* blog (March 28, 2012), she concluded, "It would be highly unusual for none of the soldiers to have had diarrhea during that period."

That's what an independent investigation looks like, thought Piarroux. Like Lanard, he questioned the value of the camp's medical log for determining diarrhea. Later, Lantagne mentioned it was highly plausible that troops with diarrhea would have avoided going to the clinic for care, and she admitted the medical log was probably not a good source of diarrhea data.[17] Of course, this implied the log was also not a good source for cholera data.

Perhaps there was another way to assess whether diarrhea had affected those Nepalese peacekeepers—procurement and inventory analysis. The clinic's medical unit would have been expected to have a supply of what is needed to treat diarrheal diseases, such as the Interagency Diarrheal Disease Kits developed in early 2009 as a standard for "agencies working in crisis situations" and given to battalions with medical units, as found at Annapurna Camp. The kits contain oral rehydration salts (ORS), infusion sets for advanced dehydration, and an assortment of antibiotics, all useful for treating hundreds of suspected cholera cases.[18]

The use of oral rehydration therapy—often home-based—had long been promoted in Nepal.[19] ORS packets could have been given to the Nepalese soldiers with symptoms of mild or even moderate cholera. Handing them out for personal use wouldn't have been recorded in the medical log, and troops in their quarters would have simply mixed ORS with bottled, boiled, or chlorinated water, drunk that for two days or so, and continued to use the base latrines or toilets—potentially filling the septic tanks with cholera-rich feces. Only more advanced cholera cases would have entered the clinic and been treated with intravenous fluids and antibiotics. But even if those cases had been deliberately omitted from the log, the UN panel should have reviewed the camp procurement books to learn whether the kits had been ordered and replaced. They made no mention of doing so.

Even if by chance MINUSTAH didn't use the kits, the panel could have reviewed the medical clinic's inventory and ordering forms for past use of intravenous fluids, ORS, and the four most effective antibiotics cited in Nepal for treating cholera—ampicillin, tetracycline, ciprofloxacin, and erythromycin.[20] A simple review of inventory and ordering forms should have revealed past usage, perhaps pointing to unrecorded diarrhea or cholera among the troops.

As the UN panel conducted its investigation around Haiti, the number of inconsistencies and missed opportunities to find evidence grew. Lantagne said, for instance, that they were told a sample of eighty Nepalese troops was tested for cholera in Haiti right after Piarroux told the UN's Edmond Mulet in mid-November 2010 that the epidemic's explosive early phase was likely caused by many symptomatic cholera cases in the MINUSTAH camp. All were found negative, as Alain Le Roy stated at his December 15 press conference.[21]

Piarroux assumed the standard fecal tests had been ordered to impugn his assertion of cholera in the camp. Their timing made no sense otherwise. The initial October cholera cases among Nepalese troops would already have been treated or resolved by November, leaving no residual evidence of *Vibrio cholerae* in their stools. Could this obvious bias explain why the panel didn't even bother to mention these late tests in its report?

The panel visited three hospitals in Haiti—in Mirebalais, Deschapelles, and Saint-Marc—and relied on medical records from the hospital registries, looking for patients hospitalized in October 2010 for diarrhea and dehydration. Those records, though, were insufficiently detailed, and so the panel used the more general category "hospitalizations due to severe diarrhea" as a proxy for cholera cases.

At the community hospital in Mirebalais, panel members learned of the first hospitalized death from dehydration on October 17, 2010, the date in the MSPP October 21–24 report. Staff said the first cholera cases came from Mèyé near the MINUSTAH camp, but the panel never cross-checked this information with the Haitian epidemiologists. It did, though, visit the large public market in Mirebalais to determine whether fish or shellfish products were sold—following the *MMWR* editors' false trail of ships' ballast water in coastal Saint-Marc. None from the coast were found, and local women told them none were *ever* sold. Local people did not eat fish. At least that fact made it into the panel's report: the population "in Mirebalais was not exposed to *Vibrio cholerae* from possibly contaminated seafood."

At Albert Schweitzer Hospital in Deschapelles, Artibonite département, the panel again reviewed admission records and based its observations about cholera on "severe diarrhea" cases—noting that the first such cases were seen on October 20, 2010. This confirmed what Ian Rawson had blogged. The number of cases increased dramatically after that date, making exact record keeping more difficult.

Finally, the UN panel visited Saint-Nicolas Hospital in Saint-Marc, again reviewing medical records and noting in September and October a consistent low number of diarrhea cases until October 20, when an explosive outbreak of apparent cholera occurred. The 404 recorded hospitalizations and 44 deaths on that date came from fifty communities throughout the Artibonite River delta, although only 9 of the 404 (2.2%) came from the city of Saint-Marc, where cargo ships in the harbor drained water ballast—a strong rebuttal of *MMWR*'s insinuation. While cholera struck all ages, those twenty to twenty-four years made up the largest group at the hospital, which the staff surmised was due to "cholera transmission in agricultural workers exposed to Artibonite River irrigation water in the rice paddies and fields."

Even before Piarroux's coauthored article appeared in *Emerging Infectious Diseases*, the journal published a study for which the authors had received nineteen fecal samples from a Haitian hospital cited as "St. Mark's Hospital, Artibonite" but was likely Saint Nicolas Hospital in Saint-Marc, Artibonite département.[22] The authors processed the samples within a month of the epidemic's beginning and found sixteen positive for *V. cholerae* O1 Ogawa El Tor, the same organism previously reported in Haiti.[23] By November 9, when the specimens arrived at the University of Florida Emerging Pathogens Institute, the epidemic was already well under way. The Haitian MSPP had recently reported a cumulative total of 11,125 cholera hospital admissions and 725 cholera deaths.[24] Thus the sixteen specimens represented a small sample drawn from a much larger population of cholera patients.

Still, the study drew an important conclusion. The authors used a sophisticated molecular typing technique for detecting differences in rapidly changing areas of the cholera genome. Had cholera been in Haiti for many years, as proponents of the environmental hypothesis claimed, the researchers would have found multiple strains of the organism with different genetic profiles—diversification observed in countries where cholera has long resided in environmental reservoirs. They observed only one cholera strain, however, thus confirming Piarroux's insistence that human activity had brought the single cholera strain to Haiti.

At the end of its investigation, even the UN panel had to dismiss the environmental hypothesis, writing, "The most likely cause of the outbreak was the consumption of contaminated water from the river." The report declared that an "explosive cholera outbreak began on October 20, 2010, in the Artibonite River delta, indicating that cholera had spread throughout the Artibonite River delta within two to three days of the first cases being seen in the upstream region."

Epidemiologists and students of epidemics are expected to use clues and logic to help explain causes on the basis of facts. Understanding the dynamics of the Artibonite River was central to unraveling the epidemiological puzzle. If the epidemic had indeed begun near Mirebalais, how did cholera microbes manage to infect so many in communities throughout the lower Artibonite valley days later?

To explain this, Piarroux and his *EID* coauthors focused first on the fact that a person needs to ingest about one hundred thousand cholera vibrios to become infected and develop cholera disease. So the first premise was that a one-liter container of contaminated water consumed from the river would need to hold at least one hundred thousand vibrios. Next they focused on the downriver communities, an area covering 1,500 square kilometers more than 25 kilometers from Mèyé, where many people had developed cholera at about the same time. The cholera organisms entered the river at the starting point and a day or two later simultaneously infected people in those communities. After an incubation period of one to two days following infection, an explosive cholera epidemic appeared. With the river as transmitting agent, every liter of water during a three-hour passing time likely contained at least a hundred thousand vibrios.

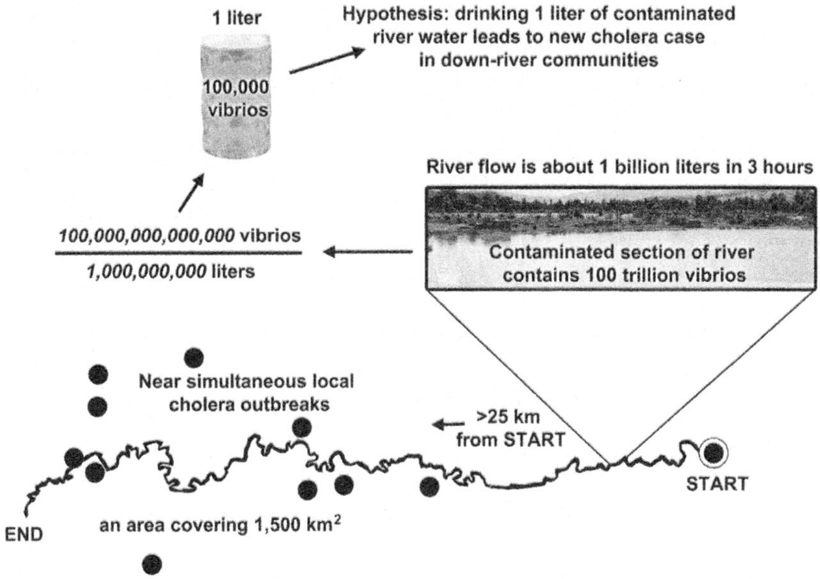
1 liter
100,000
vibrios
Hypothesis: drinking 1 liter of contaminated
river water leads to new cholera case
in down-river communities
River flow is about 1 billion liters in 3 hours
100,000,000,000,000 vibrios
1,000,000,000 liters
Contaminated section of river
contains 100 trillion vibrios
Near simultaneous local
cholera outbreaks
>25 km
from START
START
END
an area covering 1,500 km²

FIGURE 18.1. First epidemiological clues and logic to explain explosive phase of the epidemic. Created by Ralph R. Frerichs.

Prior research allowed Piarroux and his colleagues to estimate the flow rate of the Artibonite at about one billion liters in three hours. Thus, a contaminated three-hour section of the river would have (100,000 vibrios) × (1,000,000,000 liters) or one hundred trillion vibrios. With such a large contaminated plume, enough vibrios would flow downriver to start a widespread cholera epidemic simultaneously in several communities (see figure 18.1).

The UN panel also estimated the Artibonite's flow. Daniele Lantagne, the panel's environmental engineer, twice visited Péligre dam, about ten kilometers upstream from Mirebalais, and the downriver Canneau dam near Deschapelles, where the river splits into irrigation canals for the Artibonite valley's small farms. She spoke with dam and water- and electricity-related organizations and related that in the dry season (January to August) the Artibonite River flow volume was about fifty cubic meters per second, equivalent to fifty thousand liters of water per second. The panel report stated that once the water reached Canneau dam, about forty cubic meters per second were diverted to the left bank canal system and ten cubic meters per second to the right. More important for investigating the cholera source was the volume of flow in the wet season (August to November), when the outbreak occurred. The "flow rate increases," the UN panel wrote, not having more specific information.

Information on U.S. river flow typically comes from government-maintained stream gauges verified with monthly in-person flow testing, providing seasonal information over many years. No stream gauges were used along the Artibonite River, so Lantagne felt uncomfortable estimating flow data for October 2010.

Piarroux estimated, and even cited a reference, that during October of the wet season the flow usually exceeded one hundred thousand liters per second (i.e., one hundred cubic meters per second).[25] Much earlier, the U.S. Army Corps of Engineers had suggested that the Artibonite River contained even more water and that during the wet season from May to October might flow from Mirebalais to the Gulf of Gonâve at rates between five hundred thousand liters and five million liters per second (i.e., five hundred to five thousand cubic meters per second).[26] Those estimates were ten to one hundred times greater than the "dry season" flow volume reported by the UN panel. Assuming a higher flow volume, there would need to have been even more cholera microbes coming into the Artibonite near Mirebalais to overcome the dilution effect as the river flowed towards the delta communities.

The panel report also focused on the time it took for water to flow from one location to another. One Haitian group told Lantagne it took one and a half to two days for water released from Péligre dam to reach Canneau dam in both the dry and wet seasons. Another said it took a day during the wet season. Lantagne also learned it took a day for water to flow from Canneau dam through the canal system to the Caribbean Sea. These observations were among the most important facts in the report, since they helped estimate how long it would take for a cholera plume to float from the Mirebalais region to the coast.

But what good were estimates of flow volume and time without a discussion—missing from the panel report—of how contaminated sewage was linked to river water and then to disease? Cholera-laden sewage leaked or poured into a river is diluted over time; concentration depends on the river flow volume. Knowing how many cholera organisms are needed to cause disease, an investigator could work backwards, estimating how much cholera-contaminated sewage would need to be leaked or poured into the river to overcome the dilution effect of flow volume and transport enough vibrios downriver to transmit the disease. Going through this mathematical exercise with a range of river flow volume estimates would have alerted the UN panel that a few asymptomatic cholera cases in Mèyé—or even a few symptomatic cases—could never have generated enough cholera vibrios to cause an explosive downriver outbreak. Instead, there had to have been many symptomatic cases with heavy fecal loads of cholera organisms.

Two panel members were physicians experienced with clinical cholera. Surely they knew the number of cholera microbes defecated by a typical cholera case—but in any case, Piarroux made sure they had had that information before they left for Haiti. With the *Nature Reviews* article he provided, plus Lantagne's range of river flow volumes, the panel should have been able to estimate a high and low number of cholera cases needed to overcome river dilution and infect drinking water in the delta communities. The report contained no such estimates.

Of course, the flow was important only insofar as the disease actually traveled via the river. The panel visited Annapurna Camp and took note of the nearby waterways. Two branches of the Mèyé tributary system flow past the camp and an adjacent area used for waste disposal. They come together just north of the camp as the Mèyé River, which then joins another tributary just south of Mirebalais and flows on to the Artibonite at Mirebalais. The panel authors noticed "significant human activity along this tributary, with women washing, people bathing, people collecting water for drinking, and children playing." Further, "it was reported that the Mirebalais city water supply system was not operating for a few weeks, and recipients relied on alternate water sources until repairs were completed"—although the panel didn't provide exact dates.

Camp personnel did not use the river water but drew water from a deep borehole "treated on-site using a high-quality process chain including filtration, reverse osmosis, and chlorination"—a system "most recently refurbished on October 26, 2010." That was only five days after the Haitian government and PAHO first reported the cholera outbreak. Why the refurbishment? The panel said nothing, but Piarroux figured it was to cover the UN's tracks. Sanitation problems might have persisted without the repairs, leaving the proverbial smoking gun.

Most important for cholera transmission is the handling of wastewater. The UN panel expressed concerns over black-water sewage at Annapurna Camp, which contained human waste from toilets and latrines and thereby could have a high concentration of cholera microbes. The panel also noted that pipes at the camp appeared "haphazard" and there was a risk of cross-contamination from "pipes that run over an open drainage ditch" and flowed directly into the southwestern branch of the Mèyé tributary system. Cross-contamination could occur between the black-water pipes and those carrying gray water from bathing, doing laundry, and washing dishes. These haphazard pipes were observed four months after the cholera epidemic had started and two months after the UN-sponsored sanitation team visited Haiti. If that was the cleanup view, what must conditions have been like in mid-October?

"It was evident from inspection, as well as reported by local Haitians," the panel wrote, "that recent (post October 2010) construction work in this area had been undertaken"—that is, removal of the pipes directly connecting the overflow of septic tanks with the passing stream used by the Mèyé villagers. Despite this work, the flow of septic fluids to the river had still not been resolved.

The UN panel confirmed that a truck came "from Port-au-Prince to collect the waste from the fiberglass tanks in the camp using a pump. The waste is then transported across the street and up a residential dirt road to a location at the top of the hill, where it is deposited in an open septic pit." There was no fence around the pit. Children played and animals roamed in the immediate area. The southeast branch of the Mèyé tributary system was "a short walk down the hill." The panel calculated it would take two to eight hours for water to flow from near the septic pit to the junction with the Artibonite River.

To Piarroux, the exact schedule for emptying the tanks of black water was important information. A thorough investigation would try to determine links by comparing that schedule, the Nepalese troop arrival dates, and the dates of new cholera cases. Lantagne said the panel had asked MINUSTAH for this information: a MINUSTAH spokesman had stated in a press conference the previous October that there were "documents that show how many times the private company trucks come to the base."[27] But Lantagne said the "data appeared highly inaccurate, and were not sufficient for analysis,"[28] so the panel relied on the word of MINUSTAH staff members that the contractor emptied the tanks twice per week when called. That contradicted the once-a-week answer given in the press conference.[29]

In summary, the UN panel determined there was potential for feces to enter into and flow from the drainage canal running through the camp directly into the southwestern branch of the Mèyé tributary system, and for waste from the open septic disposal pit to contaminate the southeastern branch of the Mèyé tributary system either by overflow during rainfall or by contamination via animal transport. As the panel wrote,

> Given the velocities of the water in the Meille/Mèyé tributary system, and the flow of water reported by operators along the Artibonite River, contamination in the Meille/Mèyé tributary system could have reached the Canneau dam within one to two days, and would have been fully distributed in the canal system in the Artibonite River Delta within a maximum of two to three days. This timeline is consistent with the epidemiological evidence indicating that the outbreak began in Mirebalais and within two to three days, cases were being seen throughout the Artibonite River Delta. This timeline verifies that river transport was the likely transmission route for cholera to spread from the mountains of Mirebalais to the Artibonite River Delta.

Okay, thought Piarroux, so far, so good. The panel members seemed to have gotten close to the truth. Still, though, there was no mention of UN involvement or of the associated linkage with cholera specimens in Nepal described by Nair in his section of the UN report. Nair, through personal connections, had learned that the International Vaccine Institute (IVI) in Korea had recently received from the National Public Health Laboratory in Kathmandu multiple strains of *Vibrio cholerae* O1, isolated in Nepal between 2007 and 2010 (see chapter 17). Among these, Nair wrote, "the strains isolated in Haiti and Nepal during 2009 were a perfect match." Did this mean the Nepal isolates of 2009 were the same as the Haiti isolate of 2010? To clarify, I wrote to Dong Wook Kim of IVI and learned that "2009" in the UN report was a mistake that should have read "2010."[30] Thus the "perfect match" of the IVI analysis was among Nepal and Haiti isolates, all collected in 2010.

Even setting the mistake aside, why, wondered Piarroux, had the panel acknowledged the Korean findings that the cholera strain in Haiti was genetically identical with the cholera strain in Nepal but then said no more?

Piarroux's mission report was barely acknowledged, but the panel did cite him in writing that "although residents report contractor trucks dumping feces into the septic pit, it has been suggested there might have been an unauthorized feces dumping directly into the Meye Tributary System." It was Piarroux who had suggested that in his report. The panel added that this "proposition could not be independently confirmed" and there would be no speculation about missing pieces of evidence.

To its credit, the panel dismissed the environmental theory and acknowledged that the cholera outbreak was "a result of human activity." Furthermore, its members agreed with Piarroux that the explosion had begun with the contamination of the Mèyé tributary of the Artibonite River and that the disease was a "pathogenic strain of current South Asian type *Vibrio cholerae*." But the UN panel was unwilling to name the likely culprits—unlike Piarroux and his coauthors in their *Emerging Infectious Diseases* article.

Piarroux and his colleagues had begun where disease detectives typically begin: describe the outbreak, tally the distribution of new cases over time, and then use that information to look for associated factors (often termed "risk factors") that might explain the observed patterns. To address what caused the outbreak, they focused their attention on the earliest days in mid-October when the cholera patients first appeared. CDC scientists had stated that *Vibrio cholerae* was likely introduced into Haiti in one event,[31] so Piarroux and his colleagues looked for that one event and human activity clues, arriving at Annapurna Camp and the Nepalese peacekeepers. While a handful of troops might have been asymptomatic cholera carriers or incubating the disease when they left Nepal for Haiti, some probably became symptomatic en route or shortly after arriving.

The Piarroux group also addressed the curious finding that a few days after the epidemic began in Mirebalais commune, a large number of cases suddenly occurred nearly simultaneously throughout the delta region of the Artibonite River—skipping over three communes near Mirebalais and appearing suddenly in seven more distal communes. The authors noted that the explosive epidemic had occurred in the downriver communes at almost the same time, as if cholera had descended all at once on the area.

This pattern was far different from the usual occurrence in cholera epidemics. Typically, cholera comes to an area and then progressively moves through the population as family members and others are exposed to infected food and water. The explosive and simultaneous pattern seemed almost as if a mighty hand of pestilence in one dramatic action had strewn microbes throughout the delta area. But the investigation revealed that after the initial few cases a second event had taken place several more days after the UN troops arrived at Annapurna Camp, scattering microbes in one dramatic gesture in downriver communities.

The value of Jean Gaudart's addition to the research team became readily apparent. He used special software to study mathematically the occurrence of cholera cases in space and time and identified clearly two statistically significant clusters of cases, one in the commune of Mirebalais from October 16 to 19 and a second in several communes near the Artibonite delta from October 20 to 28 (see figure 18.2). The two space-time clusters appeared unrelated,

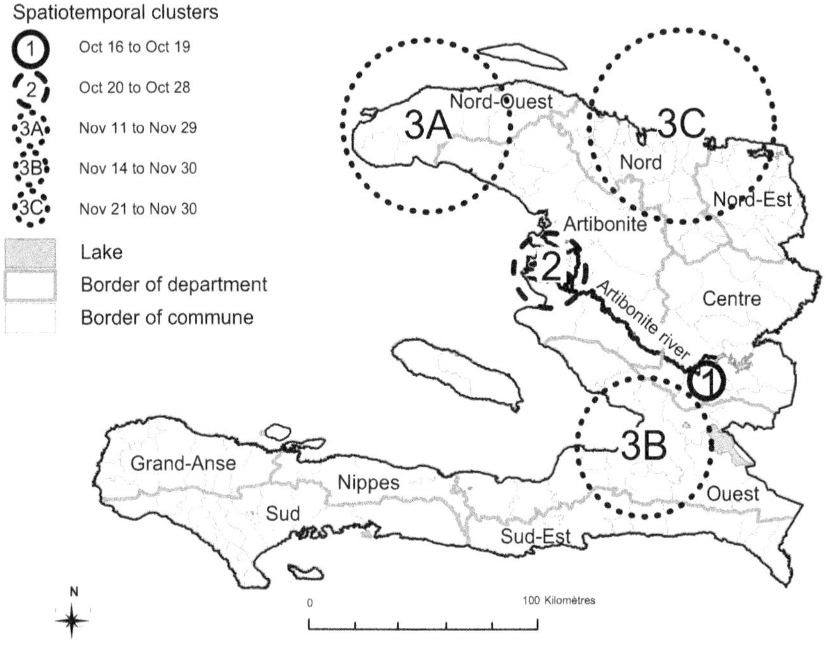

FIGURE 18.2. Space and time clusters of cholera cases during October–November 2010, Haiti. Other départements were affected later. Based on Piarroux et al., "Understanding the Cholera Epidemic."

meaning that cholera had moved from the Mirebalais area to the delta communities but skipped over populated areas along the way. If the cholera pathogens had gradually spread with human traffic along Haiti's paths, roads, and highways, there would have been no distinct space-time clusters suggesting separate outbreaks.

Gaudart's analysis supported the hypothesis that disease-causing microbes moved as a single mass along the quick-flowing Artibonite River from Mirebalais through lesser exposed areas to the communes in the river delta—just as Piarroux had suspected in his initial investigation. After an incubation period of one to two days, new cholera cases appeared on October 19–20 (but were not reported until October 20) in the downriver cluster, with a pattern that resembled a common-source outbreak. By mid- to late November, the cholera had spread north to Nord-Ouest département, south to Ouest département (where Port-au-Prince is located), and north to Nord département (see figure 18.2).

But there was more to the analysis. Gaudart looked for risk factors for the spread of the disease in three early-infected départements—Ouest, Centre, and Artibonite—using a statistical regression model that accounted for population size and spatial variability. His regression analysis provided even more evidence of the river's involvement in the cholera debacle. The "spread of cholera during the peak that occurred from October 20–28 was strongly linked to the Artibonite River and not to the proximity to Mirebalais, as would be expected for road-dependent propagation." The analysis pointed to the contamination of the Artibonite River, concluded the authors, "in a way that could infect thousands, and kill hundreds, of persons within a few days." Adding to this conclusion were the near-simultaneous cholera outbreaks in seven communes of the Artibonite delta on October 20–21 (see figure 4.3).

The statistician also considered the presence of internally displaced persons (IDP) camps established for people made homeless by the January 2010 earthquake, since some had expressed concern that cholera might be spreading in those camps.[32] In fact, IDP camps turned out to be a preventive factor thanks to better "access to food, safe water, and sanitation," with 90 percent lower population-adjusted risk. Conversely, living in a commune partially or totally located in the coastal plain was a strong risk factor, where such persons had a 4.6 times higher adjusted risk of becoming a cholera case than those living in communes elsewhere in the three early-infected départements.

Finally, Gaudart analyzed whether the epidemiological cholera curves in the communes bordering the Artibonite River were in or out of sync, suggesting a common or different origin. He observed a strong correlation among the epidemic curves of the Artibonite delta communes but a much weaker correlation of the downriver communes with the epidemic curve in upriver Mirebalais. The strongest correlation was between Saint-Marc and Grande-Saline, the two coastal communes bordering the main branch of the Artibonite River. This indicated "a specific mechanism was responsible for the onset of cholera in Lower Artibonite distinct from continuous spread from the primary focus" in the Mirebalais commune.

How could the supposedly independent UN panel have failed to identify the humans responsible for the Haiti's cholera outbreak? Was there some logic behind this omission?

In the epidemiology section, the panel report focused on two groups: the Nepalese peacekeepers in three MINUSTAH camps at Mirebalais, Terre Rouge, and Hinche (only the Mirebalais camp was visited, although all three camps sent sewage to the Mirebalais pit) and a contingent of Bangladeshi police supposedly stationed in September–October 2010 in Hinche and Mirebalais. Though it has not been officially reported to WHO, cholera is present in Bangladesh. Yet after mentioning the Bangladesh police, the panel failed to investigate their significance; this suggested that the comment was a red herring, and thus it offered more confusion than light.

Most striking, perhaps, was reviewing the Annapurna Camp medical log and then stating as fact that no clinical cases of cholera had occurred in the camp. So, while acknowledging that the first cases had occurred as a result of human activity, the panel claimed that the specific humans, although considered blameless, could not be identified and certainly could not be linked to the camp. "The Independent Panel concludes that the Haiti cholera outbreak was caused by the confluence of circumstances . . . and was not the fault of, or deliberate action of, a group or individual."

Although humans in the UN camps were deemed not at fault, the panel did not hesitate to assign some blame to Haitians and to their local public health environment. "The introduction of this cholera strain as a result of environmental contamination with feces could not have been the source of such an outbreak without simultaneous water and sanitation and health care system deficiencies," wrote the panel. Its members reasoned that the explosive nature of the initial spread of the outbreak was due to mass exposure to cholera-contaminated Artibonite River water, including the offshoot canals in rice paddies; lack of immunity to cholera in the population; poor water and sanitation conditions; and the spread of disease by infected persons who assembled near treatment facilities after receiving inadequate treatment and when fleeing to their home communities. In other words, the blame belonged with the Haitian people themselves, their sanitary environment, and their medical care providers. The implication: cholera was the Haitians' fate rather than an undeserved incursion from outside the country. And even the bacterium itself was at fault—after all, the type of *Vibrio cholerae* that struck the fated Haitians, the panel noted, was more pathogenic than other strains.

Piarroux was disgusted. The panel's mandate had been to "investigate and seek to determine the source of the 2010 cholera outbreak in Haiti."[33] It was a specific charge from the UN secretary-general. Instead of fulfilling it, though, the panel had worked to shift blame away from the likely source and toward the Haitians—and while rejecting the environmental theory, still hinted at it. "The canal system and delta of the Artibonite River provided optimal environmental conditions for rapid proliferation of *Vibrio cholera*," the panel wrote, describing the remaining reason for the explosive initial disease spread. It was the word "proliferation" that immediately caught Piarroux's eye. Proliferation, in the microbiologic sense, means reproduction of microorganisms. With *Vibrio cholerae*, reproduction of pathogenic strains occurs in the human gut, possibly at a low level in untreated river water,[34] or with some nonpathogenic strains in estuarial water. Suggesting that cholera had arrived in an asymptomatic human, that there were no further infections in Annapurna Camp, and that the organism had then actively reproduced in nearby river water kept the environmental theory alive.

Later, Daniele Lantagne, the panel's water and sanitation expert, was asked whether the panel thought a single asymptomatic carrier really could have contaminated the water and started the spread of the outbreak. "It was the opinion of all three of the other members," she replied, "and I deferred to their expertise."[35] She made the same point in media interviews.[36]

The UN panel report was released on May 4, 2011. The online version of the *Emerging Infectious Diseases* article by Piarroux et al. appeared two days later. A week after that, Martin Enserink of *Science* magazine published a comparative assessment of the two investigations.[37] "Although the [UN panel] study finds fault with the sanitation at three [MINUSTAH] camps . . . ," he wrote, "it is careful not to apportion blame; it also says there is no evidence that anyone within the camps ever suffered from cholera." He quoted Cravioto: "The entire catastrophe may have started with a single carrier: an infected person who wasn't sick himself but shed the bacteria in his stool."

Enserink pointed out that the UN panel report was "starkly at odds" with Piarroux's study. He outlined the logic Piarroux and his colleagues had used and quoted Piarroux: "What happened in this river is something I have never seen in all of my experience with cholera." But it was Enserink's opening sentence about the UN peacekeepers that resonated with Piarroux perhaps more than anything in the article. "They came to the island with the best of intentions—only to sow disease and death."

19

QUARANTINE AND ISOLATION

On July 2, 2009, a Chilean soldier with flu symptoms arrived in Haiti for his UN peacekeeping assignment. He was quarantined—isolated from others until formally diagnosed. The disease agent was soon confirmed as H1N1, more popularly known as "swine flu."[1] Another Chilean peacekeeper became infected, followed by a twenty-three-year-old Haitian who had not been outside the country.[2]

Swine flu had shown up in Mexico and the United States a few months earlier. Dr. Margaret Chan, director-general of the World Health Organization, declared the outbreaks a "public health emergency of international concern."[3] Soon swine flu became a pandemic.

The next time a UN spokesman mentioned "quarantine" was in mid-November 2010, but this time he was talking about cholera. Nick Birnback, chief of MINUSTAH's public affairs section, assured a reporter that "if a soldier or any other UN personnel showed symptoms of cholera they would be quarantined and treated." But, insisted Birnback, "According to the Nepalese battalions that are there, none of the soldiers have shown any symptoms of cholera. The tests of the premises and the [water and sanitation] outputs have consistently proven negative."[4]

Since 1951, cholera has been one of six quarantinable diseases given special attention by WHO, founded in 1948 as a UN agency to address health issues. The WHO protocol then was that a person with any of the six diseases was to be removed, isolated, and treated until deemed safe by a health authority. Even travelers simply exposed to the disease agent were to be kept under surveillance for the duration of the maximum incubation period to see whether they developed the disease. Persons coming by either boat or plane from a cholera-infected area were deemed healthy only if cleared by a medical examination.[5]

The WHO regulations were changed in 1969, mainly to reduce the six diseases to three. Cholera remained on the list. The 1969 regulation made clear that if cases of quarantinable diseases were "imported or transferred into a non-infected area," all information on the origin of infection was to be reported. The WHO publication *Weekly Epidemiological Record* would provide yearly updates of reported and imported cholera cases.[6]

By the mid-1990s, new knowledge spurred changes in international cholera prevention and control strategies. For instance, because there was no documented evidence, WHO no longer considered the importation of cholera-infected foods a risk.[7] In addition, travel and trade restrictions between countries were deemed ineffectual at preventing the introduction of cholera, as were quarantine and border controls.[8] WHO reasoned that most cholera cases presented no symptoms or had only mild diarrhea and that the main cause of disease spread was "healthy cholera carriers"—the large group of infected persons who were asymptomatic. Given the difficulty of identifying and isolating them, WHO deemed traveler restrictions both ineffectual and too costly.

Also considered ineffective was requiring travelers to be treated preventively with antibiotics or other drugs. WHO reasoned that therapeutic drugs were typically effective for only one to two days, so reinfection could easily occur. In addition, the agency worried that mass use of drugs would lead to antibiotic resistance.

In the 1990s, WHO established the Global Task Force on Cholera Control to assist countries with disease surveillance, case management, safe water and sanitation, and health education programs—all aimed at within-nation cholera control.[9] No mention was made, however, of charging the task force to help nations limit cholera importation.

The next changes in the regulations were more dramatic. Between 2007 and 2012, nations were expected to assess their existing disease detection-and-response capacities and implement new WHO requirements "which avoid unnecessary interference with international traffic and trade." Quarantinable diseases were no longer mentioned, but rather the notification category includes "illness or medical condition, irrespective of origin or source, that presents or could present significant harm to humans." Individual rights would be considered. Travelers suspected of carrying a contagious disease were to be subjected to "the least intrusive and invasive medical examination that would achieve the public health objective of preventing the international spread of disease," and they would have to give their express informed consent before any examinations. Refusal, though, could result in being denied entry to the country. Finally, there was a stipulation that authorities must also provide or arrange "for adequate food and water, appropriate accommodation and clothing, protection for baggage and other possessions, appropriate medical treatment, [and] means of necessary communication if possible in a language that they can understand and other appropriate assistance."[10]

With these changes, WHO had gradually shifted its emphasis from limiting cholera spread between countries to controlling the disease within countries, emphasizing clean water and proper sanitation, health education, and good food hygiene. The new thinking, widely distributed in 2010, offered few practical suggestions for Haitian public health officials.[11] WHO wrote that quarantine was "ineffective in the control of cholera" and therefore unnecessary. Requiring proof of vaccination for entry into a country was deemed no longer useful in preventing the international spread of cholera. WHO reasoned that current cholera vaccines had low protective efficacy and resulted in a high occurrence of severe adverse reactions. And finally, the agency continued to advise against requiring prophylactic administration of antibiotics or proof of such administration for travelers coming from or going to a country affected by cholera because it "has been demonstrated to have no effect on the spread of cholera, but can have adverse effects by increasing antimicrobial resistance and provides a false sense of security."

In its 2010 summary cholera data, WHO reported nearly that 180,000 cases had occurred in Haiti. None were listed as imported. While Canada and the United States were cited as having imported cholera cases, there was no mention of origin for Haiti's cases.[12]

Seven months after the Haiti epidemic began, the global task force wrote, "The first cholera cases in Haiti started to be reported on 14 October 2010 in the department of Artibonite from where the outbreak rapidly spread along the Artibonite river affecting several departments."[13] No mention was made of cholera's originating in upriver Centre département near Annapurna Camp.

Details on the source were also omitted from the WHO 2013 *Weekly Epidemiological Record* when the scientific facts were clearly known. The publication merely stated, "The explosive nature of the [cholera] outbreak was linked to lack of immunity to *V. cholerae* as well as the limited access to safe drinking-water and basic sanitation, and internal migration that followed the earthquake in January 2010."[14]

WHO regulations have long stipulated that "all information available on the origin of infection" must be reported.[15] While the term "imported" is still used in the most recent 2005 IHR modification,[16] information on the origin country or locale of cholera, beyond being "imported," is no longer required. With these changes, when it came to Haiti, WHO apparently was able to give its UN sponsor a pass.

20

THE WALL CRACKS

In October 2011, Piarroux was in Mozambique in southern Africa for a cholera workshop. There he spoke with Eric Mintz, a CDC epidemiologist who had been closely following the Haiti epidemic since its beginning a year earlier. The discussion gave Piarroux a better understanding of how some CDC epidemiologists felt torn between their professional interest as scientists to seek the source of the epidemic and their fear of becoming involved in political turmoil.

That same month, CDC posted "Cholera in Haiti: One Year Later" on its website.[1] It mentioned the date the laboratory-confirmed cholera microbe was first identified in Haiti but nothing about the source of the initial outbreak.

Two sides in this debate had been established with the publication of Piarroux's *Emerging Infectious Diseases* article and the laboratory *Mbios* article describing the identical nature of *V. cholerae* in Nepal and Haiti[2] versus the supposedly independent UN panel's report. The pressing coming task, thought Piarroux, was getting help to those in Haiti who needed it and ultimately eliminating cholera from the country. Yet the seminal epidemiological and laboratory articles did not end the scientific debate, carried on by journalists and others. So he realized the first wave of research was not enough—he had to reenter the fray.

He invited two colleagues to join a small team to publish a summary of the available evidence: Robert Barrais, the Haitian epidemiologist he had worked with in the field, and me, since I had been compiling an extensive collection of documents and articles on various aspects of the epidemic as it evolved. We added Paul Keim, the Arizona microbiologist who had helped analyze some of the samples sent around the world by Nepal's National Public Health Laboratory. Prominent for his groundbreaking work helping the FBI solve the U.S. anthrax outbreak in 2001,[3] Keim liked a good mystery and was happy to join the group. His was just the kind of detective thinking our team wanted.

In short order, the team assembled a review article, "Evidence for the Nepalese Origin of Cholera in Haiti," that presented epidemiological and molecular-genetic evidence and even some of the evidence from journalists. Getting it published proved challenging. The *New England Journal of Medicine* turned it down. The *Lancet Infectious Diseases* said no to a shortened version. *PLoS Neglected Tropical Diseases* rejected a version with further cuts but offered limited space for a considerably shortened opinion piece in the "Viewpoint" section. The team declined.

Clinical Microbiology and Infection (*CMI*) had recently accepted a separate article by Piarroux and a colleague slated for publication a few months later.[4] It described how human-borne transmission, rather than resurgent environmental strains, had driven deadly cholera epidemics in Africa and Haiti and included a policy note suggesting that cholera borne by humans might be more easily controlled than cholera arising from ubiquitous environmental contamination. If epidemiologists were to develop local cholera control strategies, the authors wrote, they needed to learn more about the origin of outbreaks and epidemics and not just assume they arose from a contaminated environment.

Clearly understanding the importance of questioning environmental initiation, a *CMI* editor wrote in the same issue of the journal,

> Cholera is a disease that is both infectious and vectored by water. Major work carried out by John Snow in London in the 19th century showed very quickly that water, contaminated by the feces of patients, was the source of cholera. Multiple environmental theories have been suggested since then, because of the presence of *Vibrio cholerae* in many watery environments. However, the epidemic in Haiti shows that this remains a contagious disease whose source is infected people and not the inert environment. It also demonstrated that neglecting isolation and quarantine strategies led to a catastrophe in a country already suffering from a natural disaster.[5]

CMI accepted the new article too. The team decided to abandon the review approach and revise the piece to include new findings on the evolution of cholera cases in Haiti during the first weeks of the epidemic and then resubmit it as an original article. The journal accepted the revised version and even offered to publish some of the evidence online as "supplemental information" to provide a complete assessment of what had taken place in Haiti. The full article appeared first online in April and then in the June 2012 edition of the journal. To correct the record, we unambiguously titled the article "Nepalese Origin of Cholera Epidemic in Haiti."[6]

On November 3, 2011, two human rights attorneys—Mario Joseph of the Bureau des Avocats internationaux in Port-au-Prince and Brian Concannon Jr. of the Institute for Justice and Democracy in Haiti in Boston—filed a petition for relief against MINUSTAH. The attorneys represented "over 5,000 individual claimants [in Haiti] who died or were injured from cholera," The first paragraph of the document contended, "The cholera outbreak is directly attributable to the negligence, gross negligence, recklessness and deliberate indifference for the health and lives of Haiti's citizens by the United Nations . . . and its subsidiary, the United Nations Stabilization Mission in Haiti ('MINUSTAH')."[7] The petition argued that the UN had failed to comply with both its own regulations and international human rights law.

The petitioners recounted the events that had contributed to the origin of cholera in Haiti and the latest scientific evidence. Their demands were clear.

> In this petition and others to follow, the victims seek effective remedy. They seek a fair and impartial hearing. They seek monetary compensation for their losses. They also seek redress in the form of the UN's commitment to prevent the further spread of cholera in Haiti. To this end, the victims request that the UN, in partnership with the Government of Haiti, fund and establish a comprehensive sanitation, potable water, and medical treatment program to protect Haitians' health and lives. Finally, they seek a public acknowledgement by the UN and MINUSTAH of responsibility for the cholera outbreak and its associated harms. Such recognition will signal to the Haitian people and the world that the UN honors accountability in principle and in practice.

At a November 8 press conference in New York, Martin Nesirky—spokesperson for the secretary-general—addressed the petition.[8] "The Secretary-General has taken this matter very seriously from the outset." He reminded reporters that the UN-appointed "panel of independent scientific experts" had determined "it was not possible to be conclusive about how cholera was introduced into Haiti."

When he tried to move on to other issues, reporters persisted. The panel "report speaks for itself," replied a somewhat exasperated Nesirky, reiterating that "the Haiti cholera outbreak was caused by the confluence of circumstances as described in the report, and was not the fault or deliberate action of a group or individual person."

When a reporter asked whether it would be correct to state that the panel's conclusion was the UN's position on the petition, Nesirky became a bit testy. "As I have said—no. What I said is that the Secretary-General commissioned this independent panel of experts. They presented their findings and conclusions to the Secretary-General. The Secretary-General has shared that report with the Government of Haiti and beyond that has made it publicly available. And the report speaks for itself."

Reporters were not giving up, however. The conversation went back and forth as Nesirky tried to dodge attributing a specific position to the UN and the reporters continued to push. One referred to the petition directly. "But [the petitioners] also say there are also four other independent reports that point out that the strain came from South-East Asia. Is it the UN's suggestion that someone else introduced this strain into . . . I mean, how else would it get there if not through the UN?"

Nesirky parried and then employed the same focus-shifting tactic his MINUSTAH counterpart had used with reporters more than a year earlier. "Our focus has to be on seeking to stop the spread and helping to treat those who have been hit with cholera."

Piarroux had nothing to do with the petition for relief. He had no relationship with the two attorneys, although a year later he met Mario Joseph to explain his research findings. Nonetheless, the petition cited his report on the very first page. He certainly supported any effort to confront the United Nations with facts and evidence, because the facts put the issue of origin at the center of the discussion—which had important implications not only for how to fight cholera in Haiti but also worldwide.

In their *EID* article, Piarroux and his coauthors wrote that an accurate field investigation helps health workers manage the epidemic. Assessing causation, however, is more complicated. The authors recognized that individual epidemiological studies are typically suggestive rather than definitive. They may *point* toward the truth, but without additional evidence they typically do not *guarantee* truth. Ultimately, "identifying the source and the responsibilities falls within the scope and competence of legal authorities."

Piarroux hoped the petition for relief would open a dialogue and get lawyers and judges involved with the evidence. That needed to unfold in the context of medical ethics and the fundamental principle of all assistance efforts: *primum non nocere*—first, do no harm.

The UN remained committed to the conclusions of the panel report in the months following its release, but political pressure mounted as more people learned about the petition for relief. The monolithic wall the UN built around determining the origin of cholera in Haiti began to crumble. In early 2012, when members of the UN panel themselves began to speak out, Piarroux could only wonder whether their views had been different all along or whether they had evolved as evidence came into sharper focus.

On February 21, 2012, Daniele Lantagne e-mailed other panel members asking whether they would be comfortable stating that "the evidence is clear that the most likely route of importation of cholera into Haiti was staff associated with the UN MINUSTAH facility in Mirebalais. However, it is not possible with certainty to pinpoint the actual individual or individuals who imported the cholera, and if they were associated with the UN."[9] The other panel members agreed.

Piarroux was pleased to learn the panel was open to the possibility of multiple infected persons with its statement "individual or individuals," not just a single asymptomatic person—but this communication was made only in an internal e-mail.

Two weeks later, Lantagne was interviewed on Al Jazeera English.[10] "Based on the summation of the circumstantial and scientific evidence," she said, "the most likely scenario is that someone associated with the UN-MINUSTAH facility was the person responsible." She pointed specifically to Annapurna Camp. It was the first public acknowledgment of a changed position, and it was big. Lantagne linked the importation of cholera to a human—but not multiple humans as stated by Piarroux—in the UN camp.

In late March 2012, Deborah Sontag of the *New York Times* wrote in an in-depth article, "Epidemiologic and microbiologic evidence strongly suggests that United Nations peacekeeping troops from Nepal imported cholera to Haiti, contaminated the river tributary next to their base through a faulty sanitation system and caused a second disaster."[11] Sontag also quoted Keim and Piarroux. "'It was like throwing a lighted match into a gasoline-filled room,' said Dr. Paul S. Keim, a microbial geneticist whose laboratory determined that the Haitian and Nepalese cholera strains were virtually identical." And "Renaud Piarroux was more pointed regarding the UN, stating, 'In telling the truth, the UN could have gained the trust of the population and facilitated the fight against cholera. But that was bungled.'"

Despite the cracks in the wall, though, the UN stood firm. "The United Nations maintains that an independent panel of experts determined the evidence implicating its troops to be inconclusive," Sontag wrote. "Questioned for this article, though, those same experts said that Dr. Keim's work, conducted after their own, provides 'irrefutable molecular evidence' that Haiti's cholera came from Nepal, in the words of G. Balakrish Nair, an Indian microbiologist."

Nair, like Lantagne, abandoned the UN monolith—publicly. Two panel members down, thought Piarroux, and two to go before the truth was fully embraced.

Sontag's article continued, quoting Lantagne. "When you take the circumstantial evidence in our report and all that has come out since, the story now I think is stronger: the most likely scenario is that the cholera began with someone at the Minustah base."

The UN remained insistent. "Even so, Anthony Banbury, a United Nations assistant secretary general, said last week, 'We don't think the cholera outbreak is attributable to any single factor.'"

Sontag even learned that Nepalese troops were no longer at the UN camp, having been replaced in early 2012 with peacekeepers from Uruguay. "Nepal's troop strength is being cut by two-thirds, more than any other country's. United Nations officials said that this was unrelated to tensions over cholera."

Sontag's dispatch was from Mirebalais itself. "But people here think otherwise," she continued. "'If they hadn't left, we would have burned it down,' Deputy Mayor Moise said of the base."

There was no UN comment in the article about panel members changing their minds. And at the next briefing after Sontag's article appeared, spokesperson Nesirky stuck to his guns, reiterating that the UN was studying the petition claims and the panel's conclusion that "it was not possible to be conclusive about how cholera was introduced to Haiti." Then he refused further comment, "including on the *New York Times* story."[12] When a reporter asked a question about the revelation that some of the panelists "no longer stand behind the idea that it can't be proved," Nesirky said, "Any other questions?"

In her *Times* article, Sontag quoted two lawyers from Bureau des Avocats Internationaux. In a separate article of their own, the lawyers said the UN had a "simple" choice: "It can rise to the occasion and demonstrate that the rule of law protects the rights of poor Haitians against one of the world's most powerful institutions, or it can shrink from the challenge and demonstrate that once again in Haiti, 'might makes right.'"[13]

Six months earlier, Piarroux and his colleague Benoît Faucher had expressed similar sentiment in the French newspaper *Le Monde*, reminding readers of a passage in the UN's own 1948 Universal Declaration of Human Rights: "*Tous les êtres humains naissent libres et égaux en dignité et en droits*" ("All human beings are born free and equal in dignity and rights"). Don't the people of Haiti deserve the same? the authors asked.

> We all agree that no one deliberately introduced cholera into Haiti, but that is no excuse for not establishing in detail the individual and institutional responsibilities. When a plane crashes, a systematic investigation is conducted even when it is obvious that neither the pilot, the airline, nor the manufacturer deliberately caused the accident. Is it so incongruous to ask the same thing in memory of the 6,000 Haitian people who have died of cholera? No one would have questioned the need for such an investigation had similar conduct occurred in Europe or the United States.[14]

A chorus of news outlets began to comment on—and challenge—the UN's continued stonewalling. The *Wall Street Journal* reported on the screening of *Baseball in the Time of Cholera* at New York City's Tribeca Film Festival.[15] The directors, two aid workers living in Haiti, set out to document the emergence of Haiti's first Little League baseball team but shifted their focus when one player's mother suddenly died of cholera. "Our film," they told the *Journal*, "aims to 'put a face' on the epidemic. Instead of lecturing that cholera killed thousands of people, we want to show the viewer what cholera has done to one boy and his family. And most of all, we want people to realize that the cholera epidemic is not the fault of the Haitian people. It was brought to Haiti by foreigners and despite very clear evidence pointing towards the United Nations as the carrier, the U.N. still denies responsibility for the outbreak."

The American actress Olivia Wilde, one of the film's executive producers, made clear that the film was part of an emerging campaign to pressure the UN. Writing in the *Huffington Post*, she called it

> an important piece of advocacy in the struggle to stop another devastating outbreak of cholera as the rainy season descends this month. We made this film because it is simply not an option to let the 7,000 men, women and children killed disappear into the cold swamp of statistics. I felt gutted by helplessness watching a small child die of cholera, but with this film, and with our collective voice, we have a chance to save thousands of lives by forcing the UN to make clean water and sanitation their priority in Haiti.[16]

In late April, the *Economist* ran an editorial titled "The UN in Haiti: First, Do No Harm."[17] Stating that "studies have all but established MINUSTAH's role as fact," it strongly rebuked the UN's "dodge" of responsibility. "MINUSTAH's agreement with the government states that bigger disputes should be handled by a special tribunal. So far, however, none has been set up. Since the force and its troops enjoy immunity from local courts—which most countries demand before offering soldiers to the UN—cholera victims have no other formal legal recourse. As a result, their lawyers are threatening to challenge MIINUSTAH's immunity in the Haitian courts if the UN does not address their claims. That could affect peacekeeping operations worldwide."

The next month, the *New York Times* also editorialized, "The United Nations bears heavy responsibility for the outbreak: its own peacekeepers introduced the disease through sewage leaks at one their encampments. Before that, cholera had not been seen in Haiti for more than a hundred years."[18]

The UN was losing the battle to keep opinion makers on its side. In the scientific community, though, where judgment tends to be more reserved than in the media, supporters of the environmental theory who had been silent during this particular debate were preparing a new offensive.

Back in early November 2010, just after Hurricane Tomas had battered Haiti—adding to the misery already caused by the earlier earthquake and the ongoing cholera epidemic—a group of Bangladeshi scientists and clinicians from the ICDDR,B in Dhaka had gone to Haiti to share their experience with epidemic cholera. It was a well-publicized assistance mission that included a briefing with President René Préval.[19] Piarroux, in Haiti during most of that time, had met members of the group on November 16 at an evening roundtable organized by the Haitian Medical Association, where they talked about their medical care and education sessions for local health care providers.

During this same period, Rita Colwell and colleagues from the University of Maryland were conducting a study in Haiti in collaboration with Alejandro Cravioto, then director of ICDDR,B and later chair of the UN panel. Colwell alluded to the investigation in a late-November telephone interview with *Humanosphere*; she said she and her colleagues had water samples from the Haiti outbreak and were doing their own analyses.[20] It was a rare breach in the code of silence.

What was the Colwell-Cravioto Haiti research all about? It would have been reasonable to assume that Colwell, a fervent and outspoken proponent of the environmental hypothesis, was looking for scientific support for her career-defining theory. Many ICDDR,B scientists also favored the theory. But the investigation had been kept quiet, perhaps to avoid provoking public anger over a theory that let the Nepalese peacekeepers off the hook.

No one associated with the Colwell-Cravioto field study ever spoke to Piarroux or his Haitian colleagues about the investigation. There were no Haitian scientists working back in Maryland with the samples. Cravioto never even hinted at the study with Colwell when he later corresponded with Piarroux.

Then, nearly two years later in early June 2012, Colwell presented the research at a genome analysis conference,[21] and soon thereafter an advance copy of her scientific article appeared on the Web and was then published a month later in the prestigious *Proceedings of the National Academy of Sciences USA* (*PNAS*).[22] Colwell, the corresponding author, used her strong connections and academy status to get the article accepted as a "contributed submission," which allowed her to appoint the two reviewers rather than having anonymous reviewers selected by the editor—the norm for scientific journals. Cravioto was among the coauthors. It helped explain to Piarroux why Cravioto had kept quiet while two members of his panel broke ranks with the official story.

The Colwell-Cravioto article reiterated that *Vibrio cholerae* O1, Ogawa, El Tor was present in Haiti. New, however, was the discovery of a second group, *Vibrio cholerae* non-O1/non-O139, commonly found in aquatic environments.

Many forms of the cholera organism do not cause disease—a fact commonly overlooked. There are actually hundreds of serogroups of *Vibrio cholerae*, but only two groups—O1 and O139—produce cholera toxin and cause epidemic cholera. The remaining serogroups are typically lumped together in a third group, non-O1 and non-O139 *Vibrio cholerae*.[23] Some members of this group, if they have disease-causing components, may cause sporadic cases of diarrhea but not epidemic cholera. Colwell's article reported finding no such disease-causing components within the *V. cholerae* non-O1/non-O139 in Haiti.

Since non-O1/non-O139 forms of *Vibrio cholerae* usually do not cause disease, finding them in aquatic environments in the weeks following Hurricane Tomas may be of scientific interest but is not typically *news*. They've been reported in the coastal waters of Venezuela,[24] and CDC regularly reports finding them in U.S. coastal regions.[25] Scientists found non-O1/non-O139 cholera microbes in Louisiana's Lake Pontchartrain, redistributed from Gulf of Mexico waters in the churning rain and wind of Hurricanes Katrina and Rita in 2005.[26] But none had virulence-associated genes, suggesting no clinical cholera impact. When Hurricane Tomas battered Haiti in 2010, non-O1/non-O139 forms of *Vibrio cholerae* could well have been brought from the Caribbean by the swirling winds, but that didn't mean the winds brought *epidemic disease*, already tallied at about 6,700 hospitalized cholera cases and nearly 450 deaths since the start in mid-October.[27]

Colwell and Cravioto, though, very much needed to make a point that the role of *V. cholerae* non-O1/non-O139 in the Haiti epidemic "either alone or in concert with *V. cholerae* O1, cannot be dismissed." To support the environmental theory, they chose to ignore the disease-causing role of cholera *toxin*.

The article went to great lengths to make the case for the environmental theory and draw a connection between clinical cholera and non-O1/non-O139 cholera. The authors' clinical definition for cholera was "exhibiting symptoms of profuse watery diarrhea, vomiting, and dehydration with varying severity." Finding only *V. cholerae* non-O1/non-O139—the environmental strain of the cholera microbe—in 17 of 81 "clinical cholera" samples, Colwell later stated that the team considered this form of *Vibrio cholerae* to be the sole pathogen causing clinical disease, or at least according to the cholera definition they employed. But Colwell's team omitted (and Colwell later confirmed)[28] in its original article the fact that they had not cultured the 17 specimens for other enteric pathogens, including viruses, bacteria, and parasites that could well have caused some of the apparent symptoms. Those likely included rotavirus, shigella, or salmonella, which had emerged as the relevant pathogens in an extended survey in Haiti of hospital patients with acute diarrhea conducted by CDC and Haitian investigators from April 2012 to March 2013.[29] Testing more than 1,600 specimens for the likely cause of acute diarrhea, those investigators found that 40 percent had no detected pathogen. Among the remaining specimens, *V. cholerae* O1 was the overwhelming (94%) microbe, but they also found rotavirus (especially prevalent among hospitalized patients under age five), shigella, and salmonella. They did not identify even a single isolate with *V. cholerae* non-O1/non-O139.

Digging deeper would have rendered their environmental theory altogether useless in the Haitian context, so Colwell, Cravioto, and their coauthors omitted any mention of disease severity in the persons who provided the 81 clinical specimens. Even more unusual, they left out the most common variable in population studies—age. Diarrhea is especially prevalent among children under five. One study reported that among those young Haitian children seen in cholera treatment centers, diarrhea-causing pathogens—notably shigella, enterotoxigenic *Escherichia coli*, rotavirus, *Giardia*, and the microscopic parasite *Cryptosporidium*—were even more common than *Vibrio cholerae*.[30] Since the Colwell-Cravioto group didn't gather age data, there was no way to rule out that many of the 17 specimens in question came from young children who were just sick from common childhood pathogens.

While there was much to debate scientifically, Colwell and her colleagues seemed to accept that the deadly cholera bacteria had been imported to Haiti by "outside visitors" but were not convinced that the visitors were Nepalese UN soldiers. The intent of her group's research—"contribute to the understanding of the origin of the outbreak as indigenous or introduced"—was certainly laudable. Furthermore, her team agreed with Piarroux and others that the Haiti outbreak strain of *Vibrio cholerae* O1 was indeed clonal—that is, descended from a single progenitor and thus implying a single source. Where they differed was in the significance of the non-O1/non-O139 *V. cholerae* her team found in some patients' stools. While admitting that the local *V. cholerae* non-O1/non-O139 organisms were not clonal, the Colwell-Cravioto group emphasized that some of the environmental vibrios contained potential disease-causing components. If these components were rearranged by a complex process of "genomic recombination," new cholera vibrios might be generated that add cases and deaths to the Haitian epidemic. Did such genomic recombination actually occur in Haiti? The authors did not say, instead letting the intriguing thought float in the wind.

The vague assertions and apparent logical flaws were too much for Piarroux. There had to be a response.

21

ANSWERS

Perceiving logic flaws and omissions, Piarroux and his colleagues could not leave the Colwell-Cravioto article unanswered. He and his writing team wrote a letter to the *PNAS* journal that had published the article, adding another author to bolster their already high credibility: Dr. Jacques Boncy, director of Haiti's National Public Health Laboratory.[1]

In five paragraphs, Piarroux's team showed that *V. cholerae* non-O1/non-O139 was uncommon to nonexistent among specimens gathered and processed in Boncy's laboratory in October–November 2010; these findings were different from those reported by Colwell, Cravioto, and their coauthors. The letter's main focus, though, was the Colwell et al. opinion that "a definitive statement of source attribution [i.e., cause of cholera's origin in mid-October, 2010] cannot yet be made." Colwell and her coauthors had omitted substantial epidemiological findings obtained early in the epidemic by Piarroux and his colleagues, and either overlooked or intentionally omitted the accumulated evidence on the epidemic's origin, including additional findings published in April 2012.[2] The letter ended straightforwardly: the *PNAS* authors had "provided no evidence to counter that cholera was brought to Haiti by a contingent of Nepalese United Nations peacekeeping troops."

In the same issue of *PNAS*, a letter to the editor from John Mekalanos, the prominent Harvard University cholera expert, and some of his colleagues expressed shock at the Colwell-Cravioto group's statement that "assignment of attribution [for cholera in Haiti] remains controversial" and challenged the basic science.[3] They questioned the assertion that *V. cholerae* non-O1/non-O139 had in some manner increased the disease-causing ability of *V. cholerae* O1, concluding, "We find no evidence that indigenous non-O1 *V. cholerae* contributed any genetic material to the toxigenic Haitian O1 outbreak strain." That is, there was no sign of pathogenic genomic recombination.

The statements of Colwell, Cravioto, and their colleagues "obscure the true origin of the 2010 Haitian cholera epidemic." The Mekalanos group could not have made it any clearer.

PNAS let the Colwell-Cravioto team respond.[4] They countered on some points but retreated on others. Responding to Piarroux and his team, they insisted their special collection method for the cholera microbes was "sensitive and discriminating, but more expensive and labor- and time-intensive" than that of Haiti's National Public Health Laboratory. This, they claimed, allowed them to uncover *V. cholerae* non-O1/non-O139 in greater numbers than with conventional cholera collection methods. This did not address the fact that they had omitted a wide array of readily available epidemiological, laboratory, and journalistic evidence that made clear the true source of Haiti's epidemic. And to fit their environmental agenda, they claimed the source could not be identified definitively without extensive study of the worldwide distribution of *Vibrio cholerae*, including population sampling in many settings. How convenient to set the evidence bar so high, thought Piarroux, and to insist on laboratory findings exclusively.

Notably, in their response to the Mekalanos group, the Colwell-Cravioto group stated that their intent had been to report "diversity and not attribution," implying their article was more descriptive in nature, telling about varied strains of *V. cholerae* appearing in Haiti. They didn't bother to explain why "attribution" statements were repeatedly included in the beginning and ending sections of their article.

Rita Colwell certainly talked a lot about attribution to the news media, pressed by savvy journalists who had read her *PNAS* article. Immediately after the article appeared online, Richard Knox of National Public Radio wrote about it and interviewed Colwell.[5] Did she think "one strain was introduced by the Nepalese soldiers and the other was native to Haiti, or at least predated the current epidemic?" he asked.

Colwell replied, "The introduction [from Nepal] can't be ruled out but it can't be proven either. I think the evidence is at best circumstantial, and it is not sufficient to account for the entire epidemic."

If the evidence was circumstantial, Knox persisted, then what did Colwell think caused the Haitian cholera epidemic? She gave a rather telling answer: the country's explosive cholera epidemic was "most likely explained by the 'perfect storm' of three converging factors." First was the impact of the massive January 2010 earthquake. Colwell explained that Haiti's geology is limestone and that became very alkaline from the earthquake's disrupting effects. She had long contended that *Vibrio cholerae* thrives in alkaline waters.

Next was temperature. Colwell mentioned that Haiti had had one of the hottest summers on record prior to the epidemic, and high temperatures warmed the coastal estuaries where cholera likes to breed in copepods, or tiny crustaceans, helping the organism gain traction.

The third converging factor seemed especially odd to Piarroux, given the epidemic's timing. She told Knox that Hurricane Tomas skirted Haiti, causing heavy rain and flooding, and thus was a factor. This came after the warming of the estuaries. "With all the river systems churned up with nutrients and warm water and proper alkalinity," she said, "it would be ideal for the organism to become quite dominant."

Colwell didn't bother to mention Hurricane Tomas had hit three weeks after the epidemic began, and after 6,742 cholera hospitalizations and 442 reported deaths.[6]

Knox also interviewed David Sack, Colwell's noted environmental theory ally. Sack, too, focused on timing, telling Knox he believed "the epidemic exploded too soon after the Nepalese peacekeepers reportedly arrived in Haiti" for them to have been the origin. Instead, according to Sack, the non-O1/non-O139 strain "might have been hiding in Haiti's environment, waiting for Colwell's perfect storm." In his opinion, we might "never know how the South Asian strain of cholera got into Haiti."

At least their views were consistent, Piarroux noted, recalling that they had both espoused essentially the same ones in the weeks immediately following the cholera outbreak. Back then, Colwell had postulated that the aquatic environment conditions produced by a strong La Niña in 2010 "may have made cholera flare up in Haiti for the first time in 50 years."[7]

Colwell's tour through the media continued, including an interview with *Science* magazine. "A just-published study," wrote Kai Kupferschmidt of the Colwell-Cavioto article, "is set to reignite the politically sensitive debate about the origins of the cholera epidemic that has killed some 7000 people in Haiti and sickened another half-million since 2010. The disease, which is still raging in the island nation, is widely thought to have been introduced to Haiti by United Nations peacekeepers, but some contest that verdict."[8]

Sack showed up again as well, supporting Colwell's view and stating, "All the pieces needed to explain the epidemic in Haiti have not yet been fit together."

The *Science* reporter, though, wasn't satisfied with what Colwell and Sack had to say. He wanted more perspectives and spoke with the Piarroux team. Paul

Keim observed that the Colwell-Cravioto study offered no explanation whatsoever for how a pathogenic strain of cholera had first come to Haiti—a minimum requirement for an epidemiological investigation of a disease's outbreak. I seconded Keim in a separate interview. And Piarroux questioned the clinical diagnosis of cholera done for the study by a local physician and nurse, especially among cases with *V. cholerae* non-O1/non-O139 as the sole identified pathogen. The two health workers, employed by a local NGO, had gathered most of the specimens using a special environmental collection method assigned for all isolates. Piarroux explained that the laboratory team might have overlooked other causes of diarrhea, including viruses that coexisted with the newly discovered environmental strain of *V. cholerae* non-O1/non-O139.

Colwell and her colleagues stuck to their guns. Nowhere were their efforts appreciated more than at the UN and among Nepalese government officials.

Shortly after the *PNAS* and NPR pieces came out, the *UN Dispatch* took on the topic.[9] Sponsored by the United Nations Foundation and not formally representing the official views of the UN, the publication is nevertheless widely read and cited by UN personnel.

The opening sentence was cautious: "United Nations peacekeepers might not be the sole source of Haiti's cholera epidemic, according to a university research group." The reporter then acknowledged, "It is now almost universally believed that the peacekeepers [were] the source of the outbreak." But the point was to sow doubt, so back to "However, that might not be the whole story, at least according to new work coming out of a group of University of Maryland researchers and reported by NPR."

Piarroux knew that many people would equate the words "reported by" a reputable news outlet as synonymous with the truth.

The *UN Dispatch* article explained the key points Colwell and her colleagues had made about "not one, but two strains of cholera" existing in Haitian patients and her insistence to the NPR reporter that contrary evidence was "at best circumstantial" and "not sufficient to account for the entire epidemic."

The Nepalese had something to say, too. Several weeks after the *PNAS* article appeared online, Kashish Das Shrestha described the findings in a Nepalese newspaper piece that combined news, history, and opinion.[10] He mentioned Colwell's prominence as a scientist and quoted her and Sack from Knox's NPR report. His main conclusion: the new study established that the Nepalese troops "may not have been at fault for thousands of deaths [in Haiti]." But then Shrestha changed direction, adding insight into the government's reaction. He recounted his off-the-record conversation with a high-ranking Nepalese official attending the UN's annual assembly in New York City. The diplomat said the issue of Nepal's role in the cholera epidemic had officially faded and was no longer discussed in government circles.

But it was an earlier article by the same author that interested Piarroux even more. In December 2010, Shrestha had traveled to Haiti and was given access to Nepalese peacekeepers. He spoke with some of them about cholera and learned that they had largely ignored the allegations about their role. Back then, Shrestha interpreted the posture of these "inattentive" troops as confidence that the allegations were not true, although he noted that the troops he spoke with seemed embarrassed for Nepal.[11]

Piarroux was concerned that the Colwell-Cravioto journal article and the mixed messages about "attribution" Colwell was giving in interviews were sowing confusion. Colwell's "perfect storm" hypothesis seemed scientifically inaccurate to Piarroux and would give Haitians the false sense they were fated to combat cholera for decades or longer. He felt it was wrong to attribute cholera in Haiti to a massive earthquake, coupled with a very hot summer, topped off with a hurricane. And so he felt the need to speak out again, and this time to a wider readership. So he published an op-ed in the *Caribbean Journal*, the region's leading digital newspaper.[12]

Piarroux wrote, "In reality, the epidemic started in an area spared by the earthquake, following a summer which was not especially hot and, last but not least, at the time Hurricane Tomas struck the country, thousands of cholera cases and hundreds of deaths were already recorded." It was obvious, he continued, that the Artibonite River and its canals had played a role in the spread of cholera. But he wanted to make clear that the truth demanded going beyond the river itself: "Without any sick people among peacekeepers of the United Nations, without the formation of a reservoir of bacteria in the septic tanks of the military camp and without waste discharge into the waters of a river, the epidemic could not have developed so brutally."

Precisely because he dismissed the environmental theory and Colwell's perfect storm, Piarroux could offer Haitians some hope about the future. Noting that "the cholera clone that provoked the epidemic is currently overwhelmed by other bacteria" in Haiti's watery environment, "including *Vibrio cholerae* that do not produce toxin and that are not able to provoke deadly epidemics in humans," he wrote,

> Studies are underway to confirm such an observation, but this brings a message of hope with which I would like to end this article: if the environment actually was an auxiliary at the onset of this epidemic, it would seem to be not permissive enough to sustainably host a large amount of the epidemic strain that was imported in 2010.

> This enhances our hope of getting rid of cholera in Haiti, if increasing pressure is applied on current outbreaks, particularly on the often neglected outbreaks affecting inhabitants living in remote villages.
>
> Haiti is not the first island territory to have been affected by cholera epidemic; others, like Madagascar, got rid of cholera after experiencing severe outbreaks in the early 21st century.
>
> Hopefully everything will be done in order for this to happen in Haiti as well.

Criticism of Colwell, who was still active in a long and distinguished career, was mounting in the scientific community and media. She was determined to defend herself. In a feature article about her life in the University of Maryland alumni magazine, she insisted that the *PNAS* article "simply presented our scientific data" and did not challenge anyone claiming the Nepal strain of cholera was the sole cause of the epidemic.[13]

"As scientists," she said, "we should stand fearlessly behind our work and let the implications of the data play themselves out, however strong the opposition." She accentuated the point by comparing her travails to those faced by some of the great scientists of the past—Louis Pasteur, Robert Koch, Charles Darwin, and Galileo Galilei—who "illustrate a basic point, perhaps the true essence of scientific research. A scientist, no matter the discipline, must fearlessly follow where the data lead. Fretting over the reception of that data or over the negative consequences risks the validity of that research."

Piarroux respected that perspective. It was, after all, a guiding principle for a good epidemiologist: follow the clues wherever they may lead. But he was also aware that steely, fearless determination sometimes leads to clouded judgment, and Colwell's environmental theory was particularly susceptible to that when it came to Haiti. He mulled this over for a few days, and then his wife made a curious discovery.

Martine Piarroux—physician and cartographer—helped her husband analyze scientific articles dealing with cholera epidemics. As she read the Colwell-Cravioto article several times, something bothered her, but she couldn't quite put her finger on it. One morning, it suddenly became clear. The first figure in the article included an epidemiological map that was at least partly familiar. Searching the Web, Martine found the original version, published in October 2010 by OCHA, the UN agency that deals with humanitarian affairs (see figure 21.1).[14]

Piarroux looked at the two maps. The original OCHA map, with its shaded legend, focused on Internally Displaced Persons, showing where in Ouest and

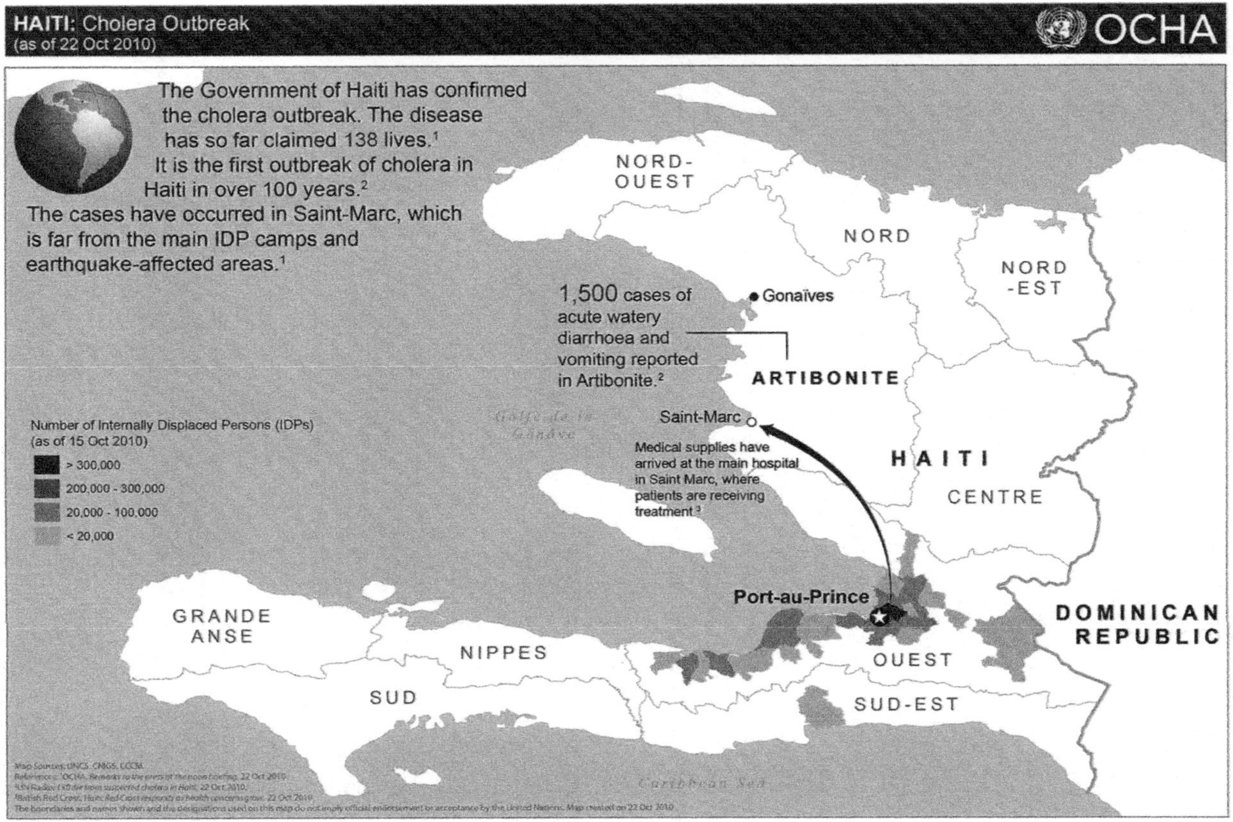

FIGURE 21.1. Haiti cholera outbreak map. From OCHA, "Haiti: Cholera Outbreak (as of 22 Oct 2010)."

Sud-Est départements they were housed in tents and other temporary dwellings after the January 2010 earthquake. It also pointed specifically to "1,500 cases of acute watery diarrhea and vomiting reported in Artibonite" and included a large arrow extending from Port-au-Prince to Saint-Marc to explain that "medical supplies have arrived at the main hospital in Saint-Marc, where patients are receiving treatment." At the top, OCHA stated explicitly that "the [cholera] cases have occurred in Saint-Marc, which is far from the main IDP camps and the earthquake affected areas."

Obviously, the OCHA map was put to a different use in the *PNAS* article, and without a source attribution. The original map legend was replaced with new text, and added circles showed the location of isolates gathered in the Colwell-Cravioto study. But the shading for the IDP areas remained, giving a false impression that these were cholera locations at the time of the study. Colwell and her colleagues had apparently altered the OCHA map rather than making their own—the norm for original research in a scientific publication (see figure 21.2). Was it to direct readers' attention to where earthquake damage had been considerable along the Ouest and Sud-Est département coasts? To claim this was where cholera had first spread

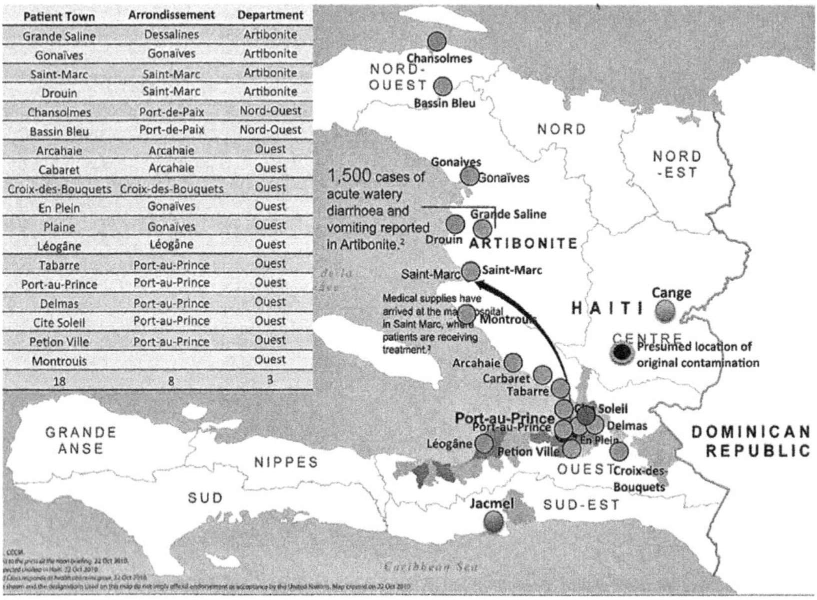

Patient Town	Arrondissement	Department
Grande Saline	Dessalines	Artibonite
Gonaïves	Gonaïves	Artibonite
Saint-Marc	Saint-Marc	Artibonite
Drouin	Saint-Marc	Artibonite
Chansolmes	Port-de-Paix	Nord-Ouest
Bassin Bleu	Port-de-Paix	Nord-Ouest
Arcahaie	Arcahaie	Ouest
Cabaret	Arcahaie	Ouest
Croix-des-Bouquets	Croix-des-Bouquets	Ouest
En Plein	Gonaïves	Ouest
Plaine	Gonaïves	Ouest
Léogâne	Léogâne	Ouest
Tabarre	Port-au-Prince	Ouest
Port-au-Prince	Port-au-Prince	Ouest
Delmas	Port-au-Prince	Ouest
Cite Soleil	Port-au-Prince	Ouest
Petion Ville	Port-au-Prince	Ouest
Montrouis		Ouest
18	8	3

FIGURE 21.2. Isolates collected during 2010 Haiti cholera outbreak for Colwell-Cravioto *PNAS* article. From Hasan et al., "Genomic Diversity of 2010 Haitian Cholera Outbreak Strains," E2011.

before reaching the equally traumatized Port-au-Prince area? To imply a link between earthquake-ravaged areas and the epidemic? If so, that would fit the first factor in Colwell's perfect storm theory.

Piarroux wanted to give Colwell, Cravioto, and their colleagues the benefit of the doubt that their reuse of the OCHA map was just scientific sloppiness, not done deliberately to create a false impression.

Colwell wasn't finished buttressing her perfect storm theory, this time the third factor—that heavy rainfall had caused the river systems to churn up nutrients, warm water, and proper alkalinity. Piarroux was surprised when, a few months later, she and her team published a new article claiming that a climatic anomaly—heavy rainfall in September 2010 (a full month before the epidemic onset)—might have played a role in the proliferation of *Vibrio cholerae* in Haiti's environment and thereby helped trigger the cholera epidemic.[15] That form of a disease-causing mechanism, they wrote, "is markedly different from endemic cholera where tidal intrusion of seawater carrying bacteria from estuary to inland regions, results in outbreaks." In other words, now they were postulating an expansion of the original environmental argument. It no longer depended on a coastal estuarine origin.

The only heavy rain Piarroux knew of, though, came with Hurricane Tomas, which hit Haiti three weeks after the cholera epidemic had started. It was odd for Piarroux and his colleagues to have missed a heavy September rainfall, especially since his group had used the same climatic data set as the Colwell group. While investigating in Artibonite département, Piarroux had even asked residents about possible flooding before the epidemic's onset. No one reported any. In fact, Piarroux's team could not find a single episode of heavy rainfall during September 2010 in the meteorological data set.

Disturbed by what they considered a misleading argument, Piarroux and his colleagues submitted a journal letter taking on Colwell's claim directly. It showed a frequency graph with daily rainfall from the beginning of September to the end of November 2010.[16] It seemed clear: excessive rainfall leading to flooding occurred only on November 6 in Haiti as a whole and on November 6 and 7 in the Artibonite basin, all as a result of one event—Hurricane Tomas—three weeks after the cholera epidemic was first reported.

Colwell's team responded with a letter of its own.[17] It didn't answer Piarroux's direct challenge and ignored the daily rainfall amounts. Instead, it focused on ways to analyze climate data with multiyear averaging and standard deviations.

As Colwell continued to promote her environmental theory, the views of UN panel members continued to evolve. Nair and Lantagne, in early 2012, had already identified Annapurna Camp as the place where the "human activity" occurred. Lantagne was even more direct with the BBC later that year.[18] Yet by the time of a 2013 Earth Day presentation at Tufts University, her academic home, she added a curious statement, saying, "None of the organizations on the ground in October chose to investigate the source of cholera. They deliberately decided not to look into it."[19]

Piarroux, of course, knew better. He had sent the UN panel the MSPP October 21–24, 2010, report on the outbreak conducted immediately by Haitian investigators.

What panel members said to journalists and in public presentations was not always consistent with their scientific publications. The day before Lantagne's BBC comments came out, the *Journal of Disaster Research* formally accepted for publication a scientific article by the panel members that was more closely aligned with the panel's original May 2011 report.[20] The authors cited the research articles of Piarroux et al. and Hendriksen et al. and mentioned Piarroux's conclusion about the importation of cholera, but they still rejected Piarroux's findings. He had to stifle a chuckle as he traced the panel's rejections of his work based on insufficient evidence. Earlier, the panel had written that his evidence did not support his conclusions "with reasonable certainty."[21] Now in its more recent article, the panel wrote that his conclusions could not be accepted with "absolute certainty." What evidence criteria would come next? Piarroux wondered.

The authors, however, were more accepting of the Hendriksen group's conclusions, writing that the near-perfect match of three Nepal cholera isolates and three Haiti isolates were "consistent with Nepal as the origin of the Haitian outbreak of cholera." But still, in concluding, the panel members largely repeated what they had written in their initial report for the UN—no mention of Annapurna Camp or Nepalese peacekeepers. The UN continued to be absolved of any responsibility.

How could Lantagne and Nair put their names to this new article while telling reporters the Nepalese peacekeepers were the likely source of cholera in Haiti? The inconsistency deeply troubled Piarroux. At least Cravioto was consistent.

But even Cravioto's loyalty didn't last. In 2014 (online access May 2013), panel members published a chapter in *Current Topics in Microbiology Immunology* with a further evolution of their collective view.[22] "The preponderance of the evidence and the weight of the circumstantial evidence does lead to the conclusion that personnel associated with the Mirebalais MINUSTAH facility were the most likely source of introduction of cholera into Haiti," they wrote. "We do not feel that this was a deliberate introduction of cholera into Haiti; based on the evidence we feel that the introduction of cholera was an accidental and unfortunate confluence of events."

It came as a short and direct statement through a spokesperson, but on February 21, 2013, Ban Ki-moon formally addressed the legal claim for compensation filed against the UN in 2011 on behalf of Haitian cholera victims:

> Today, the United Nations advised the claimants' representatives that the claims are not receivable, pursuant to Section 29 of the Convention on the Privileges and Immunities of the United Nations. The Secretary-General telephoned Haitian President Michel Martelly to inform him of the decision, and to reiterate the commitment of the United Nations to the elimination of cholera in Haiti.[23]

The statement mentioned UN efforts to provide treatment and improve conditions in the country, and the secretary-general again expressed "his profound sympathy for the terrible suffering caused by the cholera epidemic."

That same month, the physician epidemiologist Ezra Barzilay and others at CDC, PAHO, and the Haitian MSPP described the impact of the epidemic's first two years in a major article in the influential *New England Journal of Medicine*. Official statistics documented the enormous suffering and loss from cholera: 604,634 reported cases of infection; 329,697 hospitalizations; 7,436 deaths. This, the authors noted, was the "world's largest national cholera epidemic in recent memory."

Something was missing, but by then Piarroux had come to expect the omission. The epidemiologist authors wrote nothing of how the disease had first appeared other than that the epidemic was due to an "inadvertent introduction of toxigenic *V. cholerae* into Haiti in October 2010."[24] Piarroux's article with colleagues in *Emerging Infectious Diseases* was acknowledged but not the findings.

Well, thought Piarroux, at least the victims have the sympathy of UN's Ban Ki-moon.

The *NEJM* article was accompanied by a post on January 9 at the *Now@NEJM* blog by Sushrut Jangi, who interviewed Barzilay, the article's lead author and a CDC epidemiologist since 2004.[25] When the cholera epidemic had first appeared in Haiti, Barzilay was deputy incident manager for the Haiti Cholera Response—the CDC's second in command. He did most of the talking in the interview, but his junior colleague and coauthor Nicholas Schaad also took part.

Midway through, Jangi began to focus on the outbreak's early days. "What part of the country was affected first?" he asked.

Barzilay responded, "It became clear to us that the first cases were among communities along the Artibonite River."

Jangi followed up. "Can you say the river led to the spread of the infection?"—a simple question requiring a simple "yes" answer. Schaad jumped in.

"We can say there was an association with communities along the river," declared Schaad. "We can't say the river was a cause."

As he read, Piarroux could barely believe his eyes. Even the UN panel, which had worked overtime to keep blame away from the Nepalese peacekeepers, had determined the river spread the infection.

Later, Jangi asked a question at the very heart of what epidemiologists do. "Was a patient zero ever identified?"

The term "patient zero" was made famous in Randy Shilts's book *And the Band Played On* about the early AIDS epidemic in North America, later made into a film by HBO.[26] It has come to be used widely, especially in the press, to designate the first case in an infectious disease outbreak.

Again, Schaad answered. "Not that I know of." Barzilay followed with "no."

Had early actions been different, CDC officials might have answered the question about patient zero. But time is the enemy when searching for a source, and it was the friend of those who wanted to avoid identifying cholera's origin. Anywhere else in the world, Piarroux surmised, CDC would have immediately gone to the location that Haitian public health officials and journalists identified as the source place of an outbreak. Given its power and connections, surely CDC could have gained entry into Annapurna Camp to conduct an investigation. Instead, though, CDC claimed it had been too busy to investigate the source—an excuse that had long failed to move Piarroux.

It would have been straightforward enough: go to Mirebalais and use the medical, microbiological, and serological approaches epidemiologists had developed decades earlier that were being put to good use throughout the world. In 1982, researchers demonstrated that in "an area with non-endemic cholera, a single serum specimen" with both a vibriocidal antibody test and an ELISA antitoxin test "virtually confirms a recent infection with *V. cholera*"—as long as the investigation is "conducted not much more than one month after the outbreak."[27]

Piarroux believed CDC's leadership had made a conscious choice not to go to the camp, for political reasons. Five months later, CDC instead used those same tests to conduct a seroepidemiological survey of cholera in about 2,500 persons in downriver Grande-Saline commune, far from Mirebalais.[28] Meanwhile, the Nepalese troops in the upriver Annapurna Camp who could have been tested had returned home.

Time had conveniently run out for anyone hoping to find patient zero.

Most, but not all, of the pieces of the origin puzzle had fallen into place when Piarroux was back in Haiti in February 2013. One missing piece was how the second wave of early cases had begun—causing the explosive outbreak that engulfed communities along the Artibonite River.

The origin of the first wave was pretty clear. One or more of the soldiers arriving on October 9 or 12 must have been infected with cholera prior to departing Nepal. As any epidemiologist could have discerned, additional soldiers in the first or second arrival group might have become infected in an airplane's close quarters, on the bus to Annapurna Camp, or in the initial days in camp. Some cholera-infected soldiers experienced explosive diarrhea, others had mild diarrhea, and still others had no diarrhea, but they all harbored *Vibrio cholerae* of varying concentrations in their stools. The nearby stream was contaminated, no matter how the vibrios got into the water. Piarroux was well aware that the passing stream was used for household water and bathing by local villagers. The first confirmed cholera case—a resident of the village of Mèyé—developed symptoms of the disease on October 14, a few days after infection, having passed through a brief incubation period. So began the first wave.

The missing puzzle piece about the second wave was unveiled on Saturday evening, February 23, 2013. Piarroux and his French colleague Stanislas Rebaudet were having dinner at the home in Haiti of Alex Larsen, who had been the country's minister of health during Piarroux's 2010 investigation. The discussion turned to the epidemic's beginnings, and Larsen solved the mystery of precisely *how* cholera-contaminated waste from Annapurna Camp got into the Artibonite River.

Larsen had learned that on October 17, 2010, a replacement driver from the sanitation company made a routine trip to the camp. When he drove the fecal waste across the highway and up the dirt road, he found the hilltop septic pit that overlooked the passing river already overflowing. The driver telephoned his boss back in Port-au-Prince and asked what to do; he was told that because it was late in the day, he should just dispose of the waste wherever he could. He chose the passing stream. In went the infectious contents.

A large septic plume of cholera-laden feces flowed north to the Artibonite River, passing Mirebalais in the late afternoon to evening hours. The plume floated on during the night to the Artibonite Valley, where on October 18–19 it infected water drinkers as it flowed to the coastal Golfe de la Gonâve. A day or two later, cholera cases began to appear at local hospitals and clinics—the second wave of new cholera, soon to become the largest such epidemic in the world.

About seven months after that dinner with Alex Larsen, another startling bit of news arrived. Timothy McGirk and others from the Investigative Reporting Program at the University of California, Berkeley Graduate School of Journalism, were examining the UN's response to cholera in Haiti. Piarroux and I had been in touch with McGirk's team since June 2013. When Piarroux later gave a presentation at UCLA, McGirk and an assistant conducted a lengthy interview

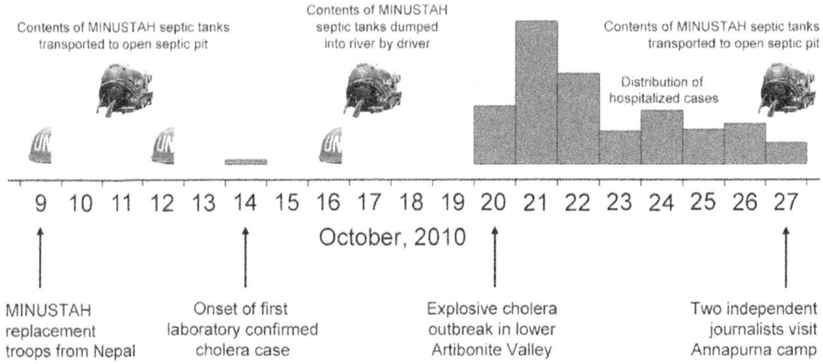

FIGURE 21.3. Events related to origin of cholera outbreak in Haiti. Created by Ralph R. Frerichs.

with him. They exchanged information from their distinct and independent investigations.

A year later, McGirk e-mailed Piarroux with an update on the project's progress—which included a startling development. In 2013, the team went to Mèyé and interviewed Haitians who worked at Annapurna Camp when cholera first appeared. As McGirk explained,

> We conducted the interviews in Creole through a Haitian journalist-translator we brought with us.
>
> In [Mèyé] . . . we found one former employee who was working at the base in mid-October 2010. Separately, in the larger nearby town of Mirebalais, we interviewed a second ex-employee. Both knew each other, both had menial jobs inside the base. Their stories matched up. They both reported seeing "many" soldiers—they didn't specify how many—who were vomiting and sick. Both these employees say they got cholera, one of them twice.
>
> We also interviewed the family of another young Haitian—supposedly one of the first victims—who sold soap and snacks inside the base. One day, soon after the arrival of the Nepali contingent, he was invited to share food with the Nepalese with whom he'd become friendly. That night he contracted fever and had bouts of vomiting and diarrhea. He was taken to Mirebalais on the back of a motorcycle and died there. His family had its own spring, so didn't draw water from the river. It seems that he contracted cholera directly from the soldiers.[29]

There it was: contaminated sewage dumped into the river and apparent symptomatic cholera among Nepalese soldiers. The information from Larsen and McGirk was, in a sense, the last piece of the cholera puzzle.

Over time, extensive investigation by scientists and journalists uncovered the etiological pathway, stretching to the limits what was possible given the lack of MINUSTAH access and cooperation. What remained missing, however, was an international judicial inquiry to assess the mountain of evidence and legally determine the truth, something the UN had wanted to avoid at all costs. While the reputation of the United Nations may have been spared, the considerable obfuscation had unwelcome consequences in the continued battle against the epidemic.

22

SANITATION, WATER, AND VACCINATION

When he was first in Haiti in November 2010, Piarroux's mission was to solve a disease puzzle—both the origin and the spread of the cholera outbreak. Doing both steps is at the heart of epidemiology, defined as "the study of the occurrence and distribution of health-related events, states and processes in specified populations, including the study of the determinants influencing such processes, and the application of this knowledge to control relevant health problems."[1] While many epidemiologists conduct research focusing on the former part of the definition, they understand that the ultimate point is to use the knowledge for disease control. Piarroux's first inclination, as he saw the situation unfold and get increasingly worse with time, was to focus on control by slowing down the epidemic. But then, on the basis of his experience in Africa, he realized that eliminating cholera from Haiti might be possible—under the right circumstances.

Piarroux was well aware of the measures advocated by various agencies and officials. In 1990, the United Nations Development Programme had issued the New Delhi Statement, writing, "Safe water and proper means of waste disposal are essential for environmental sustainability and better human health, and must be at the center of integrated water resource management."[2] The words "better human health," could just as well have been written "reduction and elimination of cholera."

Twenty years later, when the Haiti cholera epidemic began, the quality of sanitation and water in the country remained among the worst in the Western Hemisphere.[3] An improved sanitation facility is typically defined as one that hygienically separates human excreta from human contact; such facilities were available only to 10 percent of Haitians in rural areas and 24 percent of urban residents. About half of those living in rural regions practiced open defecation, using no facility for fecal waste. It was the same among 9 percent of Haitians in urban areas.

The drinking water situation was equally dire. An improved water source is one protected from outside contamination—particularly from fecal matter—by virtue of its construction or through some active intervention. In rural Haiti, 49 percent had no access to improved water sources, including 21 percent who used only surface water—water that collects on the ground or is the top layer of a body of water. In urban areas of Haiti, the situation was much better, but still problematic—15 percent had no access to improved water and 4 percent drank only surface water.

Efforts to improve water and sanitation intensified after cholera arrived. Assuming the cost to be $746 million to $1.1 billion—a figure later doubled—officials of PAHO, CDC, and the UN opined in the *Lancet* that such funds would "decrease the burden of cholera and other diarrheal diseases and prevent the further spread of cholera beyond the island of Hispaniola" (twenty million people divided equally between Haiti and the Dominican Republic).[4] They believed a solution was at hand for about $37 to $55 per person. It was a good idea, but the estimates were way off.

In 2013, the Haitian government, in collaboration with CDC, UNICEF, and PAHO, released its own ten-year plan to eliminate cholera in Haiti.[5] "The country is taking a second breath," wrote Dr. Florence Guillaume, Haiti's new minister of health, and was moving forward in collaboration with the Dominican Republic to address cholera with "water and sanitation [improvements], epidemiological surveillance, health promotion for behavior change, and care of infected persons in health institutions."

The plan seemed to support Piarroux's elimination strategy: "The elimination of cholera from the island entails interrupting its transmission." Yet the plan also appeared to support those who favored the environmental presence of cholera: "Because the bacteria [*Vibrio cholerae*] are in the environment, sporadic cases will always be detected." Piarroux wondered what they meant. Were they espousing that environmental non-O1/non-O139 forms of *Vibrio cholerae* present in some Haitian waters might convert by genomic recombination to a virulent form, as suggested by Colwell and colleagues? Or did the plan authors have another environmental theory in mind, believing the toxigenic form of *Vibrio cholerae* O1 that caused the Haitian epidemic had now become comfortable in Haiti's water environment? Piarroux remained convinced that *Vibrio cholerae* non-O1/non-O139 did not play a role in the epidemic. On the basis of field studies in Haiti and experiences in Africa, he also felt that toxigenic *Vibrio cholerae* O1 would not remain in Haitian waters once all human cases were eliminated. But science is full of surprises. Like others, he would need to await additional research, continuing to learn more about the epidemiology of the disease.

The Haitian elimination program's total cost over ten years was estimated at $2.2 billion, or $220 per person in the country, with $1.6 billion expected from DINEPA, Haiti's national organization for water supply and sanitation; $270 million from MSPP; and $373 million from other Haitian ministries. That cost seemed reasonable to Piarroux, although he was quite troubled by the suggestion that cholera's elimination would take another decade of Haitians suffering disease and death.

Piarroux also wondered where the funds would come from. To reach the $2.2 billion goal, the Haitian government would need international financial assistance. After all, Haiti's estimated gross national income was only $810 per capita per year (compared with $43,550 in France and $54,070 in the United States).[6] But everyone knew it would take more than money. As the plan stated, "While clinical and curative health services are clearly necessary during major emergency situations, it is also just as important to invest at the government level in order to ensure that the Ministry of Public Health has the capacity to efficiently manage the health system on a national scale, as well as the local capacity to be able to supervise hospital and health clinic services that are handled by NGOs." The reluctance of outside agencies to provide that kind of support, and the consequences, were well described by Jonathan Katz, former AP reporter who helped break the story of the Nepalese peacekeepers and cholera.[7]

In January 2014, the UN announced a two-year plan to assist Haiti for the first fifth of its decade-long strategy to eliminate transmission of cholera.[8] The plan stated, "The persistence of cholera is mainly due to the lack of access to clean water and appropriate sanitation facilities." Member nations were asked for $70 million to fund the plan—well short of the $448 million actually budgeted for the first two years, let alone the considerable funds required for the entire ten-year plan.

In December 2013, to assist with fund-raising and offer support for the two-year plan, UN Secretary-General Ban Ki-moon appointed Pedro Medrano Rojas of Chile to serve as senior coordinator for the cholera response in Haiti.[9] Some months later, Rojas met with Piarroux, first in New York and then in Paris, to discuss an alternative plan for cholera elimination—one more closely aligned with the human activity theory.

Addressing water and sanitation is one strategy for controlling cholera. Another is mass vaccination. Scientists who subscribe to the environmental theory embrace vaccination for different reasons than do those who believe cholera spreads from human activity. People susceptible to the disease, argue the environmental theorists, need to be personally protected from the ever-present cholera monster, ready to strike if provoked by weather, an earthquake, or whatever. Piarroux, though, understood that pathogenic *Vibrio cholerae* O1 was a foreign intruder whose survival in Haiti would require human amplification. The more human immunity to cholera created by vaccination, the less chance for that amplification—making elimination much easier.

Both cholera vaccines, Dukoral and Shanchol, require two oral doses and a booster dose two years later, all kept cold before use.[10] Dukoral has an added benefit: it uses a structurally similar toxin of enterotoxigenic *Escherichia coli*, another important cause of bacterial diarrhea, and gives added protection from that disease as well. Neither vaccine, however, protects against a broad array of gastrointestinal diseases that improved sanitation and water help control.

Even before cholera struck Haiti, WHO had recommended against vaccinating entire populations in endemic countries, assuming cholera would remain ever present in the environment but at a lower level. Some months earlier the agency had written that to reduce cholera to a manageable level, "vaccination should be targeted at high-risk areas and population groups. The primary targets for cholera vaccination in many endemic areas are preschool-aged and school-aged children. Other groups that are especially vulnerable to severe disease and for which the vaccines are not contraindicated may also be targeted, such as pregnant women and HIV-infected individuals. Countries should also consider vaccinating older age groups if funding is available." Piarroux was surprised that WHO included preschool-age children in the primary target group for vaccination, since the cholera vaccine was known to have low efficacy in children under five.

WHO estimated the cost of the vaccine at $1.50 per delivered dose, or $3.00 per vaccinated person for the first two doses, followed by a booster dose two years later and every two years thereafter. Refrigeration or cold boxes would also have to be available—contributing to the expense. A few years later, those cost estimates would nearly double.

WHO advised that "periodic mass vaccination campaigns are probably the most practical option for delivering cholera vaccines. Schools, health care facilities, religious institutions and other community settings may be appropriate venues for vaccination campaigns."

It was not until November 2011, however, that WHO gave prequalification approval to one of the vaccines—Shanchol, developed by the International Vaccine Institute in South Korea, the same nonprofit that had received cholera samples from Nepal for analysis.[11] After the UN panel had issued its report, several of the panel members had notable connections with IVI. Panel member Claudio F. Lanata and UN consultant David A. Sack were appointed to IVI's scientific advisory group, joining former UN panel member G. Balakrish Nair.[12] Alejandro Cravioto, the panel chair, became IVI's chief scientific officer in October 2012, charged with overseeing the institute's scientific affairs and "lend[ing] his expertise and advice on matters relevant to vaccine science and technology and potential opportunities."[13]

Five months after WHO gave prequalification approval to Shanchol, the government of Haiti selected the vaccine for local evaluation.[14]

There was much talk in Haiti about vaccinating the entire population of ten million. Knowing it was often in short supply, Piarroux wondered where all that Shanchol would come from. In 2011, the Sixty-Fourth World Health Assembly called for the creation of a stockpile of vaccine as part of a comprehensive strategy for cholera prevention and control.[15] Over the next three years, the oral cholera stockpile increased in size, reaching two million doses by June 2014.[16] But that was only enough to vaccinate 10 percent of the Haitian population with two doses and would leave none for anyone else in the world.

Piarroux learned that a sizable portion of the WHO stockpile was already being employed in Haiti as part of the UN-financed effort to assist with a vaccination campaign. In 2012, two demonstration projects were implemented in urban and rural Haiti to establish the acceptability and feasibility of using the oral cholera vaccine. Partners in Health and GHESKIO, two NGOs with long-term experience in Haiti, were awarded the contract.[17] The demonstrations were conducted in urban Cité de Dieu adjacent to Port-au-Prince; [18] in rural Saint-Marc commune—specifically the community of Bocozel, where the two schoolboys Paul and Jean had died of cholera on October 19, 2010—and in the rural area of neighboring Grande-Saline commune.

When the vaccine was found to be acceptable and feasible[19] and able to induce immunity,[20] vaccination campaigns led by MSPP took place in various areas of the country, including during August–September 2014 in the three départements of Artibonite, Centre, and Ouest.[21] The program tapped into the global WHO stockpile created in 2011, requiring enough doses to vaccinate about two hundred thousand persons. The Haitian Institute for Statistics and Information, CDC, and PAHO/WHO all planned to evaluate whether the vaccine was effective in preventing the disease once the campaign ended. CDC economists had recently estimated the cost of receiving two doses of Shanchol vaccine would be $5.80, much higher than WHO's earlier $3.00 estimate.[22]

Given the actual cost of full vaccination, Haiti's population, and the limited availability of Shanchol in the WHO stockpile and elsewhere, Piarroux questioned the sense of employing a mass vaccination strategy. It seemed more logical to target vaccination aimed at stopping cholera transmission in select areas still under the threat of outbreaks. Selective vaccination—with more manageable amounts of vaccine—could become part of a broader campaign to eliminate the disease.

Piarroux understood that sanitation, clean water, and vaccination held promise for reducing, controlling, or perhaps even eliminating cholera in Haiti. But such control efforts are very costly. They take a long time. If not widespread enough, they may not work as hoped.

Relying on their understanding of human activity's role in cholera transmission, Piarroux and his colleagues moved in a different direction. They decided to focus on cholera *elimination*—a strategy that would leave Haiti once again free of the disease.

23

STRUGGLES AND ELIMINATION

"I am surely not an expert on cholera," wrote Dr. Anthony Robbins, a leading figure in public health and former president of the American Public Health Association, in late March 2014. "I have never seen a patient with the disease. And I have never been to Haiti."[1]

Nevertheless, Robbins published three pieces on cholera in Haiti that month. He acknowledged the epidemic had "infected more than 700,000 people and killed over 8,000 in Haiti over the last few years."[2] He could not ignore the mounting evidence that UN peacekeepers were the source of the disease. He wrote of the "many . . . now seeking compensation from the United Nations for illnesses and deaths. They blame the international earthquake relief operations for the epidemic. And perhaps the U.N. was negligent in the way it managed the human fecal waste of its people responding to the earthquake disaster."[3]

But from Robbins's perspective, Haiti was a powder keg awaiting its fate, some kind of spark. "An outbreak in Haiti awaited only the introduction of a communicable pathogen, in this case *Vibrio cholerae*, rather like a parched landscape awaiting a lit match."[4] The possibility of real negligence wasn't enough to assign real blame. Robbins's message focused on the higher good brought about by the UN presence in Haiti.

Robbins praised the good works of "international earthquake relief operations" but turned a blind eye to the devastating impact of the epidemic on Haitians' lives and seemed tone-deaf to their demands to understand how the epidemic began. He did, however, have a solution. He echoed the message uttered so many times by

CDC, WHO, PAHO, and the UN. "The bottom line is that all low-income countries that lack potable water and sanitation are vulnerable," he wrote. "Haiti presented an ideal environment for cholera to spread. But it might have struck other communities in other countries." His solution: "The world must invest in the infrastructure that will prevent the kind of epidemics we are witnessing in Haiti."[5] Robbins conveniently shifted the attention away from the UN peacekeepers.

While certainly laudable as a long-term aim, his suggestion offered no respite for the Haitian people, who would have to wait years for such an elusive solution. Such efforts by Haitian officials had been attempted in 1998 with an Inter-American Development Bank loan for water and sanitation infrastructure, but they were never funded because of international political differences.[6]

The call for clean water and quality sanitation systems has long been central to public health. In the 1850s, John Snow faced a similar confrontation over cholera control with Edwin Chadwick—the designer of the New Poor Law of 1834, supporter of the Public Health Act of 1848, and leader of England's sanitary reform movement.[7] The new laws established boards of guardians to guide and administer sanitary measures. The sanitarians were on a mission: they believed combining social reform and public hygiene could prevent, or at least ameliorate, all epidemic diseases while addressing broader social problems.

The popular view among sanitarians was that "epidemics were caused by inhalation of agents in the atmosphere," the miasma theory. While the sanitarians and Snow bet on different notions—the latter embraced the germ theory—they shared an ultimate goal of improved sanitation and water. Snow accepted social and sanitary reform as a grand goal, but he had more immediate concerns—as Piarroux did years later.

Snow's view of cholera control focused specifically on stopping local transmission. During the Broad Street Pump cholera outbreak of 1854, which killed hundreds of persons in London's Soho neighborhood, Snow convinced the area board of guardians to remove the handle from the public pump on Broad Street, believed to be the source of the contaminated water.[8] Since then, the image of an old handleless London pump has become dear to epidemiologists who view Snow—today considered the father of epidemiology—as a man of action who used observations and scientific reasoning to formulate a control measure.

Like Snow, Piarroux set as his goal not only to control but also to eliminate cholera in Haiti. He preferred to leave the social and sanitary reforms to others more adept at dealing with the vagaries of the political and financial arenas.

While Robbins was presenting his Haiti views, investigators from the University of Florida who had been studying cholera in Ouest département for the past few years reported finding toxigenic *V. cholerae* O1 in local waters.[9] Their discovery seemingly suggested a second environmental theory for cholera: once an epidemic has started, the toxigenic agent is able to live in surface water and continue the epidemic. But Piarroux disagreed. While he accepted that toxigenic vibrios might be floating in surface waters of Haiti, the likely source was stools of human cholera cases, especially evident during rainy days when feces and sewage are washed into waterways. In a letter to the editor, Piarroux and a colleague noted that it is "impossible to determine whether V. cholera-positive rivers constitute perennial reservoirs of the bacteria or whether they act only as transient vectors of the pathogens."[10] The two French men knew that for this second environmental hypothesis to be tested, the disease first had to be eliminated in humans. They surmised that thereafter the toxigenic vibrios would no longer be found.

What made Piarroux so confident? In part, it was the research of two French microbiologists—described later in this chapter—but also the experience of Madagascar, another country that had been temporarily affected by cholera. The island nation is located off Africa's east coast near Comoros, where Piarroux had consulted in 1998.

Cholera had arrived in Comoros in January 1998, likely imported by air travelers from East African countries where an epidemic was occurring, especially Tanzania and Mozambique.[11] Fourteen months later, it spread to Madagascar, which had not seen cholera for decades. *Vibrio cholerae* O1 Ogawa El Tor was the causative strain, similar to the pathogen that appeared years later in Haiti. The disease first emerged in Madagascar's harbor city of Mahajanga, probably coming by maritime transport from Comoros (see figure 23.1).[12]

Cholera plagued Madagascar for three years. Local health efforts resorted to several control efforts, including a reporting system to identify suspicious cases and deaths, treatment (including intravenous rehydration), public education, and disinfection of houses. Mass immunization was never part of the weaponry. At the time, WHO felt the efficacy of the existing oral vaccine was insufficient to justify the cost.[13]

Then cholera quickly died out, with only twenty-seven cases reported to WHO in 2002, five in 2003, and none thereafter.[14] The disease left no epidemiological trace. As of this writing, not a single cholera case—either imported or linked to a putative environmental reservoir—has been documented.

Piarroux recognized the similarities between Madagascar and Haiti, two poor island nations with mainly agricultural and service industries, deficient sanitation systems, a lack of resources, and all manner of political tensions. He thought the elimination approach taken in Madagascar might work in Haiti too. Piarroux was certainly not against improved access to sanitation and potable water—far from it. Instead, it was a matter of time. He strongly believed that removing

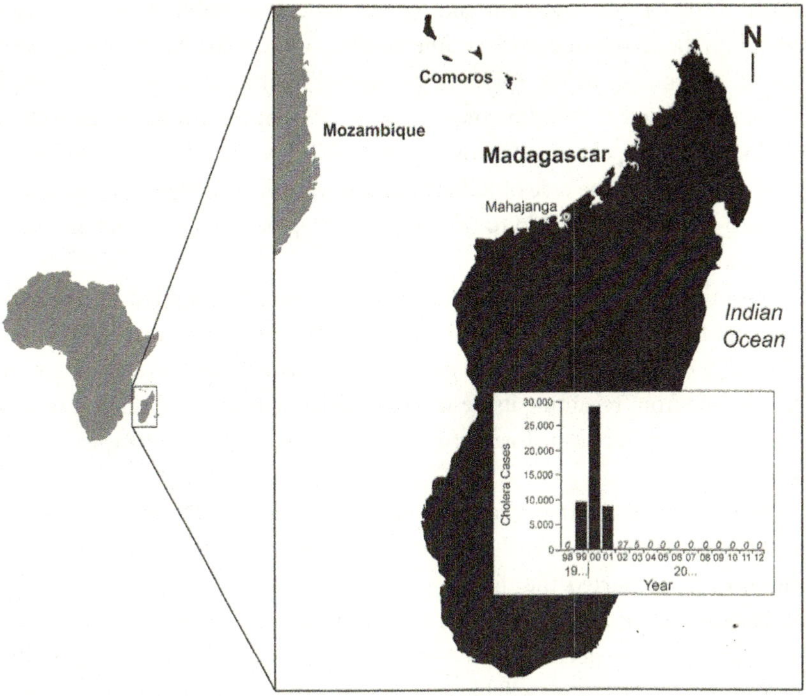

FIGURE 23.1. Cholera appearance and elimination in Madagascar. Created by Ralph R. Frerichs from data in WHO, "Cholera, 1998–2012."

cholera in Haiti could not wait for a ten-year program of sanitation and water improvement—it needed to be done now. He was convinced that with the right strategy, cholera could be stamped out altogether. Rapid case finding and treatment and encouraging health workers to treat cholera cases quickly and disinfect household environments—focusing on those should reduce or eliminate the threat of further transmission.

To succeed, however, Haiti needed to make some major changes. Piarroux was unsure he had the influence to make that happen. He had spent no extended time in the country since his initial field investigation in November 2010, only a brief stay in April 2011 to lecture on parasitology. He had lost his contacts in the Ministry of Health when the government changed in mid-2011. He hadn't spoken with the newly appointed national coordinator for cholera. Would he be able to insinuate himself back into fighting cholera in Haiti through his remaining epidemiologist contacts?

The situation had also changed since the first months of the epidemic. What remained of the anticholera campaign was a morass of unproductive routines limited to patient management and the rebroadcast of public health messages thrust into the cacophony of every other public sound. What Piarroux had feared from the beginning of the epidemic had come true. Despite the appointment of a national cholera coordinator, everyone had been reassigned to the routine activities they had performed before the epidemic. It was a particularly egregious waste of abilities in the case of Robert Barrais, who went to Marseille in 2011 on a French-funded scholarship to take courses on epidemiological surveillance at Piarroux's university.

The quality of epidemiological surveillance had deteriorated and was no longer useful for organizing control activities. At the beginning of 2012, few data were being collected. Cholera was endemic and nascent but was only one rainy season away from regaining its destructive epidemic form. And that's just what happened. After Hurricane Isaac struck Haiti in August 2012, cholera again raged forth.

Piarroux faced another challenge. As a result of the UN panel's report—despite the fact that the panel members had later acknowledged that Nepalese peacekeepers imported the disease to Haiti—most "experts" still considered the Haitian aquatic environment a cholera reservoir. In 2012, a mathematical modeling group declared that "weak sanitary infrastructures and favorable environmental conditions will likely lead to indefinite persistence of the pathogen within Haiti, suggesting that cholera will continue to be a threat for many years."[15] Also in 2012, PAHO/WHO projected that should the current situation persist, "the number of new cases in 2013 may range between 118,000 and 120,000."[16] The experts were on the same page, but their book was far different from Piarroux's.

When the rebound of new cholera cases came with the beginning of the rainy season and the hurricanes that followed, the environmental theory was touted as the explanation. Piarroux knew otherwise, but no one was asking his advice. Slowly, though, the tide began to shift.

In August 2011, the prestigious journal *Nature* published an article showing that all strains of cholera isolated in the world during epidemics belonged to a single lineage that resulted from the evolution of a single clone individualized in the mid-twentieth century.[17] This clonal lineage included all the El Tor strains of *Vibrio cholerae* O1 together with the O139 subclone found mainly in Asia. Unlike the hundreds of environmental strains, the pathogenic O1 and O139 strains shared the genetic arsenal necessary to produce disease-causing cholera toxin. This indicated that the strains circulating in humans during epidemics were derived from a clone with specific characteristics different from the many *Vibrio cholerae* environmental strains.

Piarroux had long suspected the organisms that cause cholera outbreaks and those found in the environment are two distinct microbial populations living in two separate contexts: one group of vibrios containing the cholera toxin that circulates in humans and the immediate environment (water storage caldrons, wells, and the like) and a second group found in coastal waters and occasionally lakes and rivers that cannot provoke epidemic cholera.

The *Nature* article was grist for Piarroux's mill. The Haitian environment certainly played a role when patients were infected by drinking contaminated river water, but that was a transitory phenomenon, different from having a permanent reservoir of infection. Human fecal matter with pathogenic microbes had to be floating in the river.

But while eyes may see, vision becomes opaque when the mind holds a different worldview. To Piarroux, how one sees the future of an epidemic is linked closely to the theoretical debate of human activity versus environment. Elimination is an alien concept to believers that cholera settled permanently in the Haitian environment. While they trust that improving hygiene and water and sanitary conditions will reduce cholera to a manageable level, they overlook the fact that people have been talking about improving such conditions in Haiti for a long time but to no avail. Piarroux certainly agreed with the environmental group that improved sanitation and clean water are vital for a thriving society, but he favored a different strategy to eliminate the immediate problem of cholera in Haiti.

CDC and PAHO were also in the water-and-sanitation camp, the latter seeing benefits beyond cholera: such improvements would "also help prevent other causes of waterborne, childhood-killer diarrheal diseases," according to PAHO's deputy director, Jon Andrus, and there would be "enormous" secondary benefits for Haiti along with "economic growth, higher productivity, and greater national stability."[18] On its website, CDC concurred, touting rehydration treatment, safe water, and adequate sanitation and hygiene—"the mainstay of cholera control and prevention"—and endorsing oral cholera vaccines "until long-term improvements in water and sanitation infrastructure occur."[19]

The Haitian government's ten-year plan bowed to their views. The problem was that even if this plan were to be realized—a very big if—waiting a decade for improved water and sanitation would relegate the young populace—the median age is only twenty-two[20]—to a decade of cholera. Piarroux believed in quicker elimination. First, health workers needed to determine areas where the disease was rampant and stop local cholera transmission through public awareness and detection of new cases, followed by early treatment and chlorination of local drinking water. As part of this strategy, water supply networks needed to be maintained and kept safe. Remarkable results had been achieved with a similar strategy in Comoros and Madagascar. Piarroux was convinced it could work in Haiti if implemented during the dry season when the number of outbreaks to be controlled would be much lower.

Piarroux was determined to promote his strategy for fighting the disease in Haiti. It would begin with confronting the environmental theory head on. The first step: convince the French embassy to fund an environmental study of the strains of *Vibrio cholerae* in Haiti by two French microbiologists, Jean Lesne and Sophie Baron, along with staff of Haiti's National Public Health Laboratory. The embassy agreed to the funding.

In July 2012 in the Artibonite plain and around Port-au-Prince, the investigators gathered more than four hundred *Vibrio cholerae* isolates from twenty-nine aquatic stations. None were armed with the genes that produce cholera toxin—that is, they could not cause epidemics.[21] Although the Baron and Lesne study was not designed to exclude the presence of very low concentrations of toxigenic strains, the results suggested the epidemic Haitian strains introduced into the waters with human waste had failed to multiply and persist at a high level in the aquatic environment. Taking into account the large inoculums of bacteria needed to provoke the disease, such findings were particularly reassuring about the risk of epidemic rebound from the environment.

To Piarroux and his colleagues, it appeared the *Vibrio cholerae* strains originating from patients were eventually supplanted in water settings by the nontoxigenic indigenous environmental strains. Far from being optimal for the growth of disease-causing *Vibrio cholera* O1, the Haitian environment with its own microbial flora seemed to provide some ecological protection against colonization of deadly toxin-producing strains. That meant that the strategy the Haitian government had adopted to fight the cholera scourge was misdirected. It made much more sense, Piarroux thought, to reprioritize a daily struggle to control human transmission wherever it occurred.

Piarroux's focus on elimination grew sharper. He anticipated that with the arrival of the next dry season, cholera would be on a downward slope. It was time to mobilize his elimination strategy and interrupt the disease's transmission. In early November 2012, he returned to Haiti for a ten-day stay, first meeting with French ambassador Didier Le Bret.

The ambassador was troubled by the growing problems with funding the approach advocated by WHO and CDC, as the Haitian government's plan had already begun to confront major financial difficulties. He feared that only a small fraction of the $2.2 billion needed would ever be collected from the international community. Many major donor nations were plagued by economic stagnation and employment problems at home. Even the ongoing pressure for the

UN to compensate Haitian victims—the death toll was already at seven thousand and rising—and pressure in the media and beyond would not overcome the reluctance of UN member nations to commit additional funds. Stopping the recurrent cholera outbreaks as quickly as possible was crucial, at least to help allay the anti-UN tension.

Those concerns, though, were financial and political. Piarroux was sympathetic and wished Le Bret success navigating those waters, but his singular focus had to be on the best way to end the cholera disaster in Haiti as quickly as possible.

It soon became apparent that Le Bret shared his goal; he offered to present Piarroux's written proposal to Haitian authorities, including President Michel Martelly and Prime Minister Laurent Lamothe. It was an important step but by itself not enough to convince Haitian leaders to adapt their control strategy. The fight against cholera remained deadlocked. Piarroux thought long and hard about how to convince policymakers and experts to give his views another look and complement the ten-year strategic plan with a shorter phase aimed at eliminating cholera as soon as possible. But considering the widespread skepticism among stakeholders, more scientific studies, Piarroux was convinced, would be needed to help move the needle.

Soon thereafter, Le Bret was recalled to Paris to become the director of Le Centre de Crise (the Crisis Center) at the Quai d'Orsay. In his new position, he immediately granted to Piarroux's employer—Assistance Publique-Hôpitaux de Marseille—funds for studies to help explain cholera's persistence in Haiti, which made it possible for Piarroux to return to Haiti periodically for short stays and to send a colleague for longer stays. Stanislas Rebaudet, a physician specializing in infectious and tropical diseases, was working on his PhD at Aix-Marseille University, researching the epidemiology of cholera in Africa. Piarroux was his adviser. Rebaudet had just completed fieldwork in Guinea to identify the origin and spread of cholera during the 2012 epidemic, and he was ready for a new challenge. He was ideal for the job.

Piarroux and Rebaudet were part of a larger team with a straightforward goal: refocus the elimination efforts. In France, Martine Piarroux and Jean Gaudart worked on mapping and spatial epidemiology. Sandy Moore—a new PhD student who had come from the United States to work under Piarroux's guidance—took on the epidemiological and microbiological aspects of cholera in Haiti and Africa. The team also had two highly experienced medical doctors and field epidemiologists: Pierre Gazin, based in the same Marseille research unit as Gaudart, had experience in developing countries and would spend half his time in Haiti doing field investigations; and Aaron Aruna Abedi, a former Piarroux graduate student employed by the Ministry of Health in DR Congo to investigate outbreaks of multiple diseases, would work in Marseille from time to time and also join field investigations in Haiti. Finally, the epidemiologist Robert Barrais committed to maintaining field communication as best he could given his many other professional obligations in Haiti.

It was February 2013. Piarroux and Rebaudet traveled to Haiti and first met with the new minister of health, Florence Guillaume. Having agreed to an in-depth meeting, Guillaume spoke with Piarroux about many aspects of the fight against cholera. Though interested, she seemed reluctant to embrace Piarroux's message of hope about rapidly eliminating cholera. Instead, she focused on explaining the current Haitian ten-year program. Because the incidence of cholera had decreased since 2011, the minister considered the epidemic's emergency phase over but believed cholera would remain endemic in Haiti. The strategic plan, she insisted, would enable the country to build treatment centers, integrate management of cholera cases into routine hospital activity, and organize vaccination campaigns.

It became clear to the French epidemiologist that his words and theories were at odds with what Minister Guillaume had been told by prominent cholera experts. She would not yield, but Piarroux remained optimistic that scientific proof and action would change her mind.

The two men got the same negative feelings when they met Dr. Donald François, the new national cholera coordinator. With the case-fatality then around 1 percent, François was comfortable that cholera was being adequately addressed in local treatment centers. He shared Guillaume's view that its immediate elimination was not an achievable objective, basing his views on the opinion that *Vibrio cholerae* were present in the Haitian aquatic environment. Piarroux's elimination plans simply made no sense to him.

Lesne and Baron, whose field research in the waters of Haiti the French embassy had commissioned, hadn't yet published their research; that came in September 2013. Ambassador Le Bret, however, described their findings that toxigenic *Vibrio cholerae* could not be detected in Haiti's aquatic environment in the note on Piarroux's elimination plans he sent to Haitian officials. Piarroux discussed those findings, took on the Colwell-Cravioto *PNAS* article, and explained that in every study the toxigenic strains were found in very small quantities after large sampling efforts. Piarroux was quite sure epidemic strains of cholera were not successfully adapting to the Haitian aquatic environment. But he was just as sure that Guillaume and François remained unconvinced.

Gaudart and colleagues on Piarroux's team formally analyzed the unusual first year of the cholera epidemic and published in April 2013, describing with maps and sophisticated statistical methods the dynamic movements of the disease.

"While the first principal outbreak spread centrifugally like a damping wave that suddenly emerged from Mirebalais and Lower Artibonite, a second principal outbreak erupted at the end of May 2011, concomitant with the rainy season, and displayed a highly fragmented epidemic pattern," they wrote. "The dynamics of the cholera epidemic varied from place to place as time passed, following no clearly predictable scheme."[22]

Except in the first epidemic phase when massive contamination turned the Artibonite River into a deadly waterway, there was no recurrent environmental factor identified in the spatial-temporal analysis other than periodic rainfall. An environmental reservoir of *Vibrio cholerae* either in coastal estuaries or elsewhere was nowhere to be found. Instead, "After the first phases of the outbreak, the absence of constant spatial clusters and the changing pattern of cholera distribution in Haiti argue for the need for control measures that should include intense efforts in rapid and exhaustive case tracking." These findings set the stage for what became the path toward elimination.

More studies followed. Researchers observed no signs of cholera transmission in the vast majority of Haitian communes during the February–March 2013 dry season.[23] The few communes with suspected cholera cases tended to be concentrated in a small number of areas, almost all in Haiti's northern half and often inland from coastal estuaries. Further analyses of the infected communes showed "community health activities appeared insufficient and were often inappropriately targeted." These observations suggested the ongoing cholera control program should be reinforced during the dry season, targeting active foci of the disease detected by a commune-specific surveillance system. Once cases diminished (as verified by microbiological testing), control actions could immediately provide access to clean water and free distribution of treatment products, including oral rehydration kits and antibiotics where appropriate.

Why had cholera not been stamped out in the infected communities? To answer, Rebaudet and Barrais visited forty-nine cholera areas where outbreaks were still being detected. In about three-quarters of them, they found nothing being done to combat transmission—for instance, no home distribution of chlorine tablets. Few residents had seen public health workers, even after weeks of continuous transmission, or had received health education messages on the dangers of consuming untreated water. Mostly, Haitians facing cholera in these areas were left on their own to prevent further transmission. Rapid and exhaustive case tracking alone would not do the trick; management and motivational issues were equally important. Much more effort was needed.

What Rebaudet and Barrais found was discouraging. It confirmed the lack of attention Piarroux had uncovered when he traveled with them to Saint-Marc during his February visit, along with Dr. Roc Magloire, director of the DELR, and two engineers from DINEPA. As they drove from Port-au-Prince, Barrais repeatedly tried reaching the Artibonite département epidemiologist by phone. Told the previous day that the group was coming, the epidemiologist decided instead to attend a training session at a coastal hotel, for which he would be paid. There was no extra money for joining a field investigation. Piarroux was struck by what he had thought would be a difficult choice in an impoverished country: extra pay versus the opportunity to work directly with an international team that included a prominent national figure.

Arriving at the Saint-Marc cholera treatment center, they found a fairly quiet situation—nothing like the rush of cases Piarroux had encountered two years earlier. There were some hospitalized patients, mostly from a village a few kilometers southeast in the foothill valley of the Monts Matheux. The team decided to visit.

The village was essentially several small groups of houses along a minor stream, extending for more than a kilometer. In the hills above was PVC pipe to bring clean water down to supply several hydrants villagers used to get household water. The pipe, though, was broken in several places, and villagers were forced to draw contaminated water directly from the stream. The DINEPA engineers told Piarroux the needed repairs would be easy, but there was a lot of red tape. Clearance was needed from donors, an administrative informality that could take months.

Piarroux's group held an impromptu meeting with several villagers. He asked whether an NGO or team from the département's health directorate had visited and learned that NGO workers had come by a few weeks earlier to raise hygiene awareness. Most disturbing was that villagers knew they were drinking unsafe water—that it was the most likely cause of the persistent cholera. The NGO workers told them to treat the water, but no chlorine tablets were distributed. They would have to buy chlorine themselves, but for people living in such dire poverty, a small expenditure like that is out of reach.

Billions for a national plan to eliminate cholera over ten years, Piarroux thought as they returned to Port-au-Prince, but no one could find the few dollars needed to provide chlorine tablets and repair the PVC pipe to stop cholera immediately?! Médecins Sans Frontières made the same point, writing, "More than three years after Haiti's devastating earthquake, the few public medical facilities in the country do not have the resources to meet the needs of most Haitians."[24]

Unfortunately, the experiences of those villagers were the rule, not the exception. Absent local assistance during the dry season, the coming rains would unleash the cholera scourge once again.

Rebaudet stayed behind in Haiti for another month after Piarroux returned to France in February 2013. He was asked to give a talk about the results of his and

Barrais's field survey to the Humanitarian Country Team, made up of the UN agencies with a humanitarian mandate and the main charitable NGOs working in Haiti. The reception was mixed, sometimes even hostile, frequently interrupted with harassing questions amid stony silence by PAHO representatives. Fortunately, this was offset by favorable comments from some NGOs and even from UNICEF that focused more on the possibility of improvement than on defending the backward slide in the struggle against cholera.

Edouard Beigbeder, the recently appointed UNICEF representative in Haiti, invited his fellow Frenchman Rebaudet for a longer talk. Beigbeder had worked for the UN in many countries, most recently in India and Indonesia, before coming to Haiti in June 2012. His friendly and confident manner immediately engaged Rebaudet, and the two men got along very well. Beigbeder knew the problem cholera in Haiti posed to the UN's reputation.

UNICEF was at the forefront of the UN's fight against cholera, but its control activities had become mired in the ordinary. This concerned Beigbeder. Plans were made for Piarroux to meet Beigbeder during his next visit to Haiti.

In May 2013, a curious twist of fate brought the two men together. Piarroux and Rebaudet were flying to Haiti from France with a layover at Pointe-à-Pitre International Airport in Guadeloupe. It turned out that Beigbeder was on the same plane. At an airport café, the three men shared views on cholera and elimination strategies. Then fate intervened again. A MINUSTAH plane crashed at the airport in Port-au-Prince. There were no fatalities, but all incoming flights were canceled, and the airport was closed.

In a hurry, the Frenchmen decided to fly to Santo Domingo in the Dominican Republic. They arrived there along with a small group of travelers wanting to get to Port-au-Prince without delay. The group negotiated with taxi drivers and set out for the Haitian border. Most of the journey was in the dark. Arriving at the border town at midnight, they spent the night at a cheap hotel and were picked up the next morning by UNICEF drivers who took them to Port-au-Prince.

The two days Piarroux, Rebaudet, and Beigbeder were together was long enough for them to strike a deal. Piarroux and his team would join forces with UNICEF, which would make available human and financial resources, expertise in improving access to water, and access to the network of NGOs with which it routinely collaborated. The team would support and aid the national epidemiological surveillance efforts housed in Port-au-Prince and do multiple field assessments to provide the information needed to implement targeted interventions aimed at cholera hotspots. UNICEF had been acting more or less blindly, not knowing the exact locations where its control programs should concentrate. New focus and emphasis would help invigorate the existing cholera surveillance system, which wasn't working well. The "merger" was a clear win-win.

Assertive leadership helped push aside the red tape and set things quickly in motion. The following week, Piarroux and Rebaudet attended a meeting with NGOs, many already partners of UNICEF: Médecins Sans Frontières, the Red Cross, Oxfam, Partners in Health, Action Contre la Faim, Médecins du Monde, Solidarités, and Agence d'Aide à la Coopération Technique Et au Développement (ACTED). Piarroux was surprised but heartened by the warm acceptance of his group's scientific findings, epidemiological interpretations, and recommendations. Several people thanked them for their work. He had expected criticism, considering all that had transpired. Instead, there was praise. He wondered whether change was finally in the air.

The involvement of the Piarroux team gave a boost to the NGOs, which had been languishing somewhat in their fight against the persistent cholera epidemic as donors were disengaging. With an invigorated fight, new funds could be mobilized to continue the struggle. UNICEF pledged $5.5 million to implement the targeted control strategy, and within three weeks a program incorporating all elements of the discussions and partnership agreements was signed by Piarroux's hospital back in Marseille, UNICEF, Haiti's Ministry of Health, and various NGOs in Haiti. The vast majority of the funds would be spent in Haiti, with a tiny slice for Piarroux's and Rebaudet's travel expenses. The two men committed to supporting the epidemiological surveillance of cholera in Haiti for two years and providing UNICEF any information that could help target active local outbreaks. The new activities were featured as a first part in the strategic ten-year plan. While Beigbeder, Rebaudet, and Piarroux aimed to eliminate cholera altogether, the first part of the plan was more incremental—reduce the annual incidence to 50,000 new cases by the end of 2015. Even though not the same as elimination, that figure was far lower than the 118,000–120,000 new cases PAHO/WHO had projected for 2013.

The rainy season had already returned, as did cholera in many localities. It was time to get going. The new collaborative team was able to prevent the widespread outbreak phase Haiti had experienced twice annually since the epidemic began in 2010. There were no large peaks of cases and mortality, either in July at the beginning of the rainy season or in November at its end. Instead, cholera incidence remained relatively stable, only growing slowly through the rainy season. By the end of 2013, the number of cases (58,809) and deaths (593) appeared to be notably lower than in the previous year (112,876 cases and 894 deaths). In fact, by late 2013, the annual incidence objective of the strategic plan for new cases had nearly been reached, two years before the 2015 target.

By mid-2014, it was clear the UN was fully on board. Peter de Clercq, the MINUSTAH official who had replaced Nigel Fisher as deputy special representative in Haiti,[25] told the UN News Centre that "cholera can still be totally eliminated from the country, since the disease has not become endemic, or anchored in the environment."[26] He even reiterated the human activity theory, stating, "It is still a transmission from person to person, or from temporary contamination of water points." The political winds had shifted radically from October–November 2010, when the environmental theory was widely touted and Fisher was actively denying the role of Nepalese troops.

The arrival of the next dry season provided more convincing evidence of the validity of the Piarroux team's approach. When the rains ended in mid-November 2013, cholera had declined drastically, reaching within a few weeks a level not seen since the epidemic's beginning and five times lower than during the previous year's dry season. Furthermore, when microbiological cultures were used as the definitive guide, it turned out that the vast majority of suspected cholera cases were not even cholera. The team's practical strategy in the field—using a clinical case definition for cholera—had led to overestimation of apparent cholera cases and underestimation of the true reduction of incidence. Appropriate laboratory tests corrected those numbers.

In a September 2014 progress report, Piarroux and Rebaudet compared cholera in a reference period from July 2012 through June 2013 with cholera during the same period a year later.[27] The decline was quite dramatic, reaching nearly 85 percent. The main foci of cholera in mid-2014 were now in the northern half of Haiti, while the southern peninsula départements were completely free for several months. The communes of the Central Plateau (Mirebalais, Hinche, and Lascahobas) in Centre département still reported a high incidence of the disease. Yet to Piarroux and Rebaudet, that finding was likely an artifact, since only a few of those clinical cases were laboratory-confirmed positive for cholera. The vast majority of the supposed cholera cases were false positives caused by other microbes.

Still, there was much more to do. In some of the troublesome départements, NGOs responsible for implementing the plan were not overly active, reluctant to intervene rapidly, delegating to others, and lacking supervision. For their part, the Haitian mobile response teams were slow to engage in the battle alongside NGOs. Despite significant pledges from international donors, funds either didn't arrive at their final destinations or were delayed by months. Without salary and operating monies, many Haitian mobile teams sat idle. Even with the UN now in Piarroux's corner, along with the minister of health and the national cholera coordinator—all giving the impression of wanting to work hard toward the same elimination goal—management and motivation issues kept cropping up. It was clear that NGOs and health authorities in certain areas had other priorities. Without a drastic change, the goal of local elimination would be missed.

The team continued to press forward with its elimination strategy, and there were 27,753 new cholera cases and 296 deaths between January and the end of December 2014, reducing by half the number of cases reported in 2013. What an improvement from the thousands of new cases and dozens of deaths recorded each day at the beginning of the epidemic, noted Piarroux. But he was far from satisfied. Cholera was still present and was even regaining strength in some areas. And with the rains, it would once again spread if drastic measures were not taken in time.

With UNICEF support, Piarroux and his team were determined not to let go. He resolved to keep up the fight, hoping that in 2015 they would achieve the elimination they had just missed during the 2014 dry season. It would be a challenge: so many other things competed for the world's attention—Islamic militants in the Middle East; Ebola in West Africa—and Haiti had faded in the eyes of the international community.

The scientific realm always features a lot of intellectual theorizing and discussion. Some is on target. Some floats like a will-o'-the-wisp, there for only a moment. For epidemiologists, the theorizing that ultimately matters should be supported by scientific observation. At least, that is the way Piarroux sees it. He and his scientific team used observation, research, and logic to challenge the prevailing wisdom of the environmental theory and its very powerful backers. Yet doing so defined him as an iconoclast or worse, at least to some.

John Snow in the mid-1800s was also an iconoclast. He questioned the conventional wisdom about cholera. Thomas Wakley, the powerful editor of the *Lancet*, was so irritated by Snow's theories that in 1858, upon Snow's death, he wrote an obituary considered "extraordinary in its brevity."[28] Some 155 years later, the journal recognized the error of its ways and commissioned a decent obituary of the epidemiological giant.

Curiously, in late 2010 the *Lancet* again made an unusual decision regarding cholera, but this time about the epidemic in Haiti. It refused without comment even to consider Piarroux's seminal article that first described what eventually became the world's largest cholera epidemic of the current seventh pandemic. But such rejection was not enough. When the etiological finger pointed toward UN peacekeepers, *Lancet Infectious Diseases*—a sister publication—boldly declared "blame is unhelpful."[29] Not only was blame helpful, but it was also essential for creating an effective control strategy.

Had others accepted what Piarroux determined early on in the epidemic, they might have worked together for the total elimination of cholera. Instead, for three long years, exactly the opposite happened—and thousands of Haitians lost their lives unnecessarily.

Even after the UN panel confirmed that the epidemic had been imported through human activities, a curious sentence in the report was left unchallenged—the panel "concludes that the Haiti cholera outbreak was caused by the confluence of circumstances . . . and was not the fault of, or deliberate action of, a group or individual." With these words, the panel absolved the UN of responsibility. With no "deliberate action of a group or individual," the blame for the epidemic's root causes was shifted to Haiti itself—its land, weather, people, and health care system.

By not addressing uncomfortable truths, the UN panel of *well-regarded scientists* failed to apply skilled field observation and logical analysis of evidence regarding cholera's origin and to question the thesis that the aquatic environment in Haiti was a reservoir for recurring cholera during periodic rainy seasons. The UN was likely very pleased with the panel's findings.

But the UN and its panel were not the only ones that contributed to the spread of mystification. Most disappointing to Piarroux were the renowned scientists who did not hesitate to use questionable maps and data to support their environmental theory, thereby continuing to confuse stakeholders' vision of cholera. While not as active in their obfuscation, many other experts and scientists followed this troubled path, some working at CDC, PAHO, and WHO, and others for professional journals, news organizations, and educational institutions. Their collective suggestions to scientifically unaware policymakers that the long-term persistence of cholera in Haiti was an established fact almost snuffed out the kindled flame of action in Haiti aimed at overcoming cholera in a timely manner with readily available means.

In spite of everything, though, the flame was not snuffed out. Others were sensing that cholera was not Haiti's fate but rather a burden—one that could indeed be addressed and eliminated. Momentum was gradually shifting.

24

RAPPROCHEMENT

Why is it important to know exactly how a disease outbreak began? The answer: knowing the source directs what should be done to prevent similar outbreaks in the future. That is, policy implications arise from the initial source investigation.

While the full details may never be known, Piarroux's investigation and other sources provide a clear picture of what likely occurred. The Nepalese replacement troops scheduled to come to Haiti in October 2010 had merely been asked whether they had had recent diarrhea—despite the fact that there had been a recent cholera outbreak in Nepal.

It would have been reasonable at least to test the troops' stool samples before they departed for Haiti. Alternatively, they could have been vaccinated against cholera. This seems sensible given they were moving from a cholera-endemic area to a highly vulnerable cholera-free area. But none of that was done. In October 2010, when the epidemic started in Haiti, vaccination was not being recommended by WHO and was not required by the UN. Universal antibiotic use might also have been an option but was not—and is still not—recommended because of concern with the development of antibiotic resistance.

In close contact during the time of travel or the first days in camp, one or two infected soldiers could easily have infected others following a typical cholera incubation period of one to two days, resulting in more cases in the coming week. The first symptomatic cases at the Annapurna Camp leaked to the small stream that flowed adjacent to a fence near the camp toilets, thereby infecting a handful of villagers living in Mèyé, some of whom traveled to Mirebalais for treatment.

As more troops were infected, the waste tanks within the camp filled with cholera-ridden diarrhea, or black water. On October 17, or possibly a day earlier, a sanitation truck of a company contracted by MINUSTAH emptied the Annapurna Camp waste tanks. In the late afternoon or early evening, the truck drove to the septic pit on the hilltop above Annapurna Camp to dispose of the load. Finding the pit filled, the driver dumped the contents and a large amount of fecal waste entered the local stream and flowed on to the Artibonite River. By the next morning, many in downstream communities were infected. The world's greatest cholera epidemic was soon under way.

This summary points to several actions that could have been taken and suggests policies that should be adopted. Realizing cholera's short incubation period, the newly arrived UN troops could have been visited and reviewed by MINUSTAH physicians during their first week in country. Had the physicians found symptomatic cases of cholera, the troops could have been isolated in camp until deemed no longer communicable.

Camp commanders could also have been made aware of the need for routine vigilance when new troops arrived. A symptom list—what to look out for—could have been incorporated into management training. There might have been a few cases in the nearby village had the cholera outbreak within the camp been detected early, but the disease would quickly have been localized and controlled through immediate therapy of cases and treatment of home waste and water.

The main intervention point, without a doubt, was proper in-camp waste management. Routinely treating black-water waste in the Annapurna Camp would have meant that what was dumped by the hilltop septic pit and flowed into the nearby stream would not have been infectious.

Even more troubling, during the first four years of the epidemic, neither the UN, WHO, nor CDC ever acknowledged officially how the epidemic got started. This allowed the simmering scientific debate to continue and called into question the basic tenets of cholera in Haiti: is toxigenic *Vibrio cholerae* a permanent resident of Haiti to be controlled but never eliminated, or is the organism an unwelcomed guest of human hosts that can be successfully treated and eliminated?

Despite all that has been discovered, Piarroux remains doubtful that the United Nations will ever fully acknowledge that Nepalese peacekeeping troops brought cholera to Haiti. Behind the scenes, however, a new narrative has unfolded, a more complex one revealed by the UN's own actions. Perhaps the French word *rapprocher*—bring closer—describes the appearance of new understanding, guidelines, and funding initiatives.

The UN's changing attitude became apparent in July 2014 when Secretary-General Ban Ki-moon traveled to a small village in Haiti's Centre département, not far from where the cholera epidemic had begun. He referred to the trip as a "necessary pilgrimage" in remembrance of the people who had lost their lives to cholera.[1] There, he spoke of "a moral duty" to help stem the further spread of the disease."[2]

In late September 2014, a letter of inquiry on the cholera outbreak in Haiti was sent to the secretary-general by three UN special rapporteurs, previously appointed by the UN's Commission on Human Rights to study and address matters of international importance.[3] They were joined as signatories by Gustavo Gallón of Colombia, an authority on human rights in Haiti who had served in a UN position for the previous year as an independent expert.

The four authors presented their concerns, citing allegations they had received about the situation in Haiti, including the assertion that "peacekeepers deployed under the MINUSTAH operation were responsible for the introduction of this strain of cholera to Haiti through insufficient and inadequate sanitation management and lack of reasonable precautions and measures to prevent, control and mitigate the introduction of cholera." They further noted that the United Nations still "has not formally accepted responsibility for allegedly causing the outbreak nor has it provided compensation to the victims and the survivors of the outbreak." Posing the germane human rights query, the authors asked, "Bearing in mind that the United Nations should be bound by international human rights law, what measures are being taken by the United Nations to ensure access to justice including provision of compensation to the individuals affected by the cholera outbreak in Haiti?"

Shifting their focus to prevention, the letter writers ended with questions about measures the UN had taken in violations of "human rights to water, sanitation and health" in the operation of MINUSTAH in Haiti and in ongoing and future peacekeeping operations worldwide.

Their answer came several months later in a letter from Pedro Medrano Rojas, the Chilean diplomat who since 2013 had served as the UN's senior coordinator for the cholera response in Haiti.[4] Piarroux had met Medrano twice and was well aware of the continuing efforts to bring worldwide attention to the cholera epidemic and garner support for the $2.2 billion ten-year plan to eliminate cholera and improve water and sanitation. Medrano's letter cited changes in UN policies intended to prevent recurrence of such a catastrophe. He wrote of Secretary-General Ban's trip to Haiti, reiterated the UN's willingness to take all necessary steps to eliminate cholera, and added that it "can only do so with the continued support of the international community." In other words, Medrano made clear that the goal of elimination was set but that financing largely depended on others beyond the UN.

Medrano did not acknowledge the source or epidemiological reason for cholera's explosive beginning. Instead, he cited the UN panel's 2011 more general conclusion that the "outbreak was caused by a confluence of circumstances and that it was not the fault of, or due to deliberate action by, a group or individual." This ignored the panel's 2013–14 follow-up publication, which stated that "the preponderance of the evidence and the weight of the circumstantial evidence does lead to the conclusion that personnel associated with the Mirebalais MINUSTAH facility were the most likely source of introduction of cholera into Haiti."[5] Even though his letter attempted to minimize the UN's responsibility and convince people the organization was doing everything possible, it did seem to hint at an admission of fault.

Piarroux agreed with Medrano that the UN had made efforts to clean up the mess once it was made, providing numerous on-the-ground support activities, including new treatment centers; family hygiene kits with soap, water purification tablets and oral rehydration salts; safe drinking water; and logistic and security assistance. The letter held particular interest for Piarroux when it explained that after release of the report in May 2011, Ban had convened a "senior-level integrated Task Force" to study the report and evaluate the merit of the panel's conclusions, including specific recommendations on cholera prevention and response. Two of those recommendations seemed crucial to Piarroux: cholera immunization prior to deployment of UN peacekeepers and various policies on wastewater management.

Cholera vaccination had finally become mandatory for all UN peacekeepers deploying to and from cholera-endemic areas, according to Medrano's letter. This pleased Piarroux. Yet vaccination alone is not enough, especially with much-less-than-perfect current cholera vaccines. Realizing these limitations, the panel had advocated that United Nations installations worldwide treat fecal waste using on-site systems that inactivate pathogens before disposal in septic pits or other areas. They further recommended that these systems be operated and maintained by trained, qualified UN staff or by local providers with adequate United Nations oversight.

Medrano noted that the UN had taken substantial actions to fulfill the wastewater management recommendation. In June 2011, the Department of Field Support (DFS) of the UN peacekeepers emphasized the need to reinforce existing policies and provide additional guidance on the management of wastewater. In response, the various peacekeeping missions around the world have provided action plans that include improvement and better monitoring of existing wastewater facilities, installation of independent wastewater treatment plants, and inspection and closer supervision of contractors involved in wastewater disposal. Furthermore, the UN's oversight capacity has been strengthened.

Eight months after the start of the cholera outbreak in Haiti, MINUSTAH established a fully functional environmental compliance unit (ECU), which then conducted a detailed analysis of the mission's wastewater facilities. According to Medrano, MINUSTAH had already installed thirty-two wastewater treatment plants throughout the country, and it now closely monitors the proper disposal of untreated wastewater into government-approved disposal sites.

MINUSTAH also now provides environmental briefings for all deployed military, police, and civilian personnel. The briefings cover, among other things, solid waste management, hazardous waste management, and water management.

Finally, awareness and oversight have reached the highest local level. The deputy director of mission support for MINUSTAH chairs a mission environmental committee that meets monthly and prepares quarterly reports on environmental initiatives, including specific recommendations and challenges. These reports are then sent up the administrative ladder to Medrano's office as special representative of the secretary-general.

While the various undertakings addressed in Medrano's letter implied some responsibility for the problems the UN had created, Piarroux noted that the letter accepted no blame and made no mention of any intent to pay damages to those affected by the epidemic. Nevertheless, thought Piarroux, the UN does now accept that cholera can be eliminated and thus is in close agreement with him and his group. It is also encouraging member states to support funding for both elimination and the necessary infrastructure in Haiti to ensure there are no new outbreaks of waterborne diseases. While Piarroux appreciated the apparent UN progress, he remains concerned. Back in 2012 or 2013, ridding Haiti of cholera might have seemed an important goal, garnering international support and funding. But precious time was lost to the ongoing efforts to conceal UN culpability. Other disasters such as Ebola in 2014 and the Nepalese earthquake in 2015 captured the compassionate attention of the international community, which translated into extensive support and considerable money. Timing, it seemed, was everything.

For far too long, the misinformation campaign to protect the UN and the peacekeeping program has been perpetrated not only by the UN but also by foreign experts and scientists behaving in a manner that is anathema to everything Piarroux believes about how epidemiologists and other scientists should conduct themselves. Many of these same people remain entrusted to protect the broader world, well beyond Haiti's shores, as similar biological disasters arise. Are these experts telling the truth as new epidemics such as Ebola arise? Or are they protecting their own or others' interests? And what of those who howl with the wolves without understanding what has really occurred?

New disasters will no doubt appear. When journalists, epidemiologists, and other scientists observe blameworthy acts by powerful people or agencies, blame avoidance will likely again rear its head, deflecting investigations and causing the loss of valuable time. *C'est ainsi que les hommes vivent*, thought Piarroux. That is how people live. Yet in Haiti, welcome progress was eventually made in addressing cholera. Even within the United Nations, a healthy debate was raging between pragmatists and idealists—some advocating a total blackout on errors and others demanding culpability for violations of human rights.

To Piarroux, the evocation of a "moral duty" by Ban Ki-moon during his July 2014 necessary pilgrimage to Haiti was a rapprochement of sorts. He spoke of a moral duty to help stem the further spread of cholera in Haiti, leading to eventual elimination. If this book in some way helps stimulate the UN, other international agencies, and local programs to move in a concerted direction, rapprochement may well lead to an opening of hearts, purses, and hands and thus genuinely rid Haiti of the scourge of cholera.

Epilogue

The continuing program to eliminate cholera in Haiti reached a troublesome impasse in late 2014. Cholera deaths declined during the first nine months in all départements but persisted in Artibonite and to a lesser extent in Nord and Centre.[1] In each instance, persistence of transmission was linked with cholera management issues. With the rainy season under way, the national disease toll began to reverse course in September–October, increasing in magnitude. As cholera spread again in Haiti, Port-au-Prince was the most heavily affected area.

"More than 2,000 people with symptoms of cholera have required emergency hospitalization since mid-October in Port-au-Prince, Haiti," reported Médecins Sans Frontières on November 24.[2] "The national health structures are poorly prepared to react to cholera outbreaks, despite them being predictable during the rainy season," explained the local MSF medical coordinator.

The cholera elimination program put forth by Piarroux and his colleagues remained, with its objective of reaching zero cases throughout the country during the dry season. Human transmission should have ceased if all départements—including the three laggards, Artibonite, Nord, and Centre—had cooperated and united during the dry season in surveillance, rapid treatment, and control efforts. If the goal of elimination had been achieved, there would have been no relapse in the wet season—spreading the disease to neighboring départements and beyond. Cholera in Haiti would have come to an end. But Piarroux was not dissuaded. Accompanied by team members Stanislas Rebaudet and Aaron Aruna Abedi, Piarroux returned to Haiti in January 2015 to investigate the cholera outbreaks in Port-au-Prince and in several other affected communes and plan for the next dry season, trying once more to generate national effort.

A lack of attention had allowed cholera to find its way back to the capital city in September 2014, resulting in several violent outbreaks following heavy rainfall. Piarroux and Rebaudet immediately mapped the new cholera cases and, after follow-up investigation, showed government and international officials that the outbreaks had likely been provoked by contaminated water mixing with drinking water in the distribution network of several neighborhoods south of Port-au-Prince. Their quick diagnosis restored hope in the anticholera campaign, but precious time had been lost as cholera recolonized many areas after its elimination in the first half of 2014.

Despite all the setbacks, Piarroux and his team remain optimistic and committed.

When cholera first appeared in Haiti in 2010, the World Health Organization was notably absent, other than deflecting comments being offered by the head of the organization's cholera task force (see chapter 5). Recognizing the ineffectiveness of the cholera task force, WHO formally revitalized the group in June 2014 as the Global Task Force on Cholera Control, charged—among other tasks—"to support increased implementation of evidence-based strategies to control cholera."[3] No specific mention was made, however, of the ongoing cholera elimination efforts in Haiti or of the scientific justification for the strategy. Equally curious, WHO reduced its two-year budget in 2014–15 by 51 percent for "outbreak and crisis response" emergencies, moving money instead into noncommunicable diseases, with a budget increase of 20 percent.[4] By the end of 2014, the bacterial disease cholera had killed more than 8,700 people in Haiti, and the viral disease Ebola had taken the lives of at least 8,200 in West Africa.[5]

The situation so distressed the WHO executive board that in late January 2015 representatives of the thirty-four member states guiding the agency voted unanimously to endorse a resolution "aimed at overhauling its capacity to head off and respond to outbreaks and other health emergencies."[6] Somewhat ironically, given the lack of cholera origin investigation by CDC in Haiti, Thomas Frieden—CDC director and a WHO executive board member—was quoted by the reporter as saying, "Too many times the technical is overruled by the political in W.H.O. . . . We have to reverse that."

While Piarroux had called for a judiciary review of how cholera came to Haiti, no such review ever took place. Speaking with the German newsmagazine *Der Spiegel* in November 2014, Haitian president Michel Martelly restated the same safety and security argument used previously by many others who resisted holding the UN accountable for cholera in Haiti.[7] The reporter began by noting that the UN had been blamed for introducing the deadly disease and then asked, "Do you still welcome [the UN's] presence?"

President Martelly responded,

> The UN didn't force its way in. We created a situation that demanded that the UN be there to help us establish peace and security. Unfortunately, the cholera problem appeared. Now there are two types of reactions: trying to blame or trying to solve. Instead of making enemies, we are trying to solve this problem. The Secretary General has acknowledged the UN's responsibility, and he has pledged to help us. We'd

rather have the UN help us fight the epidemic and improve our water and sanitation system than try to do it on our own.

Martelly was asked, "What do you think of the efforts of human rights groups and cholera victims to bring on lawsuits against the UN in US courts?" The president answered, "I won't tell a victim or somebody who has lost a member of his family to not go and talk to the UN or go to court and sue them. People can do what they want. But the government has the task to manage relationships, and I think we are doing a good job."

The lawsuit brought against the UN by the Institute for Justice and Democracy in Haiti on behalf of the cholera victims finally made it to court.[8] In October 2014, the suit was formally addressed in the U.S. District Court for the Southern District of New York. The UN didn't even show up to defend itself. Instead, the United States government assumed that role, with the U.S. attorney asserting the UN's absolute immunity and complete lack of legal responsibility to resolve the claim by Haitian cholera survivors and the families of cholera decedents. The implication was that the "principle" of UN peacekeeping was more important to U.S. foreign policy than the human rights of Haitians.[9]

The final decision was deferred until January 2015, when the lawsuit was formally dismissed by Judge J. Paul Oetken. He wrote, "The U.N. is immune from suit unless it expressly waives its immunity."[10] The human rights plaintiffs plan to appeal the ruling.

While maintaining that the plaintiffs had no standing to file such a lawsuit, the UN continued to express concern over cholera in Haiti. In a late 2014 resolution, the UN Security Council welcomed "the ongoing efforts by the Government of Haiti to control and eliminate the cholera epidemic.[11] Yet as of December 2014, the national ten-year plan for cholera elimination that relied on sanitation, vaccination, and clean water projects had received a mere 13 percent of the $2.2 billion requested,[12] despite the active solicitation of Pedro Medrano Rojas.[13] Absent a dramatic reversal, the less costly elimination approach advocated by Piarroux and colleagues remains the most promising.

Looking forward to 2015, the United Nations Security Council unanimously voted to remain in Haiti for an eleventh year,[14] placing MINUSTAH among the longest foreign occupiers since Haiti's 1804 independence. Only the United States exceeded MINUSTAH, with troops in Haiti for nineteen years ending in 1934.

One group of troops in Haiti, however, was dramatically reduced—those from Nepal. When cholera first appeared, Nepal had 1,075 of the 8,500 UN soldiers in Haiti. Four years later, the Nepalese accounted for only ten staff officers among five thousand total UN troops.[15] Nepalese peacekeepers, however, were not neglected by the UN. Since 2010, when the cholera epidemic began, they have increased in other regions of the world by 16 percent. Besides its own military commitments, the United States remains the major force behind worldwide UN peacekeeping operations, contributing 28 percent of the current seven billion-dollar budget.[16]

Nepalese soldiers were also on the mind of Rita Colwell as she continued to publicize her environmental views of cholera. During a major presentation at Ohio Wesleyan University in December 2014, Colwell opined as "very controversial" the view that cholera in Haiti had been brought by UN peacekeepers from Nepal.[17] To justify her remark, she cited Haiti's recent history of cholera but misrepresented key findings. Though a cholera outbreak in Nepal occurred shortly before the peacekeeping troops departed for Haiti, Colwell told the audience it had occurred two years earlier. Compounding her error, she continued, "The troops that had gone to Haiti two years later had all tested negative." She neglected to mention that the Nepalese Army's chief medical officer had clearly stated that none of the soldiers were tested for cholera before they left the country, and UN officials in Haiti said they were not tested after arrival.

Even the timing of Hurricane Tomas in Haiti was stated in a way that seemed to favor her environmental view. "Just before the outbreak occurred there was a hurricane that skirted the island and dropped a heavy amount of rain on the island," she said. Actually, the hurricane arrived on November 5, weeks after the epidemic was well under way and the Haitian government had already reported 6,742 hospitalized cholera cases and 442 cholera deaths.[18]

Colwell did acknowledge that the strain of *Vibrio cholerae* isolated in Haiti was "very similar to a Nepal cholera strain," but she made no mention that the Nepal and Haiti strains differed by only one to two base pairs out of four million base pairs in the *Vibrio cholerae* genome—a difference of a mere 0.000038 percent—less common than one typo within all characters in this book and four more copies besides. And so in some circles the debate between human activity and environment continues, although it is eroding over time.

Nowhere was the erosion of the environmental hypothesis more evident than in an end-of-the-year 2014 scientific article.[19] Having obtained a comprehensive panel of "116 serotype [*Vibrio cholerae*] O1 strains from global sources, including 44 Haitian genomes," the researchers (including listed coauthors Rene S. Hendriksen, Geeta Shakya, and Paul S. Keim) wrote, "This study provides evidence for a single-source introduction of cholera from Nepal into Haiti followed by rapid, extensive, and continued clonal expansion." With specific reference to the environmental hypothesis and genomic recombination, the authors concluded, "The results of molecular and epidemiological analyses of this [October

2010 Haiti] outbreak suggest that an indigenous Haitian source of *V. cholerae* is unlikely and that an indigenous source has not contributed to the genomic evolution of this clade."

Though Piarroux and his colleagues have waged the fight with the environmental theory, they have decided to move on, keeping their focus primarily on eliminating cholera. While ridding Haiti of cholera is Piarroux's essential goal, scientific questions about epidemic emergence and persistence continue to occupy his thoughts, regarding both Haiti and multiple African countries. Why do cholera epidemics start in regions previously free of the disease? What leads to rapid transmission in some areas but slower spread in others? Why do elimination efforts succeed among some but fail among others? Finding answers will help Piarroux understand the sometimes unusual behavior of epidemic and endemic cholera and, most important, formulate elimination programs that turn deadly rivers back into waterways that sustain the living.

Notes

INTRODUCTION

1. Associated Press, "Aid Workers Face 'Angry and Impatient' Haitians."
2. Klarreich and Polman, "NGO Republic of Haiti."
3. Colwell, "Infectious Disease and the Environment."
4. Strassburg, "The Global Eradication of Smallpox."
5. Farha et al., "On the Cholera Outbreak in Haiti since 2010."
6. Garrett, "Ebola's Lessons: How the WHO Mishandled the Crisis."

1. UPHEAVAL

1. Harris et al., "Cholera," 2466.
2. Jenson et al., "Cholera in Haiti," 2133.
3. Ibid., 2134.
4. Desvarieux and Padgett, "Haiti's Cholera Riots."
5. BBC News, "UN Appeals for Calm after Cholera Riots in Haiti."
6. Evans, "Epidemics and Revolutions," 131–32.
7. Sérant, "Haïti: Alerte au cholera."
8. U.S. CDC, "Update: Cholera Outbreak—Haiti, 2010," *MMWR* 59, no. 45; U.S. CDC, *MMWR* 59, no. 45, errata.
9. PAHO, "PAHO Responds to Cholera Outbreak in Haiti."
10. Agence France-Presse, "Choléra en Haïti: Le bilan s'alourdit, la psychose s'installe."
11. MSPP, "Rapport de Cas, Journalier et Cumulatif," October 31, 2010.

2. VIBRIO CHOLERAE

1. Chun et al., "Comparative Genomics," 15446–447.
2. Colwell, "Global Climate and Infectious Disease," 2027.
3. U.S. CDC, "Update: Cholera Outbreak—Haiti, 2010," *MMWR* 59, no. 45.
4. Jackson et al., "Seroepidemiologic Survey of Epidemic Cholera in Haiti," 659.
5. Harris et al., "Cholera," 2466.
6. Robins and Mekalanos, "Genomic Science in Understanding Cholera Outbreaks," 224.
7. Hornick et al., "The Broad Street Pump Revisited," 1186; Cash et al., "Response of Man to Infection with Vibrio Cholerae," 48.
8. WHO, "Cholera," Fact Sheet No. 107.
9. Robins and Mekalanos, "Genomic Science," 218.
10. Nelson et al., "Cholera Transmission," 695.
11. WHO, "WHO/UNICEF Joint Monitoring Programme for Water Supply and Sanitation."
12. Ministry of Health and Population (Nepal) et al., *Nepal Demographic and Health Survey 2011*.
13. U.S. CDC, "Update: Cholera Outbreak—Haiti, 2010," *MMWR* 59, no. 45.
14. Levine et al., "Duration of Infection-Derived Immunity to Cholera," 819.

15. Ali et al., "Natural Cholera Infection-Derived Immunity in an Endemic Setting," 915.

16. Pasetti and Levine, "Insights from Natural Infection-Derived Immunity to Cholera," 1707.

3. RUMORS

1. MINUSTAH, "Haïti face à une épidemie de choléra."
2. Cash et al., "Response of Man to Infection with *Vibrio cholera*," 48.
3. U.S. CDC, "Update: Cholera Outbreak—Haiti, 2010," *MMWR* 59, no. 45; U.S. CDC, *MMWR* 59, no. 45, errata.
4. PAHO, "PAHO Responds to Cholera Outbreak in Haiti."
5. Reingold, "Outbreak Investigations," 22.
6. Sérant, "Haïti: Alerte au choléra."
7. U.S. CDC, "Cholera Outbreak—Haiti, 2010," *MMWR* 59, no. 43.
8. PAHO, "Cholera Outbreak in Haiti," *EOC Situation Report* no. 4; PAHO, "Cholera Outbreak in Haiti," *EOC Situation Report* no. 6.
9. U.S. CDC, "Update: Cholera Outbreak—Haiti, 2010," *MMWR* 59, no. 45; U.S. CDC, *MMWR* 59, no. 45, errata.
10. O'Connor et al., "Risk Factors Early in the 2010 Cholera Epidemic, Haiti," 2136.
11. Katz, "Choléra."
12. Thélot, "Bêê ê ê: De ces rumeurs qui font rougir les 'casques bleus' en Haïti," 78.
13. Marcelin, "Encore la soldatesque de la MINUSTAH."
14. Kurczy, "Haiti Cholera Outbreak 'Stabilizing.'"
15. Katz, "Protesters Blame UN base for Cholera in Haiti."
16. Permanent Mission of the People's Republic of China to the UN, "Statement by H.E. Mr. Li Baodong."
17. Katz, "Protesters Blame UN Base for Cholera in Haiti."
18. Katz, "UN Probes Base as Source of Haiti Cholera Outbreak."
19. Palca, "Mysterious Life of the Cholera Bacterium."
20. Terra News Service, "Presidente do Haiti diz que surto de cólera foi 'importado.'"

4. STEALTH

1. Lakhani, "Cuban Medics in Haiti Put the World to Shame."
2. Gorry, "Haiti One Year Later," 52.
3. Llanes et al., "Letter to the Editor," 753.
4. Styger and Barison, "Introducing the System of Rice Intensification (SRI) to Haiti."
5. BBC News, "Scores Die in Haiti Cholera Outbreak."
6. Hall-Stoodley and Stoodley, "Biofilm Formation and Dispersal and the Transmission of Human Pathogens," 8.
7. Giono, *The Horseman on the Roof.*

5. HYPOTHESES

1. Gomes, "Morte de jovem haitiano gera novos protestos contra a Minustah."
2. Parker, "Cholera in Haiti."
3. Romero, "Poor Sanitation in Haiti's Camps Adds Disease Risk."
4. Ellingwood, "As Rains Approach, a Scramble to Get Latrines and Hygiene Supplies to Haiti."
5. Harris et al., "Cholera," 2466; Cravioto et al., "Final Report of the Independent Panel."
6. Constantin de Magny and Colwell, "Cholera and Climate," 119.

7. Huq et al., "Ecological Relationships between Vibrio cholerae and Planktonic Crustacean Copepods," 281.

8. Colwell et al., "Reduction of Cholera in Bangladeshi Villages by Simple Filtration," 1051.

9. Ibid., 1054.

10. Knox, "Earthquake Not to Blame for Cholera Outbreak in Haiti."

11. U.S. Department of State, "Senator Lugar Announces Three New Science Envoys."

12. Parker, "Cholera in Haiti."

13. Kristoff and Panarelli, "Haiti: A Republic of NGOs?"

14. Goesch et al., "Comparison of Knowledge on Travel Related Health Risks," 364.

15. Estrada-Garcia and Mintz, "Cholera," 462.

16. Dubois, *Haiti: The Aftershocks of History*, 211–13.

17. Robinson, *An Unbroken Agony*, 198–207.

18. Hallward, *Damming the Flood*, 232–49.

19. Heine and Thompson, *Fixing Haiti*, 160–61.

20. Bellamy, Williams, and Griffin, *Understanding Peacekeeping*, 65.

21. UN Security Council, "Resolution 1927."

22. Geffrard, ""Une maladie importée, la MINUSTAH clame son innocence."

23. *Le Nouvelliste,* "Haïti: Des malades du choléra avaient bu de l'eau potable."

24. Walker, "UN Investigates Cholera Spread in Haiti."

25. Maharjan, "Cholera Outbreak Looms over Capital."

26. Katz, "UN Probes Base as Source of Haiti Cholera Outbreak."

27. Ibid.

28. Ibid.

29. Jeanty, "SANCO clarifie."

30. Ibid.

31. Katz, personal communication with Piarroux, July 7, 2011.

32. Al Jazeera, "UN Troops Blamed for Haiti Cholera."

33. Geffrard, "Une maladie importée, la MINUSTAH clame son innocence."

6. MAPS

1. Frerichs, "John Snow."

2. PAHO, "Cholera Cases Confirmed in Paraguay."

3. PAHO, "Cholera Outbreak in Haiti," EOC Situation Report no. 1.

4. PAHO, "Cholera Outbreak in Haiti, 2010," EW 42; PAHO, "Cholera Outbreak in Haiti, 2010," EW 43.

5. OCHA, "Haiti—Cholera Situation," October 25, 2010.

6. OCHA, "Haiti—Situation de Cholera," October 27, 2010.

7. Walker, "UN Investigates Cholera Spread in Haiti"; Katz, "UN Probes Base as Source of Haiti Cholera Outbreak."

8. OCHA, "Haiti—Situation de Cholera," October 28, 2010.

9. OCHA, "Haiti—Situation de Cholera," November 10, 2010.

7. ALTERED REALITY

1. Walker, "UN Investigates Cholera Spread in Haiti"; Katz, "UN Probes Base as Source of Haiti Cholera Outbreak."

2. U.S. CDC, "Cholera Outbreak—Haiti, October 2010, *MMWR* 59, no. 43.

3. PAHO, "Cholera Outbreak in Haiti," EOC Situation Report No. 6.

4. Associated Press, "Cholera in Haiti Matches Strains Seen in South Asia."

5. Quentel and Le Bret, ""Urgent Restreint."

6. Chaaban, "Svenska ambassadören."
7. *Helsingen Sanomat*, "Cholera Situation Spiralling Out of Control in Haiti."
8. PAHO, "Cholera Outbreak in Haiti, 2010," EW 42; PAHO, "Cholera Outbreak in Haiti, 2010," EW 43.
9. Walker, "UN Investigates Cholera Spread in Haiti"; Katz, "UN Probes Base as Source of Haiti Cholera Outbreak."
10. United Nations, "Report of the Secretary-General on the Budget for the United Nations Stabilization Mission in Haiti."
11. Glass et al., "Seroepidemiological Studies of El Tor Cholera in Bangladesh," 240–41.
12. Shampo, "Bernard Kouchner."
13. Jourdaine, "Choléra en Haïti."

8. JOURNALISTS

1. Walker, "'Fatal Sickness' Outbreak in Haiti."
2. Walker, "UN Investigates Cholera Spread in Haiti."
3. Al Jazeera, "UN Troops Blamed for Haiti Cholera."
4. Alphonse, "Sur les traces du premier décès."
5. Alphonse, Louis, and Louis, "Mirebalais Cholera, Part 1" and "Mirebalais Cholera, Part 2."
6. Katz, "U.N. Worries Its Troops Caused Cholera in Haiti"; Katz, "UN Probes Base as Source of Haiti Cholera Outbreak"; Katz, "UN Troops May Have Brought Cholera"; Katz, "Haitians Protest, Threaten UN Base."
7. Katz, "UN Troops May Have Brought Cholera."
8. Hujer, "Haiti's Cholera Disaster."
9. Delva, "Haitians Attack U.N. Troops, Blame Them for Cholera."
10. Katz, "Haitians Protest, Threaten UN Base."
11. Archibold, "Officials in Haiti Defend Focus on Cholera Outbreak."
12. Terra News Service, "Presidente do Haiti diz que surto de cólera foi 'importado.'"
13. McNeil, "Cholera's Second Fever."
14. U.S. CDC, "Multistate Outbreak of Human Salmonella."
15. Associated Press, "Recall Expands to More Than Half a Billion Eggs."
16. Crumb, "Iowa Egg Producer Separates Business, Charity Work."
17. Katz, "U.N. Worries Its Troops Caused Cholera in Haiti."
18. Maharjan, "Cholera Outbreak Looms over Capital."

9. SECRECY

1. Jourdain, "Choléra en Haïti."
2. Jourdain, "Haiti: No Let-Up in Haiti Cholera One Week from Elections."
3. Maguire, "René Préval."
4. Pow, "Inside the Rituals of Haiti's 'Vodou' Faith."
5. U.S. Library of Congress, Federal Research Division, "Country Profile: Haiti."

10. OBFUSCATION

1. Doyle, "Adventure I: Silver Blaze."
2. Romero, "Poor Sanitation in Haiti's Camps Adds Disease Risk."
3. Murray, "Katrina Aid from Cuba?"
4. Doucet, "The Nation: NGOs Have Failed Haiti."
5. Knox, "Earthquake Not to Blame for Cholera Outbreak in Haiti."
6. Colwell, "Concentric Circles."

7. Brauman, "Faiblesses du dispositif anticholéra à Haïti."
8. Hecdivert and Laraque, "Rapport de Mission au Département Sanitaire du Centre."
9. MINUSTAH, "Haïti face à une épidémie de cholera."
10. Alphonse, "Sur les traces du premier décès."

11. SPECULATION

1. Klarreich and Polman, "The NGO Republic of Haiti."
2. Organization of American States, "Who We Are."
3. Center for Economic Policy Research, "Head of OAS Electoral Mission in Haiti."
4. McFadden, "Haiti's President Confirms 3-Month Term Extension."
5. *Assistance mortelle.*
6. Porter, "Haiti's René Préval Says UN Tried to Remove Him."
7. La Torra, "Doctors Take Medical Marvels to Haiti."
8. Boling, "Public Health School Hosts Haitian Leader."
9. Mission of the United States, "World Health Assembly."
10. Keating, "Is Haiti's Government Starting to Function?"
11. Lutton, "'We Are Poor . . . But We Demand Respect.'"
12. Sontag, "In Haiti, Global Failures on a Cholera Epidemic."
13. U.S. CDC, "Global HIV/AIDS at CDC."
14. MSPP, "Plan Stratégique du Réseau National de Baoratoires, 2010–2015."
15. CDC Foundation, "Haiti Buildings."
16. U.S. CDC, "Outbreak Investigations."
17. U.S. CDC, "Foodborne Outbreaks."
18. Loharikar et al., "Cholera in the United States, 2001–2011," 695.
19. U.S. CDC, "Update: Cholera Outbreak—Haiti, 2010," *MMWR* 59, no. 45.
20. Dowell et al., "Letter from Goma."
21. Fries, "Does Politics Influence the CDC?"
22. Bellamy et al., *Understanding Peacekeeping*, 52.
23. Hallward, *Damming the Flood*, 143.
24. Robinson, *An Unbroken Agony*, 99.
25. UN Security Council, "Resolution 1529."
26. UN Security Council, "Security Council Establishes UN Stabilization Mission in Haiti."
27. UN Security Council, "Report of the Secretary-General," S/2004/908.
28. UN Security Council, "Report of the Secretary-General," S/2010/446.
29. CERFAS, "MINUSTAH."
30. Bhattarai, "Contributor Profile: Nepal."
31. Gurung, "Success of Nepali Peacekeepers."
32. Cunliffe, *Legions of Peace*, 100–102.
33. U.S. Department of State, "The United States in UN Peacekeeping."
34. UN Secretariat, "Assessment of Members States' Contributions," March 25, 2010, and "Assessment of Members States' Contributions," October 24, 2012.
35. Cooper and Robbins, "U.S. Mobilizes to Send Assistance to Haiti."
36. CNN, "Numbers Tell Stories of Horror, Heroism in Haiti."

12. PANDEMICS AND SOUTH ASIA

1. U.S. CDC, "Cholera Outbreak—Haiti, 2010, *MMWR* 59, no. 45; Chin et al., "Origin of the Haitian Cholera Outbreak Strain."
2. Devault et al., "Second-Pandemic Strain of *Vibrio cholera*," 339.

3. Islam, Drasar, and Sack, "The Aquatic Environment as a Reservoir of *Vibrio cholera*," 197.

4. Mutreja et al., "Evidence for Several Waves of Global Transmission," 462.

5. Bharati and Bhattacharya, "Cholera outbreaks in South-East Asia," 88.

6. Chastel, "Le centenaire de la découverte du vibrion d'El Tor," 76.

7. Siddique et al., "Why Treatment Centres Failed," 359.

8. Ramamurthy et al., "*Vibrio cholera* O139 Bengal," 330.

9. Barua, *Cholera*, 8.

10. Lacey, "Cholera," 1410.

11. Vinten-Johansen et al., *Cholera, Chloroform, and the Science of Medicine*, 238–39.

12. CBC News, "Cholera's Seven Pandemics."

13. Howard-Jones, "Robert Koch and the Cholera Vibrio," 379.

14. WHO, "Cholera, 2010."

15. Ali et al., "The Global Burden of Cholera," 211.

16. UN Department of Peacekeeping Operations, "Fact Sheet."

17. UN Security Council, "Report of the Secretary-General on the United Nations Stabilization Mission in Haiti," S/2010/446.

13. REPORT

1. La Fontaine, "The Wolf and the Lamb."

2. Desvarieux, "Haiti's Presidential Vote."

3. Carroll, "Haiti Votes in Historic Election as Reports of Fraud Emerge."

4. Renois, "Haïti."

5. U.S. Embassy, Kathmandu, Nepal, "Security Announcement for American Citizens in Nepal"; Maharjan, "Cholera Outbreak Looms over Capital."

6. Pasmantier, "Choléra en Haïti."

7. UN Department of Public Information, "Collective Efforts in Haiti."

14. VODOU AND CHOLERA

1. DeWitte, "Selectivity of Black Death," 1436.

2. Benedictow, *The Black Death 1346–1353: The Complete History*, 98.

3. Bosin, "Russia, Cholera Riots of 1830–1831," 2877–78.

4. Renois, "Haïti."

5. Katz, "12 Killed in Haiti Cholera Witch-Hunt."

6. Valme, "Officials: 45 People Lynched."

7. McAlister, "Vodou."

8. Dubois, "Vodou and History," 94.

9. *Encyclopedia Britannica Online*, "François Duvalier."

10. *Time*, "The Death and Legacy of Papa Doc Duvalier."

11. Council on Hemispheric Affairs, "The Tonton Macoutes."

12. Simons, "Voodoo under Attack in Post-Duvalier Haiti."

13. BBC News, "Haiti Makes Voodoo Official."

14. Grimaud and Legagneur, "Community Beliefs and Fears during a Cholera Outbreak in Haiti."

15. Ibid., 27.

16. Ibid.

15. INQUIRY

1. Gurrey, "Choléra en Haïti."

2. Pasmantier, "Haiti Cholera Outbreak 'Came from UN Camp.'"

3. Nesirky, Noon Briefing, Haiti.
4. Winter, "Election Violence Flares in Haiti."
5. Beaubien, "In Haiti, Political Impasse Compounds Uncertainty."
6. Gaudart, Rebaudet et al., "Spatio-Temporal Dynamic of Cholera."
7. U.S. Department of State, "Travel Warning, Haiti."
8. Katz, "Haiti Cholera Likely from UN Troops, Expert Says."
9. MacKenzie, "Opinion, Haiti."
10. Valero, Daily Press Briefing.
11. Castro, "Cuba's Fidel Sees UN in Haiti Cholera."
12. Agence France-Presse, "Nepal Condemns Study Linking Army to Haiti Cholera."
13. BBC News South Asia, "Haiti Cholera Outbreak."
14. U.S. CDC, "Update: Cholera Outbreak—Haiti, 2010, *MMWR* 59, no. 48.
15. Chin et al., "The Origin of the Haitian Cholera Outbreak Strain."
16. Ibid., 41.
17. Ibid.
18. Ibid., 38.
19. Ibid., 41.
20. *Lancet Infectious Diseases*, editorial, "As Cholera Returns to Haiti, Blame Is Unhelpful."
21. *Lancet Infectious Diseases*, editorial, "WHO Failing in Duty of Transparency."
22. Attal, "Qui est responsable de l'épidémie de choléra en Haïti?"
23. UN News Centre, "UN in Talks to Set Up Independent Panel of Experts."
24. Al Jazeera, "UN Troops Blamed for Haiti Cholera."
25. Sack, Sack, and Chaignat, "Getting Serious about Cholera."
26. Katz, "UN Calls for Probe into Origin of Haiti Cholera."
27. UN News Centre, "Haiti: Ban Appeals for More Funds."
28. UN News Centre, "UN Urges Massive Campaign in Haiti."

16. POLITICS BEFORE SCIENCE

1. Fraser, "World Report."
2. Harris et al., "Cholera's Western Front."
3. Ivers et al., "Five Complementary Interventions to Slow Cholera."
4. *Lancet Infectious Diseases*, editorial, "As Cholera Returns to Haiti, Blame Is Unhelpful."
5. Sadowski, "Archbishop: Haitians Feel Abandoned by World amid Continuing Disasters."
6. UN News Centre, "Haiti: Ban Appoints Four Top Medical Experts."
7. *Weekly Epidemiological Record*, "Cholera in the Americas, South America."
8. Gil et al., "Occurrence and Distribution of Vibrio Cholerae in the Coastal Environment of Peru," 699.
9. Constantin de Magny et al., "Environmental Signatures Associated with Cholera Epidemics," 17676.
10. Hurtado, "Haiti's Cholera Epidemic Caused by Weather, Say Scientists."
11. Allié, " Idées: De l'importance de connaître les origines de l'épidémie de choléra en Haïti."
12. Cravioto et al., "Final Report of the Independent Panel of Experts."
13. Sack, "Consultant Report: Cholera in Haiti."
14. Chin et al., "The Origin of the Haitian Cholera Outbreak Strain."
15. U.S. CDC, "Cholera Outbreak—Haiti, October 2010, *MMWR* 59, no. 43; Karki et al., "Cholera Incidence among Patients with Diarrhea," 36.

16. Sack, "Consultant Report."
17. Pugliese, "Point de Presse des Nations Unies en Haiti."
18. Sack, "Slide Presentation: Cholera in Haiti."
19. Sack, "Consultant Report."
20. Sack, "Mapping the Progression of the Cholera Epidemic in Haiti."
21. Sack, personal communication with the author, May 17, 2012.
22. Nelson et al., "Cholera Transmission," 695, 697.
23. Cravioto et al., "Final Report of the Independent Panel of Experts."
24. Faucher and Piarroux, "The Haitian Cholera Epidemic," 479–80.

17. NEPAL

1. Agence France-Presse, "Nepal Government Raises War Death Toll."
2. Ministry of Foreign Affairs, "Nepal's Role in the UN Peacekeeping Operations."
3. Gurung, "Success of Nepali Peacekeepers."
4. IRIN News, "NEPAL: UN Peace Mission Ends amid Political Deadlock."
5. Shakya, "Antimicrobial Resistance Surveillance in Nepal."
6. Malla et al., "Challenges and Successes."
7. Nguyen et al., "Cholera Outbreaks Caused by an Altered *Vibrio cholera*," 1569–70.
8. Hendriksen et al., "Population Genetics of Vibrio cholerae from Nepal in 2010."
9. Bhattacharjee, "Paul Keim on His Life with the FBI during the Anthrax Investigation," 1416.
10. Lewis, "TIGR Introduces *Vibrio cholerae* Genome."

18. CONCEALED IN THE FIELD

1. U.S. CDC, "How to Investigate an Outbreak."
2. U.S. CDC, "Haiti Cholera Outbreak —Map of Cumulative Attack Rate with Data on Cases, Hospitalizations, and Deaths," February 17, 2011.
3. Ibid., September 2, 2011.
4. U.S. CDC, "Update on Cholera—Haiti, Dominican Republic, and Florida, 2010" *MMWR* 59, no. 50.
5. McCarthy and Khambaty, "International Dissemination of Epidemic *Vibrio cholera*," 2600.
6. Cohen et al., "Preventing Maritime Transfer of Toxigenic *Vibrio cholerae*."
7. U.S. CDC, "CDC Situation Awareness."
8. Talkington et al., "Characterization of Toxigenic Vibrio cholerae from Haiti."
9. UN Department of Public Information, "Collective Efforts in Haiti Will Be Overwhelmed."
10. Lantagne, personal communication with the author, December 24, 2012, and January 29, 2013.
11. Piarroux, personal communication with the author, January 21 and March 2, 2013.
12. Piarroux et al., "Understanding the Cholera Epidemic, Haiti."
13. Cravioto et al., "Final Report of the Independent Panel of Experts."
14. WHO, Global Task Force on Cholera Control, "Prevention and Control of Cholera Outbreaks."
15. UN Office of the Spokesperson for the Secretary-General, Daily Press Briefing.
16. Katz, "U.N. Worries Its Troops Caused Cholera in Haiti."
17. Lantagne, personal communication with the author, November 29, 2012.
18. WHO, "Interagency Diarrhoeal Disease Kits—Information Note."
19. Ghimire, Pradhan, and Maskey, "Community-Based Interventions," 216–17.
20. Karki et al., "Cholera Incidence among Patients with Diarrhea," 186.

21. UN Office of the Spokesperson for the Secretary-General, Daily Press Briefing.
22. Ali et al., "Recent Clonal Origin of Cholera in Haiti," 699.
23. U.S. CDC, "Update: Cholera Outbreak—Haiti, 2010," *MMWR* 59, no. 48.
24. PAHO, "Cholera Outbreak in Haiti."
25. Prepetit and Boisson, "Inventaire des ressources minières de la République d'Haiti."
26. U.S. Army Corps of Engineers, "L'Evaluation des ressources d'eau d'haiti."
27. Pugliese, "Point de Press des Nations Unies en Haiti."
28. Lantagne, personal communication with the author, May 9, 2013.
29. Geffrard, "Une maladie importée, la MINUSTAH clame son innocence"; Katz, "UN Probes Base as Source of Haiti Cholera Outbreak."
30. Dong Wook Kim, personal communication with the author, July 19, 2011.
31. U.S. CDC, "Update: Cholera Outbreak—Haiti, 2010," *MMWR* 59, no. 48.
32. Schuller, "Haiti's Disaster after the Disaster."
33. UN News Centre, "Haiti: Ban Appoints Four Top Medical Experts."
34. Vital et al., "Evaluating the Growth Potential of Pathogenic Bacteria in Water," 6482.
35. Lantagne, personal communication with the author, September 20, 2012.
36. Saloomey, "UN Likely to Blame for Haiti Cholera Outbreak"; Sontag, "In Haiti, Global Failures on a Cholera Epidemic."
37. Enserink, "Cholera Linked to U.N. Forces, but Questions Remain."

19. QUARANTINE AND ISOLATION

1. Associated Press, "UN Peacekeeper in Haiti Treated for Swine Flu."
2. Center for Infectious Disease Research and Policy, "H1N1 Flu Breaking News."
3. WHO Media Centre, "Swine Influenza."
4. Besheer, "UN Facilities, Peacekeepers in Haiti Test Negative for Cholera."
5. WHO, "International Sanitary Regulations."
6. WHO, *International Health Regulations* (1969), 10.
7. WHO, "Cholera—Small Risk of Cholera Transmission by Food Imports," 55.
8. WHO, "Cholera Outbreaks—Ineffective Control Measures," 291–92.
9. WHO, "Global Cholera Control Task Force," 136–37.
10. WHO, *International Health Regulations* (2005), 1, 20, 24.
11. WHO, "WHO Statement relating to International Travel and Trade."
12. WHO, "Cholera, 2010," 326.
13. WHO, "Cholera Country Profile: Haiti."
14. WHO, "Cholera, 2012," 328.
15. WHO, *International Health Regulations* (1969), 10.
16. WHO, *International Health Regulations* (2005), 12, 46.

20. THE WALL CRACKS

1. U.S. CDC, "Haiti Cholera Outbreak."
2. Piarroux et al., "Understanding the Cholera Epidemic, Haiti"; Hendriksen et al., "Population Genetics of *Vibrio cholerae* from Nepal in 2010."
3. *Frontline*, "Paul Keim."
4. Piarroux and Faucher, "Cholera Epidemics in 2010," 231–38.
5. Raoult, "Plague and Cholera in the Genomics Era," 212.
6. Frerichs et al., "Nepalese Origin of Cholera Epidemic in Haiti."
7. Bureau des Avocats Internationalaux/Institute for Justice and Democracy in Haiti, Petition for Relief.
8. UN Office of the Spokesperson, Spokesperson's Noon Briefing.
9. Lantagne, personal communication with author, August 9, 2013.

10. Saloomey, "UN Likely to Blame for Haiti Cholera Outbreak."
11. Sontag, "In Haiti, Global Failures on a Cholera Epidemic."
12. Nesirky, Spokesperson's Noon Briefing.
13. Kolovos and Lindstrom, "UN Must Take Responsibility for Haiti Cholera Outbreak."
14. Piarroux and Faucher, "Idées—Tous les êtres humains naissent libres et égaux en dignité et en droits, même les Haïtiens?"
15. *Baseball in the Time of Cholera,* directed by Bryan Mooser and David Darg; Darg and Mooser, "What the UN Won't Admit."
16. Wilde, "Baseball in the Time of Cholera."
17. *Economist,* "The UN in Haiti."
18. *New York Times,* "Haiti's Cholera Crisis."
19. ICDDR,B News, "ICDDR,B's Emergency Response Team Return from Haiti."
20. Paulson, "Experts Say UN Did Not Bring Cholera to Haiti."
21. Colwell, "Experimental Reservoirs of Human Pathogens."
22. Hasan et al., "Genomic Diversity of 2010 Haitian Cholera Outbreak Strains."
23. Harris et al., "Cholera," 2466.
24. Fernández-Delgado et al., "Vibrio cholerae Non-O1, Non-O139 Associated with Seawater," 280.
25. U.S. CDC, "Cholera—Non-O1 and Non-O139 Vibrio cholerae Infections."
26. Nigro et al., "Temporal and Spatial Variability," 5388.
27. PAHO, "Cholera Outbreak in Haiti."
28. Colwell, personal communication with author, August 26, 2013.
29. Steenland et al., "Laboratory-Confirmed Cholera and Rotavirus," 642.
30. Charles et al., "Importance of Cholera and Other Etiologies of Acute Diarrhea," 514.

21. ANSWERS

1. Frerichs et al., "Source Attribution of 2010 Cholera Epidemic in Haiti."
2. Frerichs et al., "Nepalese Origin of Cholera Epidemic in Haiti."
3. Mekalanos et al., "Non-O1 *Vibrio cholerae* Unlinked to Cholera in Haiti."
4. Hasan et al., "Reply to Mekalanos et al."; Hasan et al., "Reply to Frerichs et al."
5. Knox, "Scientists Find New Wrinkle in How Cholera Got to Haiti."
6. PAHO, "Cholera Outbreak in Haiti."
7. Hurtado, "Haiti's Cholera Epidemic Caused by Weather."
8. Kupferschmidt, "Second Bacterium Theory Stirs Haiti's Cholera Controversy," 1493.
9. Albon, "Where Did Haiti's Cholera Epidemic Come From?"
10. Shrestha, "Haiti's Cholera Outbreak."
11. Shrestha, "Haiti's Nepali UN Peacekeepers."
12. Piarroux, "Op-Ed: What Role Did the Environment Play in Haiti's Cholera Epidemic?"
13. *Terp Magazine,* "Professor Rita Colwell."
14. OCHA, "Haiti: Cholera Outbreak (as of 22 Oct 2010)."
15. Jutla et al., "Environmental Factors Influencing Epidemic Cholera," 597.
16. Gaudart et al., "Environmental Factors Influencing Epidemic Cholera."
17. Jutla et al., "In Response."
18. Doyle, "Haiti Cholera Epidemic 'Most Likely' Started at UN Camp."
19. Lantagne, "Understanding Haiti's Cholera Outbreak."
20. Lantagne et al., "The Origin of Cholera in Haiti," 760.
21. Cravioto et al., "Final Report of the Independent Panel."

22. Lantagne et al., "The Cholera Outbreak in Haiti," 162.

23. UN Department of Public Information, "Haiti Cholera Victims' Compensation Claims."

24. Barzilay et al., "Cholera Surveillance during the Haiti Epidemic," 603.

25. Jangi, "An Interview with Ezra Barzilay."

26. Shilts, *And the Band Played On*; *And the Band Played On*, directed by Roger Spottiswoode.

27. Clements et al., "Magnitude, Kinetics, and Duration of Vibriocidal Antibody Responses," 472.

28. Jackson et al., "Seroepidemiologic Survey of Epidemic Cholera in Haiti," 654.

29. McGirk, personal communication with author, September 11, 2014.

22. SANITATION, WATER, AND VACCINATION

1. Porta, *A Dictionary of Epidemiology*, s.v. "epidemiology."

2. Boisson de Chazournes and Salman, *Les ressources en eau et le droit international.*

3. WHO, "WHO/UNICEF Joint Monitoring Program."

4. Periago et al., "Elimination of Cholera Transmission."

5. Ministry of Public Health and Population (Haiti), "National Plan for the Elimination of Cholera."

6. World Bank, "Haiti—Gross National Income per Capita (Atlas Method)."

7. Katz, *The Big Truck That Went By.*

8. United Nations, "Support Plan for the Elimination of the Transmission of Cholera."

9. UN News Center, "Interview with Assistant Secretary-General Pedro Medrano Rojas."

10. WHO, "Cholera Vaccines."

11. BioQuick News, "Cholera Vaccine Prequalified by WHO."

12. International Vaccine Institute, "Announcement—2012 Board of Trustees Meeting Held in Seoul."

13. International Vaccine Institute, "Announcement—Dr. Alejandro Cravioto Joins IVI."

14. Knox, "Vaccination against Cholera Finally Begins in Haiti."

15. Martin, Costa, and Perea, "Stockpiling Oral Cholera Vaccine."

16. WHO, "Cholera—Oral Cholera Vaccine Stockpile."

17. Ivers et al., "Use of Oral Cholera Vaccine in Haiti," 617.

18. GHESKIO Centers, "Cholera."

19. Knox, "Cholera Vaccination Test Reached Targets in Haiti."

20. Charles et al., "Immunogenicity of a Killed Bivalent (O1 and O139)," 3.

21. PAHO/WHO, "Haiti Launches Cholera Vaccination Campaign."

22. Routh and Sreenivasan, "Cholera Vaccination Campaign Evaluation."

23. STRUGGLES AND ELIMINATION

1. Robbins, "What Can We Learn from the Cholera Epidemic in Haiti?"

2. Robbins, "Haitian Cholera Outbreak Highlights Need for Infrastructure, Not Blame."

3. Ibid.

4. Robbins, "Lessons from Cholera in Haiti," 135.

5. Robbins, "Haitian Cholera Outbreak Highlights Need for Infrastructure, Not Blame."

6. Bell, *Fault Lines*, 161–62.

7. Vinten-Johansen et al., *Cholera, Chloroform and the Science of Medicine*, 171–72.

8. Frerichs, "John Snow."
9. Alam et al., "Monitoring Water Sources."
10. Rebaudet and Piarroux, "Monitoring Water Sources."
11. Piarroux, "Le choléra," 346–47.
12. Duval et al., "Cholera in Madagascar."
13. Jaureguiberry et al., "Le cholera à Tamatave (Madagascar) Février-Juillet 2000," 77–78.
14. WHO, "Cholera, 1998–2012."
15. Rinaldo et al., "Reassessment of the 2010–2011 Haiti Cholera Outbreak," 6606.
16. OCHA, "Cholera Epidemic."
17. Mutreja et al., "Evidence for Several Waves of Global Transmission," 462.
18. PAHO, "Water and Sanitation Improvements Remain Key."
19. U.S. CDC, "Immunizing against Cholera."
20. U.S. Central Intelligence Agency, "People and Society."
21. Baron et al., "No Evidence."
22. Gaudart et al., "Spatio-Temporal Dynamics of Cholera."
23. Rebaudet et al., "The Dry Season in Haiti."
24. Médecins Sans Frontières, "International Activity Report—2013, USA."
25. UN Department of Public Information, "Secretary-General Appoints Peter De Clercq."
26. UN News Centre, "As Dry Season Ends in Haiti, Significant Gains Seen in Fight against Cholera."
27. Piarroux and Rebaudet, "Rapport de mission et point de situation sur le choléra en Haïti."
28. Hempel, "John Snow."
29. *Lancet Infectious Diseases*, Editorial, "As Cholera Returns to Haiti, Blame Is Unhelpful."

24. RAPPROCHEMENT

1. UN, "Secretary-General's Remarks at Church Service."
2. UN, "Secretary-General's Remarks after Visiting Family Affected by Cholera."
3. Farha et al., "Mandates of the Special Rapporteur."
4. Medrano Rojas, Letter.
5. Lantagne et al., "The Cholera Outbreak in Haiti," 162.

EPILOGUE

1. MSPP, "Rapport de Cas, Journalier et Cumulatif (2014)."
2. Médecins Sans Frontières, "Haiti: Too Few Beds."
3. WHO, "Cholera—The Global Task Force on Cholera Control."
4. WHO, Programme Budget 2014–2015.
5. U.S. CDC, "2014 Ebola Outbreak in West Africa."
6. Fink, "W.H.O." Members Endorse Resolution to Improve Response to Health Emergencies."
7. Shafy, "President Martelly."
8. Boon, "Privileges and Immunities Hearing."
9. Katz, "The U.N. Caused Haiti's Cholera Epidemic."
10. Ingram, "U.S. Judge Rules Haitians Cannot Sue U.N. for Cholera Epidemic."
11. UN Security Council, "Resolution 2185(2014)."
12. UN Office of the Special Envoy to Haiti, "Overview of Funding."
13. UN News Centre, "Interview with Assistant Secretary-General Pedro Medrano Rojas."

14. UN, "Adopting Resolution 2180 (2014)."

15. UN Security Council, "Report of the Secretary-General on the United Nations Stabilization Mission in Haiti."

16. UN Peacekeeping, "Troop Statistics"; UN Peacekeeping, "Financing Peacekeeping."

17. Colwell, "Climate and Human Health."

18. PAHO, "Cholera Outbreak in Haiti," EOC Situation Report no. 10.

19. Eppinger et al., "Genomic Epidemiology of the Haitian Cholera Outbreak," 1, 2.

Bibliography

Agence France-Presse. "Choléra en Haïti: Le bilan s'alourdit, la psychose s'installe." *Le Nouvelliste*, October 27, 2010. http://lenouvelliste.com/lenouvelliste/article/85109/Cholera-en-Haiti-le-bilan-salourdit-la-psychose-sinstalle.html.

———. "Nepal Condemns Study Linking Army to Haiti Cholera" *República*, December 8, 2010. http://archives.myrepublica.com/portal/index.php?action=news_details&news_id=25986.

———. "Nepal Government Raises War Death Toll." ReliefWeb, September 22, 2009. http://reliefweb.int/report/nepal/nepal-government-raises-war-death-toll.

Alam, Meer T., Thomas A. Weppelmann, Chad D. Weber, Judith A. Johnson, Mohammad H. Rashid, Catherine S. Birch, Babette A. Brumback, Valery E. Madsen Beau de Rochars, J. Glenn, and Afsar Ali. "Monitoring Water Sources for Environmental Reservoirs of Toxigenic *Vibrio cholerae* O1, Haiti." *Emerging Infectious Diseases* 20, no. 3 (2014): 356–63. http://dx.doi.org/10.3201/eid2003.131293.

Albon, Chris R. "Where Did Haiti's Cholera Epidemic Come From?" *UN Dispatch*, June 20, 2012. http://www.undispatch.com/where-did-haitis-cholera-epidemic-come-from.

Ali, Afsar, Yuansha Chen, Judith A. Johnson, Edsel Redden, Yfto Mayette, Mohammed H. Rashid, O. Colin Stine, and J. Glenn Morris Jr. "Recent Clonal Origin of Cholera in Haiti." *Emerging Infectious Diseases* 17, no. 4 (2011): 699–701. http://dx.doi.org/10.3201/eid1704.101973.

Ali, Mohammad, Micheal Emch, Jin Kyung Park, Mohammad Yunus, and John Clemens. "Natural Cholera Infection-Derived Immunity in an Endemic Setting." *Journal of Infectious Diseases* 204, no. 6 (2011): 912–18. http://dx.doi.org/10.1093/infdis/143.6.818.

Ali, Mohammad, Anna Lena Lopez, Young You, Young Eun Kim, Binod Sah, Brian Maskery, and John Clemens. "The Global Burden of Cholera." *Bulletin of the World Health Organization* 90, no. 3 (2012): 209–18. http://dx.doi.org/ 10.2471/BLT.11.093427.

Al Jazeera. "UN Troops Blamed for Haiti Cholera." Al Jazeera English, October 30, 2010. http://www.aljazeera.com/news/americas/2010/10/20101029213344370246.html.

Allié, Marie-Pierre. "Idées: De l'importance de Connaître les Origines de l'épidémie de Choléra en Haïti." *Le Monde*, January 12, 2011. http://www.lemonde.fr/idees/article/2010/12/21/de-l-importance-de-connaitre-les-origines-de-l-epidemie-de-cholera-en-haiti_1455778_3232.html.

Alphonse, Roberson. "Sur les traces du premier décès [In the footsteps of the first death]." *Le Nouvelliste*, November 3, 2010. http://lenouvelliste.com/lenouvelliste/article/85268/Sur-les-traces-du-premier-deces.html.

Alphonse, Roberson, Francois Louis, and Jean Samuel Pierre Louis. "Mirebalais Cholera, Part 1." YouTube video, posted by *Le Nouvelliste Haiti*. Uploaded November 7, 2010. http://www.youtube.com/watch?v=Ke4m7mtBuks.

——. "Mirebalais Cholera, Part 2." YouTube video, posted by *Le Nouvelliste Haiti*. Uploaded November 7, 2010. http://www.youtube.com/watch?v=kmieMUQPThs.
And the Band Played On. Directed by Roger Spottiswoode. New York: HBO, 1993.
Archibold, Randal C. "Officials in Haiti Defend Focus on Cholera Outbreak, Not Its Origins." *New York Times*, November 17, 2010. http://www.nytimes.com/2010/11/17/world/americas/17haiti.html?_r=0.
Assistance mortelle (*Fatal Assistance*). Directed by Raoul Peck. Arte France and Canal Overseas Production, 2013.
Associated Press. "Aid Workers Face 'Angry and Impatient' Haitians: U.N Reports Looting at Warehouses as Survivors Suffer from Thirst, Hunger." NBC News, January 15, 2010. http://www.nbcnews.com/id/34874587/ns/world_news-haiti/t/aid-workers-face-angry-impatient-haitians/#.U01Ga61dW5M.
——. "Cholera in Haiti Matches Strains Seen in South Asia, U.S. says." *New York Times*, November 1, 2010. http://www.nytimes.com/2010/11/02/world/americas/02haiti.html.
——. "Recall Expands to More Than Half a Billion Eggs." NBC News, August 20, 2010. http://www.nbcnews.com/id/38741401/ns/health-food_safety/t/recall-expands-more-half-billion-eggs/#.U4-FjJRdXDI.
——. "UN Peacekeeper in Haiti Treated for Swine Flu." *Oklahoman* (NewsOK), July 14, 2009. http://newsok.com/un-peacekeeper-in-haiti-treated-for-swine-flu/article/feed/57606.
Attal, Sylvain. "Qui est responsable de l'épidémie de choléra en Haïti?" L'Entretien, France 24, December 14, 2010.
Baron, Sandrine, Jean Lesne, Sandra Moore, Emmanuel Rossignol, Stanislas Rebaudet, Pierre Gazin, Robert Barrais, Roc Magloire, Jacques Boncy, and Renaud Piarroux. "No Evidence of Significant Levels of Toxigenic *V. cholerae* O1 in the Haitian Aquatic Environment during the 2012 Rainy Season." *PLoS Currents: Outbreaks*, September 13, 2013. http://dx.doi.org/10.1371/currents.outbreaks.7735b392bdcb749baf5812d2096d331e.
Barua, Dhiman. "History of Cholera." In *Cholera: Current Topics in Infectious Disease*. New York: Springer, 1992.
Barzilay, Ezra J., Nicolas Schaad, Roc Magloire, Kam S. Mung, Jacques Boncy, Georges A. Dahourou, PharEric D. Mintz, Maria W. Steenland, John F. Vertefeuille, and Jordan W. Tappero. "Cholera Surveillance during the Haiti Epidemic—The First 2 years." *New England Journal of Medicine* 368, no. 7 (2013): 599–609. http://dx.doi.org/10.1056/NEJMoa1204927.
Baseball in the Time of Cholera. Directed by Bryn Mooser and David Darg. 28 min. Internet Movie Database (INDb), April 21, 2012. http://www.imdb.com/title/tt2261295.
BBC News. "Haiti Makes Voodoo Official." April, 30, 2003. http://news.bbc.co.uk/2/hi/americas/2985627.stm.
——. "Haiti Protester Shot Dead by UN Peacekeepers." November 16, 2010. http://www.bbc.com/news/world-latin-america-11761941.
——. "Scores Die in Haiti Cholera Outbreak." October 22, 2010. http://www.bbc.com/news/world-latin-america-11608551.
——. "UN Appeals for Calm after Cholera Riots in Haiti." November 17, 2010. http://www.bbc.com/news/world-latin-america-11772283.
BBC News South Asia. "Haiti Cholera Outbreak: Nepal Troops Not Tested." December 8, 2010. http://www.bbc.co.uk/news/world-south-asia-11949181.
Beaubien, Jason. "In Haiti, Political Impasse Compounds Uncertainty." NPR, December 11, 2010. http://www.npr.org/2010/12/11/131971983/in-haiti-political-impasse-compounds-uncertainty.

Bell, Beverly. *Fault Lines: Views across Haiti's Divide*. Ithaca, NY: Cornell University Press, 2013.

Bellamy, Alex J., Paul D. Williams, and Stuart Griffin. *Understanding Peacekeeping*. 2nd ed. Cambridge: Polity Press, 2010.

Benedictow, Ole J. *The Black Death 1346–1353: The Complete History*. Rochester, NY: Boydell Press, 2004.

Besheer, Margaret. "UN Facilities, Peacekeepers in Haiti Test Negative for Cholera." Voice of America, November 18, 2010. http://www.voanews.com/content/un-facilities-peacekeepers-in-haiti-test-negative-for-cholera-109290984/130836.html.

Bharati, Kaushik and SK Bhattacharya. "Cholera Outbreaks in South-East Asia." *Current Topics in Microbiology and Immunology* 379 (2014): 87–116. http://dx.doi.org/10.1007/82_2014_362.

Bhattacharjee, Yudhijit. "Paul Keim on His Life with the FBI during the Anthrax Investigation." *Science* 323, no. 5920 (2009): 1416. http://dx.doi.org/10.1126/science.323.5920.1416.

Bhattacharya, Sujit K., Dipika Sur, Mohammad Ali, Suman Kanungo, Young You, Byomkesh Manna, Binod Sah et al. "5 Year Efficacy of a Bivalent Killed Whole-Cell Oral Cholera Vaccine in Kolkata, India: A Cluster-Randomised, Double-Blind, Placebo-Controlled Trial." *Lancet Infectious Diseases* 13, no. 12 (2013): 1050–56. http://dx.doi.org/10.1016/S1473–3099(13)70273–1.

Bhattarai, Rajan. "Contributor Profile: Nepal." Nepal Institute for Policy Studies, Kathmandu, August 1, 2013. http://www.providingforpeacekeeping.org/wp-content/uploads/2013/08/Nepal-Bhattarai-1-August-2013.pdf.

Bioquick. "Cholera Vaccine Prequalified by WHO." November 11, 2011. http://www.bioquicknews.com/node/680.

Boisson de Chazournes, Laurence, and Salma M.A. Salman. *Les ressources en eau et le droit international [Water Resources and International Law]*. Leiden, Neth.: Brill, 2005.

Boling, Dee. "Public Health School Hosts Haitian Leader." *New Wave*. Tulane University, New Orleans, July 7, 2010. http://tulane.edu/news/newwave/070710_publichealth_haiti.cfm.

Bompangue, Didier, Patrick Giraudoux, Pascal Handschumacher, Renaud Piarroux, Bertrand Sudre, Mosiana Ekwanzala, Ilunga Kebela, and Martine Piarroux. "Lakes as Source of Cholera Outbreaks, Democratic Republic of Congo." *Emerging Infectious Diseases* 14, no. 5 (2008): 798–800. http://dx.doi.org/10.3201/eid1405.071260.

Boon, Kristen. "Privileges and Immunities Hearing in the Haiti Cholera Case against the UN." *Opinio Juris,* October 27, 2014. http://opiniojuris.org/2014/10/27/privileges-immunities-hearing-haiti-cholera-case-un.

Bosin, Yury V. "Russia, Cholera Riots of 1830–1831" *International Encyclopedia of Revolution and Protest*. Madden, MA, Wiley-Blackwell, 2009.

Brauman, Rony. "Faiblesses du dispositif anticholéra à Haïti." *Le Monde*, November 23, 2010. http://www.lemonde.fr/idees/article/2010/11/23/faiblesses-du-dispositif-anti-cholera-a-haiti_1443887_3232.html.

Bureau des Avocats Internationalaux/Institute for Justice and Democracy in Haiti. Petition for Relief. November 3, 2012. http://ijdh.org/wordpress/wp-content/uploads/2011/11/englishpetitionREDACTED.pdf.

Canadian Broadcast Company. "Cholera's Seven Pandemics." CBC News, October 22, 2010. http://www.cbc.ca/news/technology/cholera-s-seven-pandemics-1.758504.

Carroll, Rory. "Haiti Votes in Historic Election as Reports of Fraud Emerge." *Guardian*, November 28, 2010. http://www.theguardian.com/world/2010/nov/28/haiti-presidential-election-fraud-reports.

Cash, Richard A., Stanley I. Music, Joseph P. Libonati, Merril J. Snyder, Richard P. Wenzel, and Richard B. Hornick. "Response of Man to Infection with Vibrio

Cholerae. I. Clinical, Serologic, and Bacteriologic Responses to a Known Inoculum." *Journal of Infectious Diseases* 129, no. 1 (1974): 45–52. http://dx.doi.org/10.1093/infdis/129.1.45.

Castro, Fidel. "Cuba's Fidel Sees UN in Haiti Cholera." *Havana Times*, December 8, 2010. http://www.havanatimes.org/?p=34279.

CDC Foundation. "Haiti Buildings—Division of Epidemiology, Laboratory and Research (Direction d'Epidémiologie, de Laboratoire et de Recherches or DELR)." http://www.cdcfoundation.org/haiti/buildings.

Center for Economic Policy Research (CEPR). "Head of OAS Electoral Mission in Haiti: International Community Tried to Remove Préval on Election Day." June 6, 2014. http://www.cepr.net/index.php/blogs/relief-and-reconstruction-watch/head-of-oas-electoral-mission-in-haiti-international-community-tried-to-remove-preval-on-election-day.

Center for Infectious Disease Research and Policy (CIDRAP). "H1N1 Flu Breaking News: Antivirals by Phone, Coordinating South American Response, Usefulness of Vaccine Contracts, First Case in Haiti." July 16, 2009. http://www.cidrap.umn.edu/news-perspective/2009/07/h1n1-flu-breaking-news-antivirals-phone-coordinating-south-american.

CERFAS (Centre de Recherche, de Réflexion, de Formation et d'Action Sociale). "MINUSTAH: A Financial Overview of Peacekeeping in Haiti." *Observatory on Public Policies and on International Cooperation*, Bulletin 4, July 2013, Port-au-Prince, Haiti.

Chaaban, Sebastian. "Svenska Ambassadören: 'Smittan kommer från Nepal'" [Swedish ambassador: 'The infection comes from Nepal']." *Svenska Dagbladet*, November 16, 2010. http://www.svd.se/nyheter/utrikes/svenska-ambassadoren-smittan-kommer-fran-nepal_5680337.svd.

Charles, Macarthur, Glavdia G. Delva, Jethro Boutin, Karine Severe, Mireille Peck, Marie Marcelle Mabou, Peter F. Wright, and Jean W. Pape. "Importance of Cholera and Other Etiologies of Acute Diarrhea in Post-Earthquake Port-au-Prince, Haiti." *American Journal of Tropical Medicine and Hygiene* 90, no. 3 (2014): 511–17. http://dx.doi.org/10.4269/ajtmh.13–0514.

Charles, Richelle C., Isabelle J. Hilaire, Leslie M. Mayo-Smith, Jessica E. Teng, J. Gregory Jerome, Molly F. Franke, Amit Saha et al. "Immunogenicity of a Killed Bivalent (O1 and O139) Whole Cell Oral Cholera Vaccine, Shanchol, in Haiti." *PLoS Neglected Tropical Diseases* 8, no. 5 (2014): e2828, 1–8. http://dx.doi.org/10.1371/journal.pntd.0002828.

Chastel, Claude. "Le Centenaire de la Découverte du Vibrion d'El Tor (1905) ou les Débuts Incertains de la Septième Pandémie de Choléra [The Centenary of the Discovery of the Vibrio El Tor (1905) or Dubious Beginnings of the Seventh Pandemic of Cholera]." *Histoire des Sciences Médicales* 41, no. 1 (2007): 71–82.

Chin, Chen-Shan, Jon Sorenson, Jason B. Harris, William P. Robins, Richelle C. Charles, Roger R. Jean-Charles, James Bullard et al."The Origin of the Haitian Cholera Outbreak Strain." *New England Journal of Medicine* 364, no. 1 (2010): 33–42. http://dx.doi.org/10.1056/NEJMoa1012928.

Chun, Jongsik, Christopher J. Grim, Nur A. Hasan, Je Hee Lee, Seon Young Choi, Bradd J. Haley, Elisa Taviani et al. "Comparative Genomics Reveals Mechanism for Short-Term and Long-Term Clonal Transitions in Pandemic Vibrio cholerae." *Proceedings of the National Academy of Sciences* 106, no. 36 (2009): 15442–447. http://dx.doi.org/10.1073/pnas.0907787106.

Clements, M. L., M. M. Levine, C. R. Young, R. E. Black, Y. L. Lim, R. M. Robins-Browne, and J. P. Craig. "Magnitude, Kinetics, and Duration of Vibriocidal Antibody

Responses in North Americans after Ingestion of Vibrio cholerae." *Journal of Infectious Diseases* 145, no. 4 (1982): 465–73. http://dx,doi.org/ 10.1093/ infdis/145.4.465.

CNN. "Numbers Tell Stories of Horror, Heroism in Haiti." CNN World, January 26, 2010. http://www.cnn.com/2010/WORLD/americas/01/26/haiti.by.the.numbers/ index.html?hpt=T1.

Cohen, Nicole J., Douglas D. Slaten, Nina Marano, Jordan W. Tappero, Michael Wellman, Ryan J. Albert, Vincent R. Hill, et al. "Preventing Maritime Transfer of Toxigenic Vibrio cholerae." *Emerging Infectious Diseases* 18, no. 10 (2012): 1680. http:// dx.doi.org/ 10.3201/eid1810.120676.

Colwell, Rita R. "Climate and Human Health: New Ways of Studying Infectious Diseases." Paper presented at the Sagan National Colloquium, Ohio Wesleyan University, Delaware, Ohio, December 10, 2014. http://www.youtube.com/ watch?v=8aqOIVS09mI.

——. "Concentric Circles: A Twenty-First Century Context for Climate and Health." Paper presented at the Tenth Asian Conference on Diarrhoeal Diseases and Nutrition *(ASCODD)*, Dhaka, Bangladesh, December 8, 2003.

——. "Experimental Reservoirs of Human Pathogens: The Vibrio cholerae Paradigm." Paper presented at the Seventh Annual Sequencing, Finishing, Analysis in the Future Meeting, Santa Fe, NM, June 5–7, 2012. http://www.scivee.tv/node/52157.

——. "Global Climate and Infectious Disease: The Cholera Paradigm." *Science* 274, no. 5295 (1996): 2025–31. http://dx.doi.org/10.1126/science.274.5295.2025.

——. "Infectious Disease and the Environment: Cholera as a Paradigm for Waterborne Disease." *International Microbiology* 7, no. 4 (2004): 285–89.

Colwell, Rita R., Anwar Huq, M. Sirajul Islam, K. M. A. Aziz, M. Yunus, N. Huda Khan, A. Mahmud, R. Bradley Sack, G. B. Nair, J. Chakraborty, David A. Sack, and E. Russek-Cohen. "Reduction of Cholera in Bangladeshi Villages by Simple Filtration." *Proceedings of the National Academy of Sciences (PNAS)* 100, no. 3 (2003): 1051–55. http://dx.doi.org/10.1073/pnas.0237386100.

Constantin de Magny, Guillaume, and Rita R. Colwell. "Cholera and Climate: A Demonstrated Relationship." *Transactions of the American Clinical and Climatological Association* 120 (2009): 119–28. http://www.ncbi.nlm.nih.gov/ pmc/articles/PMC2744514.

Constantin de Magny, Guillaume, Raghu Murtugudde, Mathew R. P. Sapiano, Azhar Nizam, Christopher W. Brown, Antonio J. Busalacchi, Mohammad Yunus, G. Balakrish Nair, Ana I. Gil, Claudio F. Lanata, John Calkins, Byomkesh Manna, Krishnan Rajendran, Mihir Kumar Bhattacharya, Anwar Huq, R. Bradley Sack, and Rita R. Colwell. "Environmental Signatures Associated with Cholera Epidemics." *Proceedings of the National Academy of Sciences* 105, no. 46 (2008): 17676–81. http://dx.doi.org/10.1073/pnas.0809654105.

Cooper, Helene, and Liz Robbins. "U.S. Mobilizes to Send Assistance to Haiti." *New York Times*, January 13, 2010. http://www.nytimes.com/2010/01/14/world/ americas/14prexy.html?_r=0.

Council on Hemispheric Affairs. "The Tonton Macoutes: The Central Nervous System of Haiti's Reign of Terror." March 11, 2010. http://www.coha.org/ tonton-macoutes.

Cravioto, Alejandro, Claudio F. Lanata, Daniele S. Lantagne, and G. Balakrish Nair. "Final Report of the Independent Panel of Experts on the Cholera Outbreak in Haiti." United Nations, April, 2011. http://www.un.org/News/dh/infocus/haiti/ UN-cholera-report-final.pdf.

Crumb, Michael J. "Iowa Egg Producer Separates Business, Charity Work." *Boston Globe*, September 20, 2010. http://www.boston.com/business/articles/2010/09/20/iowa_egg_producer_separates_business_charity_work.

Cunliffe P. *Legions of Peace—UN Peacekeepers from the Global South*. London: C. Hurst, 2013.

Darg, David, and Bryn Mooser. "What the UN Won't Admit: 'Baseball in the Time of Cholera.'" *Wall Street Journal*, April 21, 2012. http://blogs.wsj.com/speakeasy/2012/04/21/what-the-un-wont-admit-baseball-in-the-time-of-cholera/?mod=google_news_blog.

Delva, Joseph Guyler. "Haitians Attack U.N. Troops, Blame Them for Cholera." Reuters, November 15, 2010. http://www.reuters.com/article/2010/11/15/us-haiti-cholera-idUSTRE6AA5PC20101115.

Desvarieux, Jessica. "Haiti's Presidential Vote: Outrage over a 'Selection.'" *Time*, November 29, 2010. http://content.time.com/time/world/article/0,8599,2033387,00.html.

Desvarieux, Jessica, and Tim Padgett. "Haiti's Cholera Riots: A Plot to Stop the Elections?" *Time*, November 16, 2010. http://content.time.com/time/world/article/0,8599,2031665,00.html.

Devault, Alison M., G. Brian Golding, Nicholas Waglechner, Jacob M. Enk, Melanie Kuch, Joseph H. Tien, Mang Shi et al. "Second-Pandemic Strain of *Vibrio cholerae* from the Philadelphia Cholera Outbreak of 1849." *New England Journal of Medicine* 370, no. 4 (2014): 334–40. http://dx.doi.org/10.1056/NEJMoa1308663.

DeWitte, Sharon N., and James W. Wood. "Selectivity of Black Death Mortality with Respect to Preexisting Health." *Proceedings of the National Academy of Sciences U S A*. 105, no. 5 (2008): 1436–41. http://dx.doi.org/10.1073/pnas.0705460105.

Doucet, Isabeau. "The Nation: NGOs Have Failed Haiti." NPR, January 13, 2011. http://www.npr.org/2011/01/13/132884795/the-nation-how-ngos-have-failed-haiti.

Dowell, S. F., A. Toko, C. Sita, R. Piarroux, A. Duerr, and B. A. Woodruff. "Letter from Goma: Health and Nutrition in Centers for Unaccompanied Refugee Children—Experience from the 1994 Rwandan Refugee Crisis." *JAMA* 273, no. 22 (1995): 1802–6. http://dx.doi.org/10.1001/jama.1995.03520460086048.

Doyle, Arthur Conan. "Adventure I: Silver Blaze." In *The Complete Sherlock Holmes*. London: Collector's Library Editions, 2012.

Doyle, Mark. "Haiti Cholera Epidemic 'Most Likely' Started at UN Camp—Top Scientist." BBC News—Latin American and Caribbean, October 22, 2012. http://www.bbc.com/news/world-latin-america-20024400.

Dubois, Laurent. *Haiti: The Aftershocks of History*. New York: Metropolitan Books, 2012.

——. "Vodou and History." *Comparative Studies in Society and History* 43, no. 1 (2001): 92–100.

Duval, P., G. Champetier de Ribes, J. Ranjalahy, M. L. Quilici, and J. M. Fournier. "Cholera in Madagascar." *Lancet* 353, no. 9169 (1999): 2068. http://dx.doi.org/10.1016/S0140–6736(99)00103–8.

Economist. "The UN in Haiti: First, Do No Harm." April 28, 2012. http://www.economist.com/node/21553450.

Ellingwood, Ken. "As Rains Approach, a Scramble to Get Latrines and Hygiene Supplies to Haiti." *Los Angeles Times*, March 6, 2010. http://articles.latimes.com/2010/mar/06/world/la-fg-haiti-latrine6–2010mar06.

Encyclopedia Britannica Online, s.v. "François Duvalier." Last modified March 1, 2013. http://www.britannica.com/EBchecked/topic/174718/Francois-Duvalier.

Enserink, Martin. "Cholera Linked to U.N. Forces, but Questions Remain." *Science* 332, no. 6031 (2011): 776–77. http://dx.doi.org/10.1126/science.332.6031.776.

Eppinger, Mark, Talima Pearson, Sara S. K. Koenig, Ofori Pearson, Nathan Hicks, Sonia Agrawal, Fatemeh Sanjar, Kevin Galens, Sean Daugherty, Jonathan Crabtree, Rene S. Hendriksen, Lance B. Price, Bishnu P. Upadhyay, Geeta Shakya, Claire M. Fraser, Jacques Ravel, and Paul S. Keim. "Genomic Epidemiology of the Haitian Cholera Outbreak: A Single Introduction Followed by Rapid, Extensive, and Continued Spread Characterized the Onset of the Epidemic." *MBio* 5, no. 6 (2014): e01721–14. http://dx.doi.org/10.1128/mBio.01721-14.

Estrada-Garcia, Teresa, and Eric D. Mintz. "Cholera: Foodborne Transmission and Its Prevention." *European Journal of Epidemiology* 12 (1996): 461–69. http://link.springer.com/article/10.1007/BF00143997.

Evans, Richard J. "Epidemics and Revolutions: Cholera in Nineteenth-Century Europe." *Past and Present* 120, no. 1 (1988): 123–46. http://dx.doi.org/10.1093/past/120.1.123.

Farha, Leilani, Gustavo Gallón, Dainius Pūras, and Catarina de Albuquerque. "Mandates of the Special Rapporteur on Adequate Housing as a Component of the Right to an Adequate Standard of Living. . . ." United Nations Office of the High Commission for Human Rights (OHCHR), Ref. AL HTI 3/2014, September 25, 2014. http://spdb.ohchr.org/hrdb/28th/public_-_AL_Haiti_25.09.14_(3.2014).pdf.

Farmer, Paul. "Who Removed Aristide?" *London Review of Books* 26, no. 8 (2004): 28–31. http://www.lrb.co.uk/v26/n08/paul-farmer/who-removed-aristide.

Faucher, Benoît, and Renaud Piarroux. "The Haitian Cholera Epidemic: Is Searching for Its Origin Only a Matter of Scientific Curiosity?" *Clinical Microbiology and Infection* 17, no. 4 (2011): 479–80. http://dx.doi.org/10.1111/j.1469–0691.2011.03476.x (epub: January 24, 2011).

Fernández-Delgado, Milagro, M. Alexandra García-Amado, Monica Contreras, Virginia Edgcomb, Juana Vitelli, Pulchérie Gueneau, and Paula Suárez. "Vibrio cholerae non-O1, non-O139 Associated with Seawater and Plankton from Coastal Marine Areas of the Caribbean Sea." *International Journal of Environmental Health Research* 19, no. 4 (2009): 279–89. http://dx.doi.org/10.1080/09603120802460368.

Fink, Sheri. "W.H.O. Members Endorse Resolution to Improve Response to Health Emergencies." *New York Times*, January 25, 2015. http://www.nytimes.com/2015/01/26/world/who-members-endorse-resolution-to-improve-response-to-health-emergencies.html?_r=0.

Ford, Harvey S. "The Cholera Campaign." *Military Engineer*, June 1942. http://www.themilitaryengineer.com/tme_mag/09_10_2013/capsule/TME_June_1942.pdf.

Fraser, Barbara. "World Report: Haiti Still Gripped by Cholera as Election Looms." *Lancet* 376, no. 9755 (2010): 1813–14. http://dx.doi.org/10.1016/S0140–6736(10)62151–4.

Frerichs, Ralph. "John Snow." In *Encyclopedia Britannica Online*. Last modified July 4, 2013. http://www.britannica.com/EBchecked/topic/550563/John-Snow.

———. "John Snow—A Historical Giant in Epidemiology." www.ph.ucla.edu/epi/snow.html.

Frerichs, Ralph R., Jacques Boncy, Robert Barrais, Paul S. Keim, and Renaud Piarroux. "Source Attribution of 2010 Cholera Epidemic in Haiti." *Proceedings of the National Academy of Sciences* 109, no. 47 (2012): E3208. http://dx.doi.org/10.1073/pnas.1211512109.

Frerichs, Ralph R., Paul S. Keim, Robert Barrais, and Renaud Piarroux. "Nepalese Origin of Cholera Epidemic in Haiti." *Clinical Microbiology and Infection* 18, no. 6 (2012): E158–163. http://dx.doi.org/10.1111/j.1469–0691.2012.03841.x.

Fries, Andrew. "Does Politics Influence the CDC?" ABC News, June 1, 2007. http://abcnews.go.com/Health/Politics/story?id=3235565.

Froggatt, Peter. "John Snow, Thomas Wakley, and *The Lancet*." *Anaesthesia* 57, no. 7 (2002): 667–75. http://dx.doi.org/10.1046/j.1365–2044.2002.02656.x.

Frontline. "Paul Keim: 'We Were Surprised It Was the Ames Strain.'" PBS, October 10, 2011. http://www.pbs.org/wgbh/pages/frontline/criminal-justice/anthrax-files/paul-keim-we-were-surprised-it-was-the-ames-strain.

Garrett, Laurie. "Ebola's Lessons: How the WHO Mishandled the Crisis." *Foreign Affairs*, September–October, 2015. https://www.foreignaffairs.com/articles/west-africa/2015-08-18/ebola-s-lessons.

Gaudart, Jean, Sandra Moore, Stanislas Rebaudet, Martine Piarroux, Robert Barrais, Jacques Boncy, and Renaud Piarroux. "Environmental Factors Influencing Epidemic Cholera." *American Journal of Tropical Medicine and Hygiene* 89, no. 6 (2013): 1228–30. http://dx.doi.org/10.4269/ajtmh.13–0499a.

Gaudart, Jean, Stanislas Rebaudet, Robert Barrais, Jacques Boncy, Benoit Faucher, Martine Piarroux, Roc Magloire, Gabriel Thimothe, and Renaud Piarroux. "Spatio-Temporal Dynamics of Cholera during the First Year of the Epidemic in Haiti." *PLoS Neglected Tropical Diseases* 7, no. 4 (2013): e2145. http://dx.doi.org/10.1371/journal.pntd.0002145.

Geffrard, Robenson. "Une Maladie Importée, la MINUSTAH Clame son Innocence." *Le Nouvelliste*, October 26, 2010. http://lenouvelliste.com/lenouvelliste/article/85056/Une-maladie-importee-la-MINUSTAH-clame-son-innocence.html.

Geohive. "Haiti." Accessed October 21, 2014. http://www.geohive.com/cntry/haiti.aspx.

GHESKIO Centers. "Cholera." Accessed September 9, 2014. http://gheskio.org/wp/?page_id=248.

Ghimire, Madhu, Yasho Vardhan Pradhan, and Mahesh Kumar Maskey. "Community-Based Interventions for Diarrhoeal Diseases and Acute Respiratory Infections in Nepal." *Bulletin of the World Health Organization* 88, no. 3 (2010): 216–21. http://dx.doi.org/10.2471/BLT.09.065649.

Gil, Ana I., Valérie R. Louis, Irma N. G. Rivera, Erin Lipp, Anwar Huq, Claudio F. Lanata, David N. Taylor, Estelle Russek-Cohen, Nipa Choopun, R. Bradley Sack, and Rita R. Colwell. "Occurrence and Distribution of Vibrio cholerae in the Coastal Environment of Peru." *Environmental Microbiology* 6, no. 7 (2004): 699–706. http://dx.doi.org/10.1111/j.1462–2920.2004.00601.x.

Giono, Jean. *The Horseman on the Roof*. Translated by Jonathan Griffin. New York: North Point Press, 1981.

Glass, R. I., A. M. Svennerholm, M. R. Khan, S. Huda, M. I. Huq, J. Holmgren. "Seroepidemiological Studies of El Tor Cholera in Bangladesh: Association of Serum Antibody Levels with Protection." *Journal of Infectious Diseases* 151 (1985): 236–42. http://dx.doi.org/10.1093/infdis/151.2.236.

Goesch, J. N., A. Simons de Fanti, S. Béchet, and P. H. Consigny. "Comparison of Knowledge on Travel Related Health Risks and Their Prevention among Humanitarian Aid Workers and Other Travellers Consulting at the Institut Pasteur Travel Clinic in Paris, France." *Travel Medicine and Infectious Diseases* 8, no. 6 (2010): 364–72. http://dx.doi.org/10.1016/j.tmaid.2010.09.005.

Gomes, Thallus. "Morte de Jovem Haitiano gera Novos Protestos contra a Minustah [Death of Young Haitian Generates New Protests against MINUSTAH]." *Brasil de Fato*, September 13, 2010. http://www.brasildefato.com.br/node/233.

Gorry, Conner. "Haiti One Year Later: Cuban Medical Team Draws on Experience and Partnership." *MEDICC Review* 13, no. 1 (2011): 52–55. http://www.alfepsi.org/attachments/article/120/Haiti%20One%20Year%20Later.pdf.

Grimaud, Jérôme, and Fedia Legagneur. "Community Beliefs and Fears during a Cholera Outbreak in Haiti." *Intervention* 9, no. 1 (2011): 26–34. http://dx.doi.org/10.1097/WTF.0b013e3283453ef2.

Gurrey, Béatrice. "Choléra en Haïti : L'hypothèse Népalaise Confirmée." *Le Monde*, December 5, 2010. http://www.lemonde.fr/planete/article/2010/12/04/cholera-en-haiti-l-hypothese-nepalaise-confirmee_1449009_3244.html.

Gurung, Dipak. "Success of Nepali Peacekeepers." *República*, November 18, 2010. http:/ archives.myrepublica.com/portal/index.php?action=news_details&news_id=25304.

Hall-Stoodley, L., and P. Stoodley. "Biofilm Formation and Dispersal and the Transmission of Human Pathogens." *Trends in Microbiology* 13, no. 1 (2005): 7–10.http://dx.doi.org/10.1016/j.tim.2004.11.004.

Hallward, Peter. *Damming the Flood: Haiti, Aristide, and the Politics of Containment.* London: Verso, 2008.

Harris, Jason B., Regina C. LaRocque, Richelle C. Charles, Ramendra N. Mazumder, Azharul I. Khan, and Pradip K. Bardhan. "Cholera's Western Front." *Lancet* 376, no. 9757 (2010): 1961–65. http://dx.doi.org/10.1016/S0140-6736(10)62172-1.

Harris, Jason B., Regina C. LaRocque, F. Qadri, E. T. Ryan, and S. B. Calderwood. "Cholera." *Lancet* 379, no. 9835 (2012): 2466–76. http://dx.doi.org/10.1016/S0140-6736(12)60436-X.

Hasan, Nur A., Seon Young Choi, Mark Eppinger, Philip W. Clark, Arlene Chen, Munirul Alam, Bradd J. Haley, Elisa Taviani, Erin Hine, Qi Su, Luke J. Tallon, Joseph B. Prosper, Keziah Furth, M. M. Hoq, Huai Li, Claire M. Fraser-Liggett, Alejandro Cravioto, Anwar Huq, Jacques Ravel, Thomas A. Cebula, and Rita R. Colwell. "Genomic Diversity of 2010 Haitian Cholera Outbreak Strains." *Proceedings of the National Academy of Sciences* 109, no. 29 (2012): E2010–E2017. http://dx.doi.org/10.1073/pnas.1207359109.

Hasan, Nur A., Seon Young Choi, Munirul Alam, Alejandro Cravioto, Anwar Huq, Thomas A. Cebula, and Rita R. Colwell. "Reply to Mekalanos et al.: Genomic Diversity of Vibrio cholerae." *Proceedings of the National Academy of Sciences* 109, no. 47 (2012): E3207. http://dx.doi.org/10.1073/pnas.1213184109.

Hasan, Nur A, Seon Young Choi, Munirul Alam, Alejandro Cravioto, Anwar Huq, Thomas A. Cebula, and Rita R. Colwell. "Reply to Frerichs et al.: Chasing the genetic diversity, not source attribution." *Proceedings of the National Academy of Sciences* 109, no. 47 (2012): E3209. http://dx.doi:10.1073/pnas.1212052109.

Hecdivert, Marie-Charleine L., and Marie-José B. Laraque, "Rapport de Mission au Département Sanitaire du Centre, Bas Plateau." Ministere de la Sante Publique et de la Population (MSPP), Haiti, October 21–24, 2010.

Heine, Jorge, and Andrew S. Thompson, eds. *Fixing Haiti: MINUSTAH and Beyond.* New York: United Nations University Press, 2011.

Helsingin Sanomat (Finland)."Cholera Situation Spiralling Out of Control in Haiti." International ed., November 18, 2010. http://www.hs.fi/english/article/Cholera+situation+spiralling+out+of+control+in+Haiti/1135261737531.

Hempel, Sandra. "John Snow." *Lancet* 381, no. 9874 (2013): 1269–70. http://dx/doi.org/10.1016/S0140–6736(13)60830–2.

Hendriksen, Rene S., Lance B. Price, James M. Schupp, John D. Gillece, Rolf S. Kaas, David M. Engelthaler, Valeria Bortolaia, Talima Pearson, Andrew E. Waters, Bishnu Prasa Upadhyay, Sirjana Devi Shrestha, Shailaja Adhikari, Geeta Shakya, Paul S. Keim and Frank M. Aarestrup. "Population Genetics of Vibrio cholerae from Nepal in 2010: Evidence on the Origin of the Haitian Outbreak." *MBio* 2, no. 4 (2011): e00157-11. http://dx.doi.org/10.1128/mBio.00157-11.

Hood, Christopher. "What Happens When Transparency Meets Blame-Avoidance?" *Public Management Review* 9, no. 2 (2007): 191–210. http://dx.doi.org/10.1080/14719030701340275.

Hornick, Richard B., S. I. Music, R. Wenzel, R. Cash, J. P. Libonati, M. J. Snyder, and T. E. Woodward. "The Broad Street Pump Revisited: Response of Volunteers to Ingested Cholera Vibrios. *Bulletin of the New York Academy of Medicine* 47, no. 10 (1971): 1181–91.

Howard-Jones N. "Robert Koch and the Cholera Vibrio: A Centenary." *British Medical Journal* 288, no. 6414 (1984): 379–81.

Hujer, Marc. "Haiti's Cholera Disaster: Epidemic Underscores Lack of Progress after Earthquake." *Der Spiegel*, November 2, 2010. http://www.spiegel.de/international/world/haiti-s-cholera-disaster-epidemic-underscores-lack-of-progress-after-earthquake-a-726563.html.

Huq, A., E. B. Small, P. A. West, M. I. Huq, R. Rahman, and Rita R. Colwell. "Ecological Relationships between Vibrio cholerae and Planktonic Crustacean Copepods." *Applied Environmental Microbiology* 45, no. 1 (1983): 275–83. http://aem.asm.org/content/45/1/275.short.

Hurtado, María Elena. "Haiti's Cholera Epidemic Caused by Weather, Say Scientists." SciDev.Net, November 22, 2010. http://www.scidev.net/global/disasters/news/haiti-s-cholera-epidemic-caused-by-weather-say-scientists.html.

ICDDR,B. "ICDDR,B's Emergency Response Team Return from Haiti." December 6, 2010. http://www.icddrb.org/component/content/article/100d30-news/2200-icddrbs-emergency-response-team-return-from-haiti.

Ingram, David. "U.S. Judge Rules Haitians Cannot Sue U.N. for Cholera Epidemic." Reuters, January 10, 2015. http://www.reuters.com/article/2015/01/10/us-un-haiti-lawsuit-idUSKBN0KJ0PX20150110.

International Vaccine Institute. "Announcement—Dr. Alejandro Cravioto Joins IVI." Seoul, South Korea, October 29, 2012. http://www.ivi.int/web/www/07_03?p_p_id=EXT_BBS&p_p_lifecycle=0&p_p_state=normal&p_p_mode=view&_EXT_BBS_struts_action=%2Fext%2Fbbs%2Fview_message&_EXT_BBS_messageId=462.

——. "Announcement—2012 Board of Trustees Meeting Held in Seoul." Seoul, South Korea, July 17, 2012. http://www.ivi.int/web/www/07_03?p_p_id=EXT_BBS&p_p_lifecycle=0&p_p_state=normal&p_p_mode=view&_EXT_BBS_struts_action=%2Fext%2Fbbs%2Fview_message&_EXT_BBS_messageId=270.

IRIN News. "NEPAL: UN Peace Mission Ends amid Political Deadlock." United Nations Office for the Coordination of Humanitarian Affairs, January 12, 2011. http://www.irinnews.org/report/91605/nepal-un-peace-mission-ends-amid-political-deadlock.

Islam, M. S., B. S. Drasar, and R. B. Sack. "The Aquatic Environment as a Reservoir of *Vibrio cholerae*: A Review." *Journal of Diarrhoeal Disease Research* 11, no. 4 (1993): 197–206. http://www.jstor.org/stable/23498278.

Ivers, Louise C., Paul Farmer, Charles Patrick Almazor, and Fernet Léandre. "Five Complementary Interventions to Slow Cholera: Haiti." *Lancet* 376, no. 9758 (2010): 2048–51. http://dx.doi.org/10.1016/S0140–6736(10)62243-X.

Ivers, Louise C., Jessica E. Teng, Jonathan Lascher, Max Raymond, Jonathan Weigel, Nadia Victor, J. Gregory Jerome et al. "Use of Oral Cholera Vaccine in Haiti: A Rural Demonstration Project." *American Journal of Tropical Medicine and Hygiene* 89, no. 4 (2013): 617–24. http://dx.doi.org/10.4269/ajtmh.13–0183.

Jackson, Brendan R., Deborah F. Talkington, James M. Pruckler, Bernadette Fouché, Elsie Lafosse, Benjamin Nygren, Gerardo A. Gómez et al. "Seroepidemiologic Survey of Epidemic Cholera in Haiti to Assess Spectrum of Illness and Risk

Factors for Severe Disease." *American Journal of Tropical Medicine and Hygiene* 89, no. 4 (2013): 654–64. http://dx.doi.org/10.4269/ajtmh.13–0208.

Jangi, Sushrut. "An Interview with Ezra Barzilay—The Cholera Epidemic in Haiti, 2010–2012." Now@NEJM, January 9, 2013. http://blogs.nejm.org/now/index.php/an-interview-with-ezra-barzilay-the-cholera-epidemic-in-haiti-2010-2012/2013/01/09.

Jaureguiberry, Stéphane, Véronique Hentgen, Nicole Raholiniana, Dieudonné Rasolomahefa, and Michel Belec. "Le Choléra à Tamatave (Madagascar) février–juillet 2000: Caractéristiques épidémiologiques." *Cahiers d'études et de recherches francophones/Santé* 11, no. 2 (2001): 73–78. http://www.jle.com/en/revues/san/e-docs/le_cholera_a_tamatave_madagascar_fevrier_juillet_2000_caracteristiques_epidemiologiques_220077/article.phtml?tab=texte.

Jeanty Jr., Gérard. "SANCO clarifie." *Le Nouvelliste*, October 28, 2010. http://lenouvelliste.com/lenouvelliste/article/85168/SANCO-clarifie.html.

Jenson, Deborah, Victoria Szabo, and Duke FHI Haiti Humanities Laboratory Student Research Team. "Cholera in Haiti and other Caribbean Regions, 19th Century." *Emerging Infectious Diseases* 17 (2011): 2130–35. http://dx.doi.org/10.3201/eid1711.110958.

Jourdaine, Stéphane. "Choléra en Haïti: Huérilla urbaine contre les Casques bleus." Agence France-Presse, November 18, 2010. http://www.lapresse.ca/international/amerique-latine/201011/18/01–4344031-cholera-en-haiti-guerilla-urbaine-contre-les-casques-bleus.php.

——. "Haiti: Choléra en Haïti: L'épidémie est 'inhabituelle et sévère,' les bilans sous-estimés." Agence France-Presse, November 19, 2010. http://lenouvelliste.com/lenouvelliste/article/85845/Lepidemie-est-inhabituelle-et-severe-les-bilans-sous-estimes.html.

——. "Haiti: No Let-Up in Haiti Cholera One Week from Elections." Agence France-Presse, November 21, 2010. http://news.smh.com.au/breaking-news-world/no-letup-in-haiti-cholera-epidemic-one-week-from-elections-20101122–182sr.html.

Jutla, Antarpreet, Elizabeth Whitcombe, Nur Hasan, Bradd Haley, Ali Akanda, Anwar Huq, Munir Alam, R. Bradley Sack, and Rita Colwell. "Environmental Factors Influencing Epidemic Cholera." *American Journal of Tropical Medicine and Hygiene* 89, no. 3 (2013): 597–607. http://dx.doi.org/10.4269/ajtmh.12–0721.

——. "In Response." *American Journal of Tropical Medicine and Hygiene* 89, no. 6 (2013): 1231–32. http://dx.doi.org/10.4269/ajtmh.13-0499b.

Kabir, Shahjahan. "Critical Analysis of Compositions and Protective Efficacies of Oral Killed Cholera Vaccines." *Clinical and Vaccine Immunology* 21, no. 9 (2014): 1195–1205. http://dx.doi.org/10.1128/CVI.00378–14.

Kar, Shantanu K., Binod Sah, Bikash Patnaik, Yang Hee Kim, Anna S. Kerketta, Sunheang Shin, Shyam Bandhu Rath et al. "Mass Vaccination with a New, Less Expensive Oral Cholera Vaccine Using Public Health Infrastructure in India: The Odisha Model." *PLoS Neglected Tropical Diseases* 8, no. 2 (2014): e2629. http://dx.doi.org/10.1371/journal.pntd.0002629.

Karki, Rabindra, Dwij Raj Bhatta, Sarala Malla, and Shyam Prakash Dumre. "Cholera Incidence among Patients with Diarrhea Visiting National Public Health Laboratory, Nepal." *Japanese Journal of Infectious Diseases* 63, no. 3 (2010): 185–87.

Katz, Jonathan M. *The Big Truck That Went By: How the World Came to Save Haiti and Left Behind a Disaster.* New York: Palgrave Macmillan, 2014.

——. "Choléra: Des Haïtiens Réclament le Départ des Casques Bleus Népalais." *La Pressa*, October 29, 2010. http://www.lapresse.ca/international/amerique-latine/

201010/29/01–4337600-cholera-des-haitiens-reclament-le-depart-des-casques-bleus-nepalais.php.

——. "Haiti Cholera Likely from UN Troops, Expert Says." Associated Press, December 7, 2010. http://www.washingtontimes.com/news/2010/dec/7/haiti-cholera-likely-from-un-troops-expert-says/?page=all.

——. "Haitians Protest, Threaten UN Base." Associated Press, November 16, 2010. http://www.boston.com/news/world/latinamerica/articles/2010/11/16/haitians_protest_threaten_un_base/.

——. "Protesters Blame UN Base for Cholera in Haiti." Associated Press, October 29, 2010. http://www.huffingtonpost.com/2010/10/29/cholera-in-haiti-proteste_n_776213.html.

——. "12 Killed in Haiti Cholera Witch-Hunt." Associated Press, December 1, 2010. http://www.sbsun.com/general-news/20101202/12-killed-in-haiti-cholera-witch-hunt.

——. "UN Calls for Probe into Origin of Haiti Cholera." Associated Press, December 15, 2010. http://www.highbeam.com/doc/1A1–499b0507a0cf4b50a4446ba7c8153937.html.

——. "The U.N. Caused Haiti's Cholera Epidemic. Now the Obama Administration Is Fighting the Victims." *New Republic*, October 24, 2014. http://www.newrepublic.com/article/119976/haiti-cholera-case-begins-us-defends-un-against-victims.

——. "United Nations Still Denies Its Troops Brought Cholera to Haiti." *Daily Beast*, April 4, 2012. http://www.thedailybeast.com/articles/2012/04/04/united-nations-still-denies-its-troops-brought-cholera-to-haiti.html.

——. "UN Probes Base as Source of Haiti Cholera Outbreak." Associated Press, October 28, 2010. http://www.thejakartapost.com/news/2010/10/28/un-probes-base-source-haiti-cholera-outbreak.html.

——. "UN Troops May Have Brought Cholera." Associated Press, November 4, 2010. http://www.boston.com/news/health/articles/2010/11/04/un_troops_may_have_brought_cholera.

——. "U.N. Worries Its Troops Caused Cholera in Haiti." Associated Press, November 19, 2010. http://www.nbcnews.com/id/40280944/ns/health/t/un-worries-its-troops-caused-cholera-haiti.

Keating, Joshua. "Is Haiti's Government Starting to Function?" *Foreign Policy*, November 9, 2010. http://blog.foreignpolicy.com/posts/2010/11/09/is_haitis_government_starting_to_function.

Klarreich, Kathie, and Linda Polman. "The NGO Republic of Haiti: How the International Relief Effort after the 2010 Earthquake Excluded Haitians from Their Own Recovery." *Nation*, November 19, 2012. http://www.thenation.com/article/170929/ngo-republic-haiti#.

Knox, Richard. "Cholera Vaccination Test Reached Targets in Haiti." NPR, July 17, 2012. http://www.npr.org/blogs/health/2012/07/17/156920472/cholera-vaccination-test-reached-targets-in-haiti?ft=1&f=2100771.

——. "Earthquake Not to Blame for Cholera Outbreak in Haiti." NPR, October 26, 2010. http://www.npr.org/blogs/health/2010/10/26/130832317/earthquake-had-nothing-to-do-with-cholera-outbreak-haiti.

——. "Scientists Find New Wrinkle in How Cholera Got to Haiti." NPR, June 18, 2012. http://www.npr.org/blogs/health/2012/06/18/155311990/scientists-find-new-wrinkle-in-how-cholera-got-to-haiti.

——. "Vaccination against Cholera Finally Begins in Haiti." NPR, April 12, 2012. http://www.npr.org/blogs/health/2012/04/12/150493770/vaccination-against-cholera-finally-begins-in-haiti.

Kohn, G. C. *Encyclopedia of Plague and Pestilence: From Ancient Times to the Present*. 3rd ed. New York: Facts on File, 2008.

Kolovos, Maria-Elena, and Beatrice Lindstrom. "UN Must Take Responsibility for Haiti Cholera Outbreak." JURIST, Hotline, February 23, 2012. http://jurist.org/hotline/2012/02/kolovos-lindstrom-cholera-haiti.php.

Kristoff, Madeline, and Liz Panarelli. "Haiti: A Republic of NGOs?" United States Institute of Peace Brief 23, April 26, 2010. http://www.usip.org/events/haiti-republic-ngos.

Kupferschmidt, Kai. "Second Bacterium Theory Stirs Haiti's Cholera Controversy." *Science* 336, no. 6088 (2012): 1493. http://dx/doi.org/10.1126/science.336.6088.1493.

Kurczy, Stephen. "Haiti Cholera Outbreak 'Stabilizing'—but Could Affect Election." *Christian Science Monitor*, October 25, 2010. http://www.csmonitor.com/World/Americas/2010/1025/Haiti-cholera-outbreak-stabilizing-but-could-affect-election.

Lacey, Stephen W. "Cholera: Calamitous Past, Ominous Future." *Clinical Infectious Diseases* 20, no. 5 (1995): 1409–19. http://dx.doi.org/10.1093/clinids/20.5.1409.

La Fontaine, Jean de. "The Wolf and the Lamb." In *The Fables of La Fontaine*. Translated by Elizur Wright, Jr. London: William Smith, 1842. http://rpo.library.utoronto.ca/poems/wolf-and-lamb.

Lakhani, Nina. "Cuban Medics in Haiti Put the World to Shame." *Independent*, December 26, 2010. http://www.independent.co.uk/life-style/health-and-families/health-news/cuban-medics-in-haiti-put-the-world-to-shame-2169415.html.

Lancet Infectious Diseases. Editorial, "As Cholera Returns to Haiti, Blame is Unhelpful." Vol. 10, no. 12 (2010): 813. http://dx.doi.org/10.1016/S1473-3099(10)70265-6.

——. Editorial, "WHO Failing in Duty of Transparency." Vol. 10, no. 8 (2010): 505. http://dx.doi.org/10.1016/S1473-3099(10)70147-X.

Lantagne, Daniele. "Understanding Haiti's Cholera Outbreak: Interventions in Developing Countries and Emergency Contexts." YouTube video. Posted by Tufts School of Engineering, April 8, 2013. www.youtube.com/watch?v=9aJptv0f_1Q.

Lantagne, Daniele, G. Balakrish Nair, Claudio F. Lanata, and Alejandro Cravioto. "The Cholera Outbreak in Haiti: Where and How Did It Begin?" *Current Topics in Microbiology and Immunology* 379 (2014): 145–64. http://dx.doi.org/10.1007/82_2013_331 (epub: May 22, 2013).

——. "The Origin of Cholera in Haiti." *Journal of Disaster Research* 7, no. 6 (2012): 759–67. http://www.fujipress.jp/finder/xslt.php?mode=present&inputfile=DSSTR000700060012.xml

Largey, Michael. *Vodou Nation: Haitian Art Music and Cultural Nationalism*. Chicago: University of Chicago Press, 2006.

La Torra, Alberta. "Doctors Take Medical Marvels to Haiti." *Palm Beach Post*, October 17, 2005. http://latorra-larsen.org/pdfs/Grand-Plan-for-Health-Care-in-Desperate-Nation-Doctors-Take-Medical-Marvels-to-Haiti-from-PBP-101705.pdf.

Le Nouvelliste. "Haïti: Des Malades du Choléra avaient bu de l'eau Potable." October 27, 2010. http://lenouvelliste.com/lenouvelliste/article/85096/Haiti-des-malades-du-cholera-avaient-bu-de-leau-potable.html.

Levine, M. M., R. E. Black, M. L. Clements, L. Cisneros, D. R. Nalin, and C. R. Young. "Duration of Infection-Derived Immunity to Cholera." *Journal of Infectious Diseases* 143, no. 6 (1981): 818–20. http://dx.doi.org/10.1093/infdis/143.6.818.

Lewis, Ricki. "TIGR Introduces *Vibrio cholerae* genome." *Scientist*, August 21, 2000. http://www.the-scientist.com/?articles.view/articleNo/12986/.

Llanes, Rafael, Lorenzo Somarriba, Plácido Pedroso, Emiliano Mariscal, Carlos Fuster, and Yamila Zayas. "Letter to the Editor: Did the Cholera Epidemic in Haiti Really Start in the Artibonite Department?" *Journal of Infections in Developing Countries* 7, no. 10 (2013): 753–55. http://dx.doi.org/10.3855/jidc.3311.

Loharikar, A., A.E. Newton, S. Stroika, M. Freeman, K.D. Greene, M.B. Parsons, C. Bopp, D. Talkington, E.D. Mintz, and B.E. Mahon. "Cholera in the United States, 2001–2011: A Reflection of Patterns of Global Epidemiology and Travel." *Epidemiology and Infection* 143, no. 4 (2015): 695–703. http://dx.doi.org/10.1017/S0950268814001186.

Lutton D. "'We Are Poor . . . But We Demand Respect.'" *Jamaica Gleaner*, October 22, 2010. http://jamaica-gleaner.com/gleaner/20101022/news/news3.html.

MacKenzie, Debora. "Opinion, Haiti: Epidemics of Denial Must End." *New Scientist*, December 4, 2010. https://www.newscientist.com/article/mg20827894-900-haiti-epidemics-of-denial-must-end.

Maguire, Robert A. "René Préval." In *Encyclopedia Britannica Online.* Last modified September 25, 2013. http://www.britannica.com/EBchecked/topic/734196/Rene-Preval.

Maharjan, Laxmi. "Cholera Outbreak Looms over Capital." *Himalayan Times*, September 23, 2010. http://www.thehimalayantimes.com/rssReference.php?headline=Cholera+outbreak+looms+over+capital&NewsID=258974.

Malla, Sarala, Shyam Prakash Dumre, Geeta Shakya, Palpasa Kansakar, Bhupraj Rai, Anowar Hossain, Gopinath Balakrish Nair et al. "The Challenges and Successes of Implementing a Sustainable Antimicrobial Resistance Surveillance Programme in Nepal." *BMC Public Health* 14, no. 1 (2014): 269. http://dx.doi.org/10.1186/1471–2458–14–269.

Marcelin, Yvon. "Encore la soldatesque de la MINUSTAH." *Le Nouvelliste*, January 21, 2009. http://lenouvelliste.com/lenouvelliste/article/66463/Encore-la-soldatesque-de-la-MINUSTAH.html.

Martin, Stephen, Alejandro Costa, and William Perea. "Stockpiling Oral Cholera Vaccine." *Bulletin of the World Health Organization* 90, no. 10 (2012): 714. http://dx.doi.org/10.2471/BLT.12.112433.

McAlister, Elizabeth A. "Vodou." In *Encyclopedia Britannica Online*. Last modified February 17, 2014. http://www.britannica.com/EBchecked/topic/632819/Vodou.

McCarthy, Susan A., and Farukh M. Khambaty. "International Dissemination of Epidemic *Vibrio cholerae* by Cargo Ship Ballast and Other Nonpotable Waters." *Applied and Environmental Microbiology* 60, no. 7 (1994): 2597–2601.

McFadden, David. "Haiti's President Confirms 3-Month Term Extension." Associated Press, February 7, 2011. http://www.bet.com/news/news/2011/02/07/haitiprestermextension.html.

McNeil Jr, Donald G. "Cholera's Second Fever: An Urge to Blame." *New York Times*, November 20, 2010. http://www.nytimes.com/2010/11/21/weekinreview/21mcneil.html.

Médecins Sans Frontières. "Haiti: Too Few Beds to Treat Cholera Patients." November 24, 2014. http://www.doctorswithoutborders.org/article/haiti-too-few-beds-treat-cholera-patients.

——. International Activity Report—2013, USA. "Haiti," 2014, 48–49. http://www.doctorswithoutborders.org/sites/usa/files/attachments/msf_activity_report_2013_interactive.pdf.

Medrano Rojas, Pedro. Letter to Ms. Farha, Mr. Gallón, Mr. Pūras, and Ms. De Albuquerque, United Nations Headquarters, New York, NY, November 25, 2014. http://spdb.ohchr.org/hrdb/28th/Haiti_ASG_25.11.14_(3.2014).pdf.

Mekalanos, John J., William Robins, David W. Ussery, Brigid M. Davis, Eric Schadt, and Matthew K. Waldor. "Non-O1 Vibrio cholerae Unlinked to Cholera in Haiti." *Proceedings of the National Academy of Sciences* 109, no. 47 (2012): E3206. http://dx.doi.org/10.1073/pnas.1212443109.

Ministry of Foreign Affairs (Nepal). "Nepal's Role in the UN Peacekeeping Operations." Government of Nepal, July 26, 2014. http://www.mofa.gov.np/en/nepals-role-in-the-un-peacekeeping-operations-116.html.

Ministry of Public Health and Population (Haiti). "National Plan for the Elimination of Cholera in Haiti, 2013–2022." February 2013. http://www.paho.org/hq/index.php?option=com_docman&task=doc_view&gid=20326&Itemid=270&lang=en.

Ministry of Health and Population (Nepal), New ERA, and ICF International Inc. *Nepal Demographic and Health Survey 2011*. Kathmandu, Nepal (Ministry of Health and Population), Calverton, MD (New ERA, and ICF International), March 2012. http://dhsprogram.com/pubs/pdf/FR257/FR257%5B13April2012%5D.pdf.

MINUSTAH. "Haïti face à une épidémie de choléra [Haiti faces a cholera epidemic]." October 22, 2010. http://minustah.org/?p=27300.

——. "SRSG Specifies the Role of MINUSTAH to Human Rights NGOs in Haiti." PIO/PR/50/2004, October 28, 2004. http://reliefweb.int/report/haiti/srsg-specifies-role-minustah-human-right-s-ngos-haiti.

Mission of the United States. "World Health Assembly—Secretary Sebelius Meets with Haiti Minister of Health, Alex Larsen," May 17, 2010. http://geneva.usmission.gov/2010/05/17/readout-secretary-sebelius-bilateral-meeting-haiti.

Moore, S., N. Thomson, A. Mutreja, and Renaud Piarroux. "Widespread Epidemic Cholera Caused by a Restricted Subset of *Vibrio cholerae* Clones." *Clinical Microbiology and Infection* 20, no. 5 (2014): 373–79. http://dx.doi.org/10.1111/1469–0691.12610.

Morabia, Alfredo. "Epidemiologic Interactions, Complexity, and the Lonesome Death of Max von Pettenkofer." *American Journal of Epidemiology* 166, no. 11 (2007): 1233–38. http://dx.doi.org/10.1093/aje/kwm279.

MSPP (Ministere de la Sante Publique et del Population). "Plan Stratégique Quinquennal du Réseau National de Laboratoires, 2010–2015." Port-au-Prince, Haiti, July 2010. http://mspp.gouv.ht/site/downloads/version%20finalisee%20Plan%20Strategique.pdf.

——. Rapport de Cas, Journalier et Cumulatif, October 31, 2010. http://www.mspp.gouv.ht/site/downloads/attachments_2010_11_04.zip.

——. "Rapport de Cas, Journalier et Cumulatif," December 8, 2014. http://mspp.gouv.ht/site/downloads/Rapport%20Web_08.12_Avec_Courbes_Departementales.pdf.

Murray, Mary. "Katrina Aid from Cuba? No Thanks, Says U.S." NBC News, September 9, 2005. http://www.nbcnews.com/id/9311876/ns/us_news-katrina_the_long_road_back/t/katrina-aid-cuba-no-thanks-says-us/#.VBnS60uNhYk.

Mutreja, Ankur, Dong Wook Kim, Nicholas R. Thomson, Thomas R. Connor, Je Hee Lee, Samuel Kariuki, Nicholas J. Croucher et al. "Evidence for Several Waves of Global Transmission in the Seventh Cholera Pandemic." *Nature* 477, no. 7365 (2011): 462–65. http://dx.doi.org/10.1038/nature10392.

Muyembe, Jean Jacques, Didier Bompangue, Guy Mutombo, Laurent Akilimali, Annie Mutombo, Berthe Miwanda, Jean de Dieu Mpuruta et al. "Elimination of Cholera in the Democratic Republic of the Congo: The New National Policy." *Journal of Infectious Diseases* 208, no. S1 (2013): S86–91. http://dx.doi.org/10.1093/infdis/jit204.

Nelson, E. J., J. B. Harris, J. G. Morris, Jr., S. B. Calderwood, and A. Camilli. "Cholera Transmission: The Host, Pathogen and Bacteriophage Dynamic." *Nature*

Reviews Microbiology 7, no. 10 (2009): 693–702. http://dx.doi.org/10.1038/nrmicro2204.

Nesirky, Martin. Noon Briefing, Haiti: "U.N. Mission in Haiti Continues to Seek Information on Origins of Cholera Epidemic." UN Office of the Spokesperson for the Secretary-General, December 7, 2010. http://www.un.org/sg/spokesperson/highlights/?HighD=12/7/2010&d_month=12&d_year=2010.

——. Spokesperson's Noon Briefing. Office of the Spokesperson for the Secretary-General, United Nations, April 2, 2012. http://www.un.org/News/briefings/docs/2012/db120402.doc.htm.

New York Times. "Haiti's Cholera Crisis." May 12, 2012. http://www.nytimes.com/2012/05/13/opinion/sunday/haitis-cholera-crisis.html?_r=0.

Nguyen, Binh Minh, Je Hee Lee, Ngo Tuan Cuong, Seon Young Choi, Nguyen Tran Hien, Dang Duc Anh, Hye Ri Lee et al. "Cholera Outbreaks Caused by an Altered Vibrio cholerae O1 El Tor Biotype Strain Producing Classical Cholera Toxin B in Vietnam in 2007 to 2008." *Journal of Clinical Microbiology* 47, no. 5 (2009): 1568–71. http://dx.doi.org/10.1128/JCM.02040–08.

Nigro, Olivia D., Aixin Hou, Gayatri Vithanage, Roger S. Fujioka, and Grieg F. Steward. "Temporal and Spatial Variability in Culturable Pathogenic Vibrio spp. in Lake Pontchartrain, Louisiana, Following Hurricanes Katrina and Rita." *Applied and Environmental Microbiology* 77, no. 15 (2011): 5384–93. http://dx.doi.org/10.1128/AEM.02509–10.

OCHA (United Nations Office for the Coordination of Humanitarian Affairs). "Cholera Epidemic." *Humanitarian Bulletin—Haiti*, no. 24, November 2012, 1–9. http://reliefweb.int/sites/reliefweb.int/files/resources/Haiti%20Humanitarian%20Bulletin%20Issue%2024%20November%202012.pdf.

——. "Haiti: Cholera Outbreak (as of 22 Oct 2010)." Relief Web, October 22, 2010. http://reliefweb.int/sites/reliefweb.int/files/resources/map_436.pdf

——. "Haiti—Cholera Situation: Affected Communes in Artibonite and Centre." Relief Web, October 25, 2010. http://reliefweb.int/map/Haiti/Haiti-cholera-situation-affected-communes-artibonite-and-centre-25-oct-2010–1930.

——. "Haiti—Situation de Cholera: Communes affectées." Relief Web, October 28, 2010. http://reliefweb.int/map/Haiti/Haiti-situation-de-cholera-communes-affectées-28-oct-2010.

——. "Haiti—Situation de Cholera: Communes affectées." Relief Web, November 10, 2010. http://reliefweb.int/map/Haiti/Haiti-situation-de-cholera-communes-affectées-10-novembre-2010–1930.

——. "Haiti—Situation de Cholera: Communes affectées dans Artibonite et Centre." Relief Web, October 27, 2010. http://reliefweb.int/map/Haiti/Haiti-situation-de-cholera-communes-affectées-dans-artibonite-et-centre-27-oct-2010.

O'Connor, Katherine A., Emily Cartwright, Anagha Loharikar, Janell Routh, Joanna Gaines, Marie-Délivrance, Bernadette Fouché et al. "Risk Factors Early in the 2010 Cholera Epidemic, Haiti." *Emerging Infectious Diseases* 17, no. 11 (2011): 2136–38. http://ex.doi.org/10.3201/eid1711.110810.

Organization of American States. "Who We Are." Accessed June 23, 2014. http://www.oas.org/en/about/who_we_are.asp.

PAHO (Pan American Health Organization). "Cholera Cases Confirmed in Paraguay." *Epidemiological Alerts* 6, no. 10 (2009). http://www2.paho.org/hq/dmdocuments/2009/epi-alerts-2009-04-22-Cholera-PAR.pdf.

——. "Cholera Outbreak in Haiti." *EOC Situation Report* no. 1, October 22, 2010. http://reliefweb.int/report/haiti/paho-eoc-situation-report-1-cholera-outbreak-haiti.

——. "Cholera Outbreak in Haiti." *EOC Situation Report* no. 4, October 25, 2010. http://www.paho.org/disasters/index.php?option=com_docman&task=doc_view&gid=119.

——. "Cholera Outbreak in Haiti." *EOC Situation Report* no. 6, October 27, 2010. http://www.paho.org/hq/index.php?option=com_content&view=article&id=4372:eoc-situation-report-6-on-cholera-outbreak-haiti-&Itemid=40293&lang=en.

——."Cholera Outbreak in Haiti." *EOC Situation Report* no. 10, November 3, 2010. http://reliefweb.int/report/haiti/paho-eoc-situation-report-10-cholera-outbreak-haiti.

——. "Cholera Outbreak in Haiti." *EOC Situation Report* no. 13, November 11, 2010. http://www.paho.org/hq/index.php?option=com_content&view=article&id=4410%3Aeoc-situation-report-13-cholera-outbreak-haiti&catid=3109%3Anews-eoc-situation-reports&Itemid=40683&lang=en.

——. "Cholera Outbreak in Haiti, 2010, New Cases Reported by Epidemiological Week: EW42 (October 17–23, 2010)." http://new.paho.org/hq/images/Atlas_IHR/CholeraOutbreak/atlas.html.

——. "Cholera Outbreak in Haiti, 2010, New Cases Reported by Epidemiological Week: EW43 (October 24–30, 2010)." http://new.paho.org/hq/images/Atlas_IHR/CholeraOutbreak/atlas.html.

——. "PAHO Responds to Cholera Outbreak in Haiti." October 21, 2010. http://www.paho.org/hq/index.php?option=com_content&view=article&id=7662:paho-responds-cholera-outbreak-haiti&Itemid=39666&lang=en.

——. "Water and Sanitation Improvements Remain Key to Defeating Cholera in Haiti and the Dominican Republic." Washington, DC, March 21, 2014. http://www.paho.org/hq/index.php?option=com_content&view=article&id=9400%3Awater-and-sanitation-improvements-remain-key-to-defeating-cholera-in-haiti-and-the-dominican-republic&catid=740%3Anews-press-releases&Itemid=1926&lang=en.

PAHO/WHO (Pan American Health Organization/World Health Organization). "Haiti Launches Cholera Vaccination Campaign." September 2, 2014. http://www.paho.org/hq/index.php?id=9875%3Ahaiti-launches-cholera-vaccination-campaign&option=com_content.

Palca, Joe. "The Mysterious Life of the Cholera Bacterium." NPR, October 29, 2010. http://www.npr.org/templates/story/story.php?storyId=130916261.

Parker, Aubrey Ann. "Cholera in Haiti—The Climate Connection." *Circle of Blue Waternews*, November 11, 2010. http://www.circleofblue.org/waternews/2010/world/hold-cholera-in-haiti-the-climate-connection.

Pasetti, Marecella F., and Myron M. Levine." Insights from Natural Infection-Derived Immunity to Cholera Instruct Vaccine Efforts." *Clinical and Vaccine Immunology* 19, no. 11 (2012): 1707–11. http://dx.doi.org/10.1128/CVI.00543–12.

Pasmantier, Deborah. "Choléra en Haïti: Une épidémie importée." Agence France-Presse, November 29, 2010. http://www.lapresse.ca/international/amerique-latine/201011/29/01–4347408-cholera-en-haiti-une-epidemie-importee.php.

——. "Haiti Cholera Outbreak 'Came from UN Camp.'" Agence France-Presse, December 5, 2010. http://www.commondreams.org/news/2010/12/07/haiti-cholera-outbreak-came-un-camp.

Paulson, Tom. "Experts Say UN Did Not Bring Cholera to Haiti: It Was Already There." *Humanosphere,* November 24, 2010. http://humanosphere.kplu.org/2010/11/experts-say-un-did-not-bring-cholera-to-haiti-it-was-already-there/#more-6034

Periago, Mirta Roses, Thomas R. Frieden, Jordan W. Tappero, Kevin M. De Cock, Bernt Aasen, and Jon K. Andrus. "Elimination of Cholera Transmission in Haiti and the Dominican Republic." *Lancet* 379, no. 9812 (2012): e12–e13. http://dx.doi.org/10.1016/S0140-6736(12)60031-2.

Permanent Mission of the People's Republic of China to the UN. Statement by H.E. Mr. Li Baodong Permanent Representative of China to the United Nation at Security Council Debate on United Nations Stabilization Mission in Haiti (MINUSTAH), April 28, 2010. http://www.china-un.org/eng/gdxw/t688491.htm.

Piarroux, Renaud. "Le choléra: Épidémiologie et transmission. Expérience tirée de plusieurs interventions humanitaires réalisées en Afrique, dans l'Océan Indien et en Amérique Centrale." *Bulletin de la Société de pathologie exotique* 95, no. 5 (2002): 345–50. http://www.pathexo.fr/documents/articles-bull/T95-5-Piarroux.pdf.

——. "Op-Ed: What Role Did the Environment Play in Haiti's Cholera Epidemic?" *Caribbean Journal*, October 17, 2012. http://www.caribjournal.com/2012/10/17/op-ed-what-role-did-the-environment-play-in-haitis-cholera-epidemic/.

Piarroux, Renaud, Robert Barrais, Benoît Faucher, Rachel Haus, Martine Piarroux, Jean Gaudart, Roc Magloire, and Didier Raoult. "Understanding the Cholera Epidemic, Haiti." *Emerging Infectious Diseases* 17, no. 7 (2011): 1161–68. http://dx.doi.org/10.3201/eid1707.110059 (epub: May 6, 2011).

Piarroux, Renaud, and Benoît Faucher. "Cholera Epidemics in 2010: Respective Roles of Environment, Strain Changes, and Human-Driven Dissemination." *Clinical Microbiology and Infection* 18, no. 3 (2012): 231–38. http://dx.doi.org/10.1111/j.1469-0691.2012.03763.x.

——. "Idées—Tous les êtres humains naissent libres et égaux en dignité et en droits, même les Haïtiens?" *Le Monde*, August 29, 2011. http://www.lemonde.fr/idees/article/2011/08/29/tous-les-etres-humains-naissent-libres-et-egaux-en-dignite-et-en-droits-meme-les-haitiens_1563820_3232.html.

Piarroux Renaud, and Rebaudet Stanislas. "Rapport de mission et point de situation sur le choléra en Haïti." Report to UNICEF, Assistance Publique—Hôpitaux de Marseille, Aix-Marseille Université, Marseille, France, September 2014.

Porta, Miquel. *A Dictionary of Epidemiology*. 6th ed. New York: Oxford University Press, 2014.

Porter, Catherine. "Haiti's René Préval says UN tried to remove him." *Toronto Star*, May 13, 2013. http://www.thestar.com/news/world/2013/05/13/haitis_ren_prval_says_un_tried_to_remove_him.html.

Pow, Helen. "Inside the Rituals of Haiti's 'Vodou' Faith": Powerful Photographs Capture Priestesses as They Invoke Spirits and Perform Sacrifices." *Daily Mail* (UK), November 10, 2013. http://www.dailymail.co.uk/news/article-2499453/Anthony-Karen-Vodou-Inside-rituals-Haitis-Vodou-faith-Mesmerizing-photos-animals-sacrificed-worshipers-overcome-spirits-ceremonies-intriguing-Caribbean-religion.html.

Prepetit, C., and D. Boisson. *Inventaire des ressources minières de la République d'Haiti*, Fascicule IV, Département de l'Artibonite, Bureau des Mines et de l'Energie, Direction de la Geologie et Des Mines, Port-au-Prince (Haiti), 1992. http://www.bme.gouv.ht/mines/fascicule/F4Artibonite.pdf.

Pugliese, Vincenzo. "Point de Presse des Nations Unies en Haiti. Response to Question 3." MINUSTAH, October 28, 2010.

Obama, Barack. "Presidential Remarks on Haitian Earthquake Relief." C-Span Video. January 14, 2010. http://www.c-span.org/video/?291323-1/presidential-remarks-haitian-earthquake-relief-efforts.

Quentel, C., and Didier Le Bret. "Urgent restreint, situation politique des états/Crise interne, choléra en Haïti: Point de situation [Urgent restricted, political situation of the states/Internal crisis, cholera in Haiti: Update on the situation]." Diplomatic communiqué from French embassy in Port-au-Prince, Haiti, November 13, 2010.

Ramamurthy, Thandavarayan, Shinji Yamasaki, Yoshifumi Takeda, and Gopinath Balakrish Nair. "Vibrio cholerae O139 Bengal: Odyssey of a Fortuitous Variant." *Microbes and Infection* 5, no. 4 (2003): 329–44. http://dx.doi.org/10.1016/S1286-4579(03)00035-2.

Raoult, Didier. "Plague and Cholera in the Genomics era." *Clinical Microbiology and Infection* 18, no. 3 (2012): 212. http://dx.doi.org/10.1111/j.1469-0691.2012.03780.x.

Rebaudet, Stanislaus, Aaron Aruna Abedi, Pierre Gazin, Sandra Moore, P. Adrien, Edouard Beigbeder, Jacques Boncy, and Renaud Piarroux. "Update from the Authors on the 'Dry Season' Strategy to Fight Cholera in Haiti.'" *PLoS Currents: Outbreaks*, Comments RSS (Really Simple Syndication), June 7, 2014.

Rebaudet, Stanislas, Pierre Gazin, Robert Barrais, Sandra Moore, Emmanuel Rossignol, Nicolson Barthelemy, Jean Gaudart, Jacques Boncy, Roc Magloire, and Renaud Piarroux. "The Dry Season in Haiti: A Window of Opportunity to Eliminate Cholera." *PLoS Currents: Outbreaks* 5, version. 1, June 10, 2013. http://dx.doi.org/10.1371/currents.outbreaks.2193a0ec4401d9526203af12e5024ddc.

Rebaudet, Stanislaus, and Renaud Piarroux. "Monitoring Water Sources for Environmental Reservoirs of Toxigenic *Vibrio cholerae* O1, Haiti." *Emerging Infectious Diseases* 21, no. 1 (2015): 169–70. http://dx.doi.org/10.3201/eid2101.140627.

Reingold, A. L. "Outbreak Investigations—A Perspective." *Emerging Infectious Diseases* 4, no. 1 (1998): 21–27. http://dx.doi.org/10.3201/eid0401.980104.

Renois C. "Haïti: 12 personnes lynchées en lien avec le choléra." Agence France-Press, December 2, 2010. http://www.lapresse.ca/international/dossiers/seisme-en-haiti/201012/02/01-4348618-haiti-12-personnes-lynchees-en-lien-avec-le-cholera.php.

Rinaldo, Andrea, Enrico Bertuzzo, Lorenzo Mari, Lorenzo Righetto, Melanie Blokesch, Marino Gatto, Renato Casagrandi, Megan Murray, Silvan M. Vesenbeckh, and Ignacio Rodriguez-Iturbe. "Reassessment of the 2010–2011 Haiti Cholera Outbreak and Rainfall-Driven Multiseason Projections." *Proceedings of the National Academy of Sciences* 109, no. 17 (2012): 6602–7. http://dx/doi.org/10.1073/pnas.1203333109.

Robbins, Anthony. "Haitian Cholera Outbreak Highlights Need for Infrastructure, Not Blame." *Scientific American* (guest blog), March 25, 2014. http://blogs.scientificamerican.com/guest-blog/2014/03/25/haitian-cholera-outbreak-highlights-need-for-infrastructure-not-blame/.

——. "Lessons from Cholera in Haiti." *Journal of Public Health Policy* 35, no. 2 (2014): 135–36. http://dx.doi.org/10.1057/jphp.2014.5.

——. "What Can We Learn from the Cholera Epidemic in Haiti?" *Science Blogs—The Pump Handle*, March 25, 2014. http://scienceblogs.com/thepumphandle/2014/03/25/what-can-we-learn-from-the-cholera-epidemic-in-haiti/.

Robins, W. P., and J. J. Mekalanos. "Genomic Science in Understanding Cholera Outbreaks and Evolution of Vibrio cholerae as a Human Pathogen." *Current Topics in Microbiology and Immunology* 379 (2014): 211–29. http://dx/doi.org/10.1007/82_2014_366.

Robinson, Randall. *An Unbroken Agony: Haiti, from Revolution to the Kidnapping of a President*. New York: Basic Civitas, 2007.

Rohter, Larry. "Mission to Haiti; Haiti's Attachés: Deadly Heirs to the Tontons Macoute." *New York Times*, October 4, 1994. http://www.nytimes.com/1994/10/04/world/mission-to-haiti-haiti-s-attaches-deadly-heirs-to-the-tontons-macoute.html.

Romero, Simon. "Poor Sanitation in Haiti's Camps Adds Disease Risk." *New York Times*, February 19, 2010. http://www.nytimes.com/2010/02/20/world/americas/20haiti.html?_r=0.

Routh, Janelle, and Nandini Sreenivasan. "Cholera Vaccination Campaign Evaluation, Petite Anse and Cerca Carvajal, Haiti, 2013." Memorandum, CDC/DHHS, May 24, 2014.

Sack, David A. "Consultant Report: Cholera in Haiti, October 2010." United Nations (DPKO/DFS/MINUSTAH), January–February 2011.

——. "Mapping the progression of the cholera epidemic in Haiti and the DR: Water sampling in the DR's Artibonite River Valley" (e-mail). Haiti M.P.H.I.S.E., January 5, 2011. http://haiti.mphise.net/email-thread-water-sampling-drs-artibonite-valley.

——. "Cholera in Haiti, October 2010." Slide presentation at the Department of International Health, Johns Hopkins University, January–February, 2011.

Sack, D.A., R.B. Sack, and C.L. Chaignat. "Getting Serious about Cholera." *New England Journal of Medicine* 355, no. 7 (2006): 649–51. http://dx/doi.org/10.1056/NEJMp068144.

Sadowski, Dennis. "Archbishop: Haitians Feel Abandoned by World amid Continuing Disasters." Catholic News Service, January 7, 2011. http://www.catholicnews.com/data/stories/cns/1100064.htm.

Saloomey, K. "UN Likely to Blame for Haiti Cholera Outbreak." Al Jazeera English, March 7, 2012. http://www.youtube.com/watch?v=Pmw1b-tV09U.

Schuller, Mark. "Haiti's Disaster after the Disaster: The IDP Camps and Cholera." *Journal of Humanitarian Assistance*, December 13, 2010. http://sites.tufts.edu/jha/archives/869.

Sérant, Claude Bernard. "Alerte au cholera." *Le Nouvelliste*, October 21, 2010. http://www.lenouvelliste.com/lenouvelliste/article/84900/Alerte-au-cholera.html.

Shafy, Samiha. "Haitian President Martelly: 'I'm Trying to Re-Establish Confidence.'" *Der Spiegel*, November 5, 2014. http://www.spiegel.de/international/world/interview-with-haitian-president-michel-martelly-a-1000719.html.

Shakya, Geeta. "Antimicrobial Resistance Surveillance in Nepal for Rational Use of Antibiotics." Slide presentation at World Health Day, Institute of Medicine, Kathmandu, Nepal, April 7, 2011.

Shampo, Marc A., and Robert A. Kyle. "Bernard Kouchner—Founder of Doctors Without Borders." *Mayo Clinic Proceedings* 86, no. 1 (2011): e6. http://www.ncbi.nlm.nih.gov/pmc/articles/PMC3012640/.

Shilts, Randy. *And the Band Played On: Politics, People, and the AIDS Epidemic*. New York: St. Martin's, 1987.

Shrestha, Kashish Das. "Haiti's Cholera Outbreak: Nepal's Role Reconsidered." *República* (Kathmandu, Nepal), July 6, 2012. http://www.myrepublica.com/portal/index.php?action=news_details&news_id=37468.

——. "Haiti's Nepali UN Peacekeepers." *República*, December 17, 2010. http://archives.myrepublica.com/portal/index.php?action=news_details&news_id=26239.

Siddique, A.K., K. Akram, K. Zaman, S. Laston, A. Salam, R.N. Majumdar, M.S. Islam, and N. Fronczak. "Why Treatment Centres Failed to Prevent Cholera Deaths among Rwandan Refugees in Goma, Zaire." *Lancet* 345, no. 8946 (1995): 359–61.

Simons, Marlise. "Voodoo under Attack in Post-Duvalier Haiti." *New York Times*, May 15, 1986. http://www.nytimes.com/1986/05/15/world/voodoo-under-attack-in-post-duvalier-haiti.html.

Sontag, Deborah. "In Haiti, Global Failures on a Cholera Epidemic." *New York Times*, March 31, 2012. http://www.nytimes.com/2012/04/01/world/americas/haitis-cholera-outraced-the-experts-and-tainted-the-un.html?pagewanted=all&_r=0.

Steenland, Maria W., Gerard A. Joseph, Mentor Ali Ber Lucien, Nicole Freeman, Marisa Hast, Benjamin L. Nygren, Eyal Leshem et al. "Laboratory-Confirmed Cholera and Rotavirus among Patients with Acute Diarrhea in Four Hospitals in Haiti, 2012–2013." *American Journal of Tropical Medicine and Hygiene* 89, no. 4 (2013): 641–46. http://dx.doi.org/10.4269/ajtmh.13–0307.

Strassburg, Marc A. "The Global Eradication of Smallpox." *American Journal of Infection Control* 10, no. 2 (1982): 53–59. http://dx.doi.org/10.1016/0196–6553(82)90003–7.

Styger, Eric, and Joeli Barison. "Introducing the System of Rice Intensification (SRI) to Haiti—Report." Cornell International Institute for Food, Agriculture and Development (CIIFAD), July 9, 2010. http://sri.ciifad.cornell.edu/countries/haiti/Haiti_TripRpt_EStyger0910.pdf.

Talkington, Deborah, Cheryl Bopp, Cheryl Tarr, Michele B. Parsons, Georges Dahourou, Molly Freeman, Kevin Joyce et al. "Characterization of Toxigenic Vibrio cholerae from Haiti, 2010–2011." *Emerging Infectious Diseases* 17, no. 11 (2011): 2122. http://dx.doi.org/10.3201/eid1711.110805.

Terp Magazine. "Professor Rita Colwell." Spring, 2013. http://issuu.com/umaryland/docs/terp_s2013_final.

Terra News Service (Brazil). "Presidente do Haiti diz que surto de cólera foi 'importado.'" October 24, 2010. http://noticias.terra.com.br/mundo/america-latina/presidente-do-haiti-diz-que-surto-de-colera-foi-quotimportadoquot,aa3dbe14db92b310VgnCLD200000bbcceb0aRCRD.html.

Thélot, Fils-lien Ely. "Bêê ê ê: De ces rumeurs qui font rougir les 'casques bleus' en Haïti." *Bulletin de la Société Suisse des Américanistes*, no. 71 (2009): 77–83.

Time. "The Death and Legacy of Papa Doc Duvalier." January 17, 2011. http://content.time.com/time/magazine/article/0,9171,876967–2,00.html.

UN (United Nations). "Adopting Resolution 2180 (2014), Security Council Approves One-Year Renewal for United Nations Stabilization Mission in Haiti." Meeting Coverage and Press Releases, SC/11599, October 14, 2014. http://www.un.org/press/en/2014/sc11599.doc.htm.

——. "Support Plan for the Elimination of the Transmission of Cholera in Haiti: 2014–2015." January 2014. http://www.un.org/News/dh/infocus/haiti/UN_Support_Strategy_Elimination_Cholera%20_FEB_2014.pdf.

UN Department of Peacekeeping Operations. "Fact Sheet—United Nations Peacekeeping." DPI/2429/Rev 7, March 2010. http://www.un.org/en/peacekeeping/documents/factsheet.pdf.

——. "Financing Peacekeeping." November 2014. http://www.un.org/en/peacekeeping/.

——. *Infantry Battalion Manual*, vol. 1 (Department of Field Support). August 2012. http://www.un.org/en/peacekeeping/documents/UNIBAM.Vol.I.pdf.

——. "Troop Statistics." November 2014. http://www.un.org/en/peacekeeping.

UN Department of Public Information. "Collective Efforts in Haiti Will Be Overwhelmed without Massive, Immediate Response, Secretary-General Warns in Remarks to General Assembly." SG/SM/13294, GA/11028, IHA/1290. December 3, 2010. http://www.un.org/News/Press/docs/2010/sgsm13294.doc.htm.

———. "Haiti Cholera Victims' Compensation Claims 'Not Receivable' under Immunities and Privileges Convention, United Nations Tells Their Representatives." Secretary-General, SG/SM/14828 February 21, 2013. http://www.un.org/News/Press/docs/2013/sgsm14828.doc.htm.

———. "Secretary-General Appoints Peter De Clercq of Netherlands as Deputy Special Representative for United Nations Stabilization Mission in Haiti." SG/A/1430, BIO/4507, PKO/366, August 12, 2013. http://www.un.org/News/Press/docs//2013/sga1430.doc.htm.

UN News Centre. "As Dry Season Ends in Haiti, Significant Gains Seen in Fight against Cholera, UN official Says." May 1, 2014. http://www.un.org/apps/news/story.asp?NewsID=47703#.U3pP4l6NhYl.

———. "Haiti: Ban Appeals for More Funds to Fight Cholera, Sets Up Panel to Probe Its Origins." December 17, 2010. http://www.un.org/apps/news/story.asp?NewsID=37106&Cr=haiti&Cr1.

———. "Haiti: Ban Appoints Four Top Medical Experts to Probe Source of Cholera Epidemic." January 6, 2011. http://www.un.org/apps/news/story.asp?NewsID=37216&Cr=haiti&Cr1.

———. "Interview with Assistant Secretary-General Pedro Medrano Rojas, Senior Coordinator for the Cholera Response in Haiti." December 5, 2013. http://www.un.org/apps/news/newsmakers.asp?NewsID=99.

———. "UN in Talks to Set Up Independent Panel of Experts to Probe Origin of Cholera in Haiti." December 15, 2010. http://www.un.org/apps/news/story.asp?NewsID=37084&Cr=haiti&Cr1.

———. "UN Urges Massive Campaign in Haiti to Boost Cholera Prevention Measures." December 30, 2010. http://www.un.org/apps/news/story.asp?NewsID=37180.

UN Office of the Special Envoy to Haiti. "Overview of Funding: Summary of Bilateral and Multilateral Pledges and Disbursements in Support of the National Plan for the Elimination of Cholera in Haiti, 2013–2022, as of December 2014." http://www.lessonsfromhaiti.org/download/International_Assistance/cih-national-plan-final.pdf.

UN Office of the Spokesperson for the Secretary-General. Daily Press Briefing, Guest: Alain Le Roy, Under-Secretary-General for Peacekeeping Operations, Giving His Quarterly Press Conference. United Nations Webcast, December 15 2010. http://www.unmultimedia.org/tv/webcast/2010/12/daily-press-briefing-and-guest-alain-le-roy-under-secretary-general-for-peacekeeping-operations-2.html.

———. Spokesperson's Noon Briefing. November 8, 2011. http://www.un.org/News/briefings/docs/2011/db111108.doc.htm.

UN Secretariat. "Assessment of Member States' Contributions for the Financing of the United Nations Stabilization Mission in Haiti (MINUSTAH) from 1 July 2008 to 30 June 2009." ST/ADM/SER.B/745, March 25, 2010.

———. "Assessment of Member States' Contributions for the Financing of the United Nations Stabilization Mission in Haiti (MINUSTAH) from 1 July 2011 to 30 June 2012." ST/ADM/SER.B/843, October 24, 2012.

UN Secretary General Ban Ki-moon. "Secretary-General's Remarks after Visiting Family Affected by Cholera, Los Palmas, Haiti, 14 July 2014." http://www.un.org/sg/statements/index.asp?nid=7861.

———. "Secretary-General's Remarks at Church Service, Los Palmas, Haiti, 14 July 2014." http://www.un.org/sg/statements/index.asp?nid=7859.

UN Security Council. "Report of the Secretary-General on the Budget for the United Nations Stabilization Mission in Haiti for the Period from 1 July 2010 to 30

June 2011." United Nations General Assembly, A/65/535, October 21, 2010. http://www.un.org/ga/search/view_doc.asp?symbol=A/65/535.

——. "Report of the Secretary-General on the United Nations Stabilization Mission in Haiti." S/2004/908, November 18, 2004. http://www.un.org/en/ga/search/view_doc.asp?symbol=S/2004/908.

——. "Report of the Secretary-General on the United Nations Stabilization Mission in Haiti." S/2010/446, September 1, 2010. http://www.un.org/en/ga/search/view_doc.asp?symbol=S/2010/446.

——. "Report of the Secretary-General on the United Nations Stabilization Mission in Haiti." S/2011/183, March 24 2011. http://www.un.org/en/ga/search/view_doc.asp?symbol=S/2011/183.

——. "Report of the Secretary-General on the United Nations Stabilization Mission in Haiti." S/2014/617, August 29, 2014. http://www.securitycouncilreport.org/atf/cf/%7B65BFCF9B-6D27–4E9C-8CD3-CF6E4FF96FF9%7D/s_2014_617.pdf.

——. "Resolution 1529 (2004)—Adopted by the Security Council at its 4919th meeting, on 29 February 2004." S/RES/1529 (2004).

——. "Resolution 1927 (2010)—Adopted by the Security Council at its 6330th meeting, on 4 June 2010." S/RES/1927 (2010).

——. "Resolution 2185 (2014)—Adopted by the Security Council at Its 7317th meeting, on 20 November 2014." S/RES/2185 (2014).

——. "Security Council Establishes UN Stabilization Mission in Haiti for Initial Six-Month Period." SC/8083, April 30, 2004. http://www.un.org/News/Press/docs/2004/sc8083.doc.htm.

U.S. Agency for International Development, Bureau for Democracy, Conflict and Humanitarian Assistance (DCHA), and Office of U.S. Foreign Disaster Assistance (OFDA). "Haiti: Complex Emergency Fact Sheet no. 7 (FY2004)." March 17, 2004. http://reliefweb.int/report/haiti/haiti-complex-emergency-fact-sheet-7-fy2004.

U.S. Army Corps of Engineers, "L'Evaluation des ressources d'eau d'haiti [Assessment of Water Resources—Haiti], Représentez-en C-1. Ressources d'eau de Surface [Map of Surface Water Resources]." District and Mobile Topographic Engineering Center, August 1999. http://www.sam.usace.army.mil/Portals/46/docs/military/engineering/docs/WRA/Haiti/Combined%20Final%20Haiti.pdf.

U.S. CDC (Centers for Disease Control and Prevention). "CDC Situation Awareness—2010 Haiti Cholera Outbreak Maps. Map: Ship Ballast Discharge Evaluation, 50 Nautical Miles Buffer and 200 Meter Depth." January 24, 2011. http://www.bt.cdc.gov/situationawareness/haiticholera/map_4.asp.

——. "Cholera—Non-O1 and Non-O139 *Vibrio cholerae* Infections." Accessed August 29, 2015. http://www.cdc.gov/cholera/non-01-0139-infections.html.

——. "Cholera Outbreak—Haiti, October 2010." *Morbidity and Mortality Weekly Report* 59, no. 43 (2010): 1411. http://www.cdc.gov/mmwr/preview/mmwrhtml/mm5943a4.htm.

——. "Foodborne Outbreaks, Finding the Point of Contamination and Source of the Food." http://www.cdc.gov/foodsafety/outbreaks/investigating-outbreaks/investigations/contamination.html.

——. "Global HIV/AIDS at CDC—Overview. Countries Where We Work—Haiti." November 2013. http://www.cdc.gov/globalaids/Global-HIV-AIDS-at-CDC/countries/Haiti.

——. "Haiti Cholera Outbreak, Cholera in Haiti: One Year Later." October 2011. http://www.cdc.gov/haiticholera/haiti_cholera.htm.

——. "Haiti Cholera Outbreak—Map of Cumulative Attack Rate with Data on Cases, Hospitalizations, and Deaths." HA Cholera MSPP Data Attack Rate, CDC-SA-GRASP, February 17, 2011, v3.

——. "Haiti Cholera Outbreak—Map of Cumulative Attack Rate with Data on Cases, Hospitalizations, and Deaths." CDC-SA-GRASP, September 2, 2011. http://www.bt.cdc.gov/situationawareness/haiticholera/map_1.asp.

——. "Haiti. HIV/AIDS Assets and Strategic Focus." http://www.cdc.gov/globalaids/Global-HIV-AIDS-at-CDC/default.html.

——. "How to Investigate an Outbreak, Steps of an Outbreak Investigation." Epidemiology in the Classroom. http://www.cdc.gov/excite/classroom/outbreak/steps.htm.

——. "Immunizing against Cholera." June 13, 2014. http://www.cdc.gov/globalhealth/immunization/othervpds/cholera.html.

——. MMWR 59, no. 45, errata, pp. 1473–74. Morbidity and Mortality Weekly Report no. 59, no. 47 (2010): 1556. http://www.cdc.gov/Mmwr/preview/mmwrhtml/mm5947a5.htm.

——. "Multistate Outbreak of Human Salmonella Enteritidis Infections Associated with Shell Eggs (Final Update)." December 2, 2010. http://www.cdc.gov/salmonella/enteritidis/index.html.

——. "Outbreak Investigations, Division of Foodborne, Waterborne and Environmental Diseases." http://www.cdc.gov/ncezid/dfwed/waterborne/investigations.html.

——. "2014 Ebola Outbreak in West Africa—Case Counts, Countries with Widespread Transmission." January 6, 2015. http://www.cdc.gov/vhf/ebola/outbreaks/2014-west-africa/case-counts.html.

——. "Update: Cholera Outbreak—Haiti, 2010." *Morbidity and Mortality Weekly Report* 59, no. 45 (2010): 1473–79. http://www.cdc.gov/Mmwr/preview/mmwrhtml/mm5945a1.htm.

——. "Update: Cholera Outbreak—Haiti, 2010." *Morbidity and Mortality Weekly Report* 59, no. 48 (2010): 1586–90. http://www.cdc.gov/mmwr/preview/mmwrhtml/mm5948a4.htm.

——. "Update: Cholera Outbreak—Haiti, Dominican Republic, and Florida, 2010." *Morbidity and Mortality Weekly Report* 59, no. 50 (2010): 1637–41. http://www.cdc.gov/mmwr/preview/mmwrhtml/mm5950a1.htm.

U.S. Central Intelligence Agency. "People and Society." In *The World Factbook—Haiti*. Last updated June 22, 2014. http://www.cia.gov/library/publications/the-world-factbook/geos/ha.html.

U.S. Department of State. "Senator Lugar Announces Three New Science Envoys." September 17, 2010. http://www.state.gov/r/pa/prs/ps/2010/09/147317.htm.

——. "Travel Warning, Haiti." Bureau of Consular Affairs, December 9, 2010. http://travel.state.gov/content/passports/english/alertswarnings/haiti-travel-warning.html.

——. "The United States in UN Peacekeeping: Strengthening UN Peacekeeping and Conflict Prevention Efforts." September 23, 2010. http://www.state.gov/r/pa/prs/ps/2010/09/147828.htm.

U.S. Embassy, Kathmandu, Nepal. "Security Announcement for American Citizens in Nepal: Cholera in Nepal." September 13, 2010. http://nepal.usembassy.gov/wm-9–13–2010.html.

U.S. Government Accountability Office (GAO). "Peacekeeping: Cost Comparison of Actual UN and Hypothetical U.S. Operations in Haiti." Report to the Subcommittee on Oversight and Investigations, Committee on International Relations, House of Representatives, GAO-06–331, February 2006. http://www.gao.gov/new.items/d06331.pdf.

U.S. Library of Congress, "Country Profile: Haiti." May, 2006. http://lcweb2.loc.gov/frd/cs/profiles/Haiti.pdf.

Valero, Bernard, Daily Press Briefing, France-Diplomatie, Ministère des Affaires Étrangères, December 8, 2010.

Valme, Jean A. "Officials: 45 People Lynched in Haiti amid Cholera Fears." CNN, December 24, 2010. http://www.cnn.com/2010/WORLD/americas/12/24/haiti.cholera.killings/.

Vinten-Johansen, Peter, Howard Brody, Nigel Paneth, Stephen Rachman, and Michael Russell Rip. *Cholera, Chloroform and the Science of Medicine: A Life of John Snow.* New York: Oxford University Press, 2003.

Vital, Marius, David Stucki, Thomas Egli, and Frederik Hammes. "Evaluating the Growth Potential of Pathogenic Bacteria in Water." *Applied and Environmental Microbiology* 76, no. 19 (2010): 6477–84. http://dx.doi.org/10.1128/AEM.00794–10.

Walker, Sebastian. "'Fatal Sickness' Outbreak in Haiti." Al Jazeera English, October 22, 2010. http://www.aljazeera.com/news/americas/2010/10/20101021165045395330.html.

——. "UN Investigates Cholera Spread in Haiti." Al Jazeera English, October 27, 2010. https://www.youtube.com/watch?v=gk-2HyQHUZ0.

Weekly Epidemiological Record. "Cholera in the Americas, South America." 67 (1992): 33–40.

WHO (World Health Organization). "Cholera." Fact Sheet No. 107. February 2014. http://www.who.int/mediacentre/factsheets/fs107/en.

——. "Cholera, 1998–2012." *Weekly Epidemiological Record* (WER) 74, no. 31 (1999): 259; *WER* 75, no. 31 (2000): 251; *WER* 76, no. 31 (2001): 234; *WER* 77, no. 31 (2002): 259; *WER* 78, no. 31 (2003): 271; *WER* 79, no. 31 (2004): 283; *WER* 80, no. 31 (2005): 263; *WER* 81, no. 31 (2006): 298; *WER* 82, no. 31 (2007): 274; *WER* 83, no. 31 (2008): 270; *WER* 84, no. 31 (2009): 310; *WER* 85, no. 31 (2010): 294; *WER* 86, no. 31 (2011): 326; *WER* 87, no. 31–32 (2012): 290; and *WER* 88, no. 31 (2013): 322.

——. "Cholera, 2009." *Weekly Epidemiological Record* 85, no. 31 (2010): 293–308. http://www.who.int/wer/2010/wer8531.pdf?ua=1.

——. "Cholera, 2010." *Weekly Epidemiological Record* 86, no. 31 (2011): 325–39. http://www.who.int/wer/2011/wer8631.pdf?ua=1.

——. "Cholera, 2012." *Weekly Epidemiological Record* 88, no. 31 (2013): 321–36. http://www.who.int/wer/2013/wer8831.pdf?ua=1.

——. "Cholera Country Profile: Haiti. Global Task Force on Cholera Control." May 18, 2011. http://www.who.int/cholera/countries/HaitiCountryProfileMay2011.pdf.

——. "Cholera—Oral Cholera Vaccine Stockpile." http://www.who.int/cholera/vaccines/ocv_stockpile_2013/en.

——. "Cholera Outbreaks—Ineffective Control Measures." *Weekly Epidemiological Record* 71, no. 39 (1996): 291–92.

——. "Cholera—Small Risk of Cholera Transmission by Food Imports." *Weekly Epidemiological Record* 66, no. 8 (1999): 55–56.

——. "Cholera—The Global Task Force on Cholera Control." June 27, 2014. http://www.who.int/cholera/task_force/en.

——. "Cholera Vaccines: WHO Position Paper." *Weekly Epidemiological Record* 85, no. 13 (2010): 117–28.

——. "Global Cholera Control Task Force." *Weekly Epidemiological Record* 66, no. 19 (1991): 136–37.

——. Global Task Force on Cholera Control. "Prevention and Control of Cholera Outbreaks: WHO Policy and Recommendations." http://www.who.int/cholera/technical/prevention/control/en/index1.html.

——. "Interagency Diarrhoeal Disease Kits—Information Note." February 2009. http://www.who.int/topics/cholera/materials/en/index.html.
——. *International Health Regulations (1969)*. 3rd ed. Geneva: World Health Organization, 1983.
——. *International Health Regulations (2005)*. 2nd ed. Geneva: World Health Organization, 2008.
——. "International Sanitary Regulations, WHO Regulations No. 2, WHO Technical Report Series (41)." July 1951. http://whqlibdoc.who.int/trs/WHO_TRS_41.pdf.
——. "Outbreak News. Cholera, Haiti—Update." *Weekly Epidemiological Record* 85, no. 49 (2010): 489–90.
——. "Programme Budget 2014–2015." October 2014. http://www.who.int/about/resources_planning/PB14–15_en.pdf?ua=1.
——. "WHO Statement Relating to International Travel and Trade to and from Countries Experiencing Outbreaks of Cholera." November 24, 2010. http://www.who.int/cholera/technical/prevention/choleratravelandtradeadvice231110.pdf.
——. "WHO/UNICEF Joint Monitoring Programme for Water Supply and Sanitation—Coverage Estimates, Improved Sanitation." July 2008. http://www.wssinfo.org/documents/?tx_displaycontroller[region]=&tx_displaycontroller[search_word]=haiti&tx_displaycontroller[type]=country_files.
——. "WHO/UNICEF Joint Monitoring Program of Water Supply and Sanitation—Progress on Drinking Water and Sanitation: 2012 Update," March, 2012. http://www.wssinfo.org/fileadmin/user_upload/resources/JMP-report-2012-en.pdf.
WHO Media Centre. "Swine Influenza, Statement by WHO Director-General, Dr. Margaret Chan." April 25, 2009. http://www.who.int/mediacentre/news/statements/2009/h1n1_20090425/en.
Wilde, Olivia. "Baseball in the Time of Cholera." *Huffington Post*, April 18, 2012. http://www.huffingtonpost.com/olivia-wilde/haiti-cholera-documentary_b_1432841.html.
Winter, Damon. "Election Violence Flares in Haiti." *New York Times*, December 8, 2010. http://www.nytimes.com/2010/12/09/world/americas/09haiti.html?_r=0.
World Bank. "Haiti—Gross National Income per Capita (Atlas Method)." World Development Indicators, 1.1 Size of the economy, 2013. http://data.worldbank.org/indicator/NY.GNP.PCAP.CD/countries/HT-XJ-XM?display=default.

Index

CPSIA information can be obtained
at www.ICGtesting.com
Printed in the USA
LVOW03s0204301117
558032LV00004B/311/P

9 781501 713583